Principles of Treatment in Parkinson's Disease

Anthony H.V. Schapira, D.Sc., M.D., FRCP, FMedSci
Professor of Neurology and Chair
University Department of Clinical Neurosciences
Royal Free and University College Medical School
Professor of Neurology
Institute of Neurology
University College London
London, England

C. Warren Olanow, M.D., FRCPC
Professor and Chairman
Department of Neurology
Mount Sinai School of Medicine
New York, New York

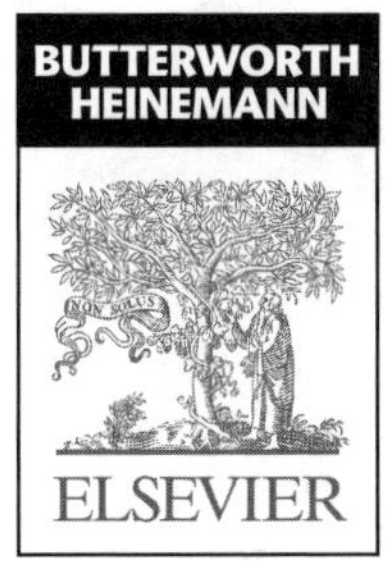

BUTTERWORTH
HEINEMANN
ELSEVIER

1600 John F. Kennedy Boulevard
Suite 1800
Philadelphia, PA 19103-2899

PRINCIPLES OF TREATMENT IN PARKINSON'S DISEASE ISBN-13: 978-0-7506-5428-9
ISBN-10: 0-7506-5428-7

NOTICE

Knowledge and best practice in this field are constantly changing. As new research and experience broaden our knowledge, changes in practice, treatment and drug therapy may become necessary or appropriate. Readers are advised to check the most current information provided (i) on procedures featured or (ii) by the manufacturer of each product to be administered, to verify the recommended dose or formula, the method and duration of administration, and contraindications. It is the responsibility of the practitioner, relying on his or her own experience and knowledge of the patient, to make diagnoses, to determine dosages and the best treatment for each individual patient, and to take all appropriate safety precautions. To the fullest extent of the law, neither the Publisher nor the Editors assume any liability for any injury and/or damage to persons or property arising out or related to any use of the material contained in this book.

ISBN-13: 978-0-7506-5428-9
ISBN-10: 0-7506-5428-7

Acquisitions Editor: Susan F. Pioli
Editorial Assistant: Joan Ryan

Printed in the United States of America.
Last digit is the print number: 9 8 7 6 5 4 3 2 1

Contributing Authors

Claire Ardouin, M.D.
Department of Neurology, J. Fourier University; Psychologist, University Hospital, Grenoble, France

Alim Louis Benabid, M.D., Ph.D.
Professor of Biophysics and Director of INSERM Unit 318, J. Fourier University; Head of Neurosurgery, University Hospital, Grenoble, France

Maria Graciela Cersosimo, M.D.
Assistant Professor of Neurology, Movement Disorders Program, University of Buenos Aires; Staff Physician, Movement Disorders Program, Hospital de Clinicas Jose de San Martin, Buenos Aires, Argentina

Stephan Chabardès, M.D.
Assistant, Department of Neurosurgery, J. Fourier University; Staff Neurosurgeon, University Hospital, Grenoble, France

Thomas N. Chase, M.D.
Chief, Experimental Therapeutics Branch, National Institutes of Health, Bethesda, Maryland

Biplob Dass, M.D.
Department of Neurological Sciences, Rush University Medical Center, Chicago, Illinois

Stanley Fahn, M.D.
Professor of Neurology and Chief, Movement Disorders Center, Columbia University Medical Center, The Neurological Institute, New York, New York

Valerie Fraix, M.D.
Assistant, Department of Neurology, J. Fourier University; Staff Neurologist, University Hospital, Grenoble, France

Jean-Michel Gracies, M.D., Ph.D.
Assistant Professor of Neurology and Assistant Attending Physician, Department of Neurology, Mount Sinai Medical Center, New York, New York

Sylvie Grand, M.D.
Assistant, Master of Conferences, Department of Biophysics, J. Fourier University; Staff Neuroradiologist, University Hospital, Grenoble, France

Peter Jenner, BPharm (Hons), Ph.D., D.Sc., FRPharms
Professor and Chairman, Division of Pharmacology and Therapeutics, King's College, London, United Kingdom

Jorge L. Juncos, M.D.
Associate Professor of Neurology (Movement Disorders), Emory University School of Medicine; Associate Professor and Staff Neurologist, Emory University Hospital, Atlanta, Georgia

William C. Koller, M.D.
Professor of Neurology, University of Miami School of Medicine, Miami, Florida

Jeffrey H. Kordower, M.D.
Department of Neurological Sciences, Rush University Medical Center, Chicago, Illinois

Paul Krack, M.D.
Professor of Neurology, J. Fourier University; Staff Neurologist, University Hospital, Grenoble, France

Jean François LeBas, M.D., Ph.D.
Professor of Biophysics, J. Fourier University; Head of Neuroradiology, University Hospital, Grenoble, France

Mara Lugassy, M.D.
Neurological Institute, Columbia University Medical Center, New York, New York

Yoshikuni Mizuno, M.D.
Professor and Chairman, Department of Neurology, Juntendo University School of Medicine; Chairman, Department of Neurology, Juntendo University Hospital, Tokyo, Japan

Hideki Mochizuki, M.D.
Assistant Professor of Neurology, Juntendo University School of Medicine, Tokyo, Japan

Melissa J. Nirenberg, M.D., Ph.D.
Fellow in Movement Disorders, Department of Neurology, Columbia University Medical Center; Assistant Attending Physician, Department of Neurology, New York-Presbyterian Hospital, New York, New York

Jose A. Obeso, M.D., Ph.D.
Professor of Neurology and Neurosurgery, University of Navarra; Consultant Neurologist and Neurosurgeon, Clínica Universitaria de Navarra, Pamplona, Spain

C. Warren Olanow, M.D., FRCPC
Professor and Chairman, Department of Neurology, Mount Sinai School of Medicine, New York, New York

Werner H. Poewe, M.D.
Professor and Chairman, Department of Neurology, Innsbruck Medical University, Innsbruck, Austria

Pierre Pollak, M.D.
Professor of Neurology, J. Fourier University; Head of Movement Disorders, University Hospital, Grenoble, France

John D. Putzke, Ph.D., MSPH
Assistant Professor of Neurology, Mayo Clinic, Jacksonville, Florida

Maria C. Rodríguez-Oroz, M.D.
Associate Professor of Neurology, University of Navarre; Consultant, Department of Neurology, Clínica Universitaria de Navarra, Pamplona, Spain

Karen A. Sawabini, D.O.
Clinical Instructor, Department of Neurology, University of Alabama School of Medicine at Birmingham, Birmingham, Alabama

Anthony H.V. Schapira, D.Sc., M.D., FRCP, FMedSci
Professor of Neurology and Chair of University Department of Clinical Neurosciences, Royal Free and University College Medical School, and Professor of Neurology, Institute of Neurology, Queen Square, London, United Kingdom

Fabrizio Stocchi, M.D., Ph.D.
Professor and Honorary Consultant of Neurology, Institute of Neurology, IRCCS Neuromed, Pozzilli, Italy

Ryan J. Uitti, M.D.
Associate Professor of Neurology and Director, Movement Disorders Center, Mayo Clinic, Jacksonville, Florida

Bradley A. Wallace, M.D., Ph.D.
Resident, Department of Neurosurgery, University of Florida College of Medicine, Gainesville, Florida; Staff Neurosurgeon, University Hospital, Grenoble, France

Ray L. Watts, M.D.
John N. Whitaker Professor and Chairman, Department of Neurology, University of Alabama School of Medicine at Birmingham; Chief, Neurology Service, University of Alabama at Birmingham Hospital, Birmingham, Alabama

Robert E. Wharen, Jr., M.D.
Associate Professor and Chair, Department of Neurosurgery, Mayo Clinic, Jacksonville, Florida

Ivana Zamarbide, M.D.
Department of Neurology and Neurosurgery, Clinical University and Medical School, University of Navarra, Pamplona, Spain

Contents

Preface

Almost 200 years have passed since James Parkinson first published his classic account of the clinical features of the disease that was later to bear his name. This seminal treatise contained an account of the phenomenology of the disease that has not been bettered. His comments on pathology were naturally limited, but he did suggest that the disease had its origins in the medulla, although that part contained within the cervical vertebrae (sic). Treatment options were recognized to be limited, but the letting of blood from the upper cervical area and the production of a purulent discharge with the use of the Sabine Liniment was thought to provide some relief. Parkinson was of the opinion that "[u]ntil we are better informed respecting the nature of this disease, the employment of internal medicines is scarcely warrantable." However, he had "sufficient reason for hoping that some remedial process may ere long be discovered, by which, at least, the progress of the disease may be stopped."

The advance of the science of medicine led to early attempts to treat patients with Parkinson's disease (PD) with belladonna, and in 1888 Sir William Gowers recommended the prescription of arsenic and Indian hemp. Surgery came into vogue in the early 20th century and included pallidotomy and thalamotomy. These were abandoned following the discovery of dopamine depletion in the brain of PD patients and the introduction of levodopa as the first successful treatment not only for the symptoms of PD, but also for any neurodegenerative disease. Indeed, PD remains the neurodegenerative disease that is most amenable to treatment and for which there are currently multiple therapeutic options that benefit patients. We hope that James Parkinson's optimism has been fulfilled and that he would be content that much has been discovered and much achieved in helping patients with this disease.

This book is intended to provide the practicing clinician with a comprehensive guide to the treatment options now available for the treatment of all stages of PD. We have tried to ensure that all aspects of disease management have been covered in detail. In addition, we have ourselves contributed chapters that have sought to put into a practical clinical context the various opportunities that exist for medical or surgical treatment. However, the book also highlights our limitations both in treating all the symptoms of PD and, most importantly, in slowing its course or preventing its progression.

It is both a privilege and a challenge to work in an area of medicine in which our knowledge is advancing so rapidly. Inevitably, this book may therefore become outdated before too long, but we hope this will be for the right reasons!

We are indebted to the hard work of all our eminent contributors, each of whom have themselves made major contributions to the field of PD. We thank them for their excellent work.

Anthony H. V. Schapira
C. Warren Olanow

Acknowledgments

First of all we wish to thank our families Laura and Sarah; Mariana, Edward, James, Alexandra and Andrew for their support, encouragement and inspiration. We thank Susan Pioli and Joan Ryan who made this book possible and who supported us with their excellent help and guidance. Finally, and once again, our thanks to all our contributors; they should take any credit and we the blame!

SECTION 1

DRUG THERAPY FOR PARKINSON'S DISEASE

1

The Role of Levodopa and Catechol-O-Methyltransferase Inhibitors

Melissa J. Nirenberg and Stanley Fahn

INTRODUCTION

Although many questions remain unanswered about the optimal management of Parkinson's disease (PD), levodopa is undoubtedly the most powerful drug available to treat this disorder. The absence of a robust response to high-dose levodopa essentially excludes the possibility of PD, whereas a marked and sustained response strongly supports this diagnosis.[1] Moreover, in spite of the numerous treatment options available in early PD, virtually all patients will eventually require levodopa therapy as the disease worsens.

Not all symptoms of PD, however, are equally responsive to levodopa. Bradykinesia and rigidity generally show the most dramatic improvement with dopaminergic therapy. Tremor has a more variable (and often incomplete) response. A number of other symptoms, including postural instability and speech disturbance, are typically unaffected by dopaminergic therapy; they are presumably due to deficits in other neurotransmitter systems. Recognition of the differential responsiveness of these symptoms to levodopa is critical for setting realistic treatment goals.

Early in the course of disease, levodopa provides a potent and effective treatment for PD, with a long-duration response that lasts continuously even with infrequent medication dosing; this is in spite of a plasma half-life of a little more than 30 minutes.[2] Adverse effects, if they occur during this "honeymoon period," usually consist of nausea, vomiting, and postural hypotension. The gastrointestinal effects are usually mitigated if a peripheral decarboxylase inhibitor such as carbidopa or benserazide is administered concurrently to prevent the synthesis of dopamine outside of the central nervous system (CNS).

As the disease progresses, more serious and chronic complications, such as "wearing off," fluctuations, and dyskinesias emerge; these motor complications affect 75% of patients after 6 years of levodopa therapy.[3] These problems markedly impair the quality of life and functional status of affected patients, and prove challenging not only for the patient, but also for the treating physician.

IS LEVODOPA NEUROTOXIC OR NEUROPROTECTIVE?

One of the most controversial questions regarding the treatment of PD is whether levodopa is neurotoxic. The results of some in-vitro studies have suggested that levodopa may be injurious to dopaminergic neurons.[4,5] These findings have raised concerns that chronic levodopa exposure might hasten disease progression in PD patients. Accordingly, some physicians and patients have opted to defer the use of levodopa for as long as possible. Other physicians have continued to use levodopa as first-line therapy, arguing that it is inappropriate to withhold the most potent symptomatic treatment for PD in the absence of clinical evidence of toxicity.[6–8]

Until very recently, there was little clinical data to support or refute the possibility of levodopa toxicity. In 2002, however, two studies were published in which functional neuroimaging techniques had been used to compare patients initially treated with pramipexole versus levodopa (CALM–PD) or ropinirole versus levodopa (REAL–PET), respectively. The CALM–PD trial used single-photon emission computerized tomography (SPECT) to look at striatal dopamine transporter (DAT) activity (β-CIT uptake) as a marker for intact axons of nigrostriatal dopaminergic neurons. This four-year trial showed a more rapid rate of decline of β-CIT uptake in the group assigned to early levodopa compared with early pramipexole treatment.[9] A similar result was found in the REAL–PET trial, which used positron emission tomography (PET) to look at putaminal ^{18}F accumulation (due to ^{18}F-Dopa uptake and decarboxylation) as a marker for functional dopaminergic terminals. This two-year study showed a more rapid rate of reduction of ^{18}F accumulation in patients who were initially treated with levodopa versus ropinirole.[10] Since there was no placebo group in either study, the findings of the two studies could be interpreted to show that dopamine agonists slow the progression of PD, levodopa hastens the progression of PD, or both. They also raise the question of whether levodopa or dopamine agonists have direct pharmacological effects on DAT or L-aromatic amino acid (dopa) decarboxylase that might confound the interpretation of these results. Thus, caution must be used in interpreting these and other studies that use imaging markers to document "neuroprotection."[11–13]

Because of ongoing controversy about whether levodopa is toxic, a large, multicenter, randomized controlled clinical trial comparing earlier versus later levodopa treatment in PD (the ELLDOPA study) was designed to address this question.[14,15] This was a double-blind, placebo-controlled, parallel-group, multicenter trial of patients with early PD who had not been previously treated with symptomatic therapy. A total of 361 patients were enrolled, and were randomized to receive treatment with either low- (150 mg/day), middle- (300 mg/day), or high- (600 mg/day) dose levodopa, or placebo. After 40 weeks of treatment, the patients underwent a three-day taper of their medications, followed by a two-week washout period during which they received no treatment for their PD. The primary outcome measure was the change in the Unified

Parkinson's Disease Rating Scale (UPDRS) score between baseline and after the washout period. The goal of the study was to determine whether levodopa treatment affects the rate of progression of PD.

At the end of the two-week washout period, the UPDRS scores of patients treated with all three doses of levodopa were lower (better) than those of the placebo-treated group, in a dose–response pattern. These findings suggest that levodopa is not neurotoxic, and may even be neuroprotective, though the possibility that patients were experiencing a longer duration of symptomatic response to levodopa could not be excluded. The highest dosage of levodopa was, however, associated with a higher incidence of motor complications, including dyskinesias and a trend to develop the "wearing off" phenomenon. Another major finding of the ELLDOPA study was that the "long-duration" benefit from levodopa starts to wane after approximately 9 months of treatment.

In addition to the clinical data, a subset of patients in the ELLDOPA trial was also evaluated with β-CIT SPECT imaging, which (as in the CALM–PD trial) was used as a marker for intact nigrostriatal dopaminergic neurons. These neuroimaging studies showed that there was a larger decrease in striatal DAT binding in patients treated with levodopa, in a dose–response pattern. Thus, in contrast with the clinical data, the imaging findings suggested that levodopa may hasten the progression of PD. As with other neuroimaging studies, however, it is possible that the observed changes in the levels of uptake of this marker reflected a pharmacological effect of levodopa on DAT activity, rather than evidence of injury to dopaminergic neurons.

Thus, intriguing as the results of the ELLDOPA study are, it remains unclear whether levodopa may (either positively or negatively) affect the natural history of PD. Given the evidence from the ELLDOPA study that the dosage of levodopa is important in the development of motor complications, it is reasonable to customize the dose of levodopa to fit the specific needs of each patient.

MOTOR AND NON-MOTOR COMPLICATIONS ASSOCIATED WITH LEVODOPA THERAPY

Motor complications can be divided into two categories: fluctuations ("off" states) and dyskinesias. There is sometimes a sensory component that accompanies these motor complications, such as pain or anxiety occurring in the "off" state. Levodopa-related motor and sensory complications can be subdivided according to the clinical phenomena that occur (Table 1.1). They can also be classified according to their temporal relationship with levodopa dosing. The latter approach is useful when discussing the treatment of motor complications (see below).

The "off" states usually consist of a return of parkinsonian symptoms such as bradykinesia, tremor, rigidity, immobility, and freezing (so-called "off freezing"). There are also other features of "off" states in many patients. "Off dystonia" is the presence of sustained contractions and spasms; these are often painful, most commonly occur in the morning on arising, and typically affect one or both feet. "Off dystonia" is an abnormal involuntary movement (dyskinesia); it is listed as such in Table 1–1, but should also be recognized as

TABLE 1.1 Major fluctuations and dyskinesias as complications of levodopa

Motor fluctuations ("offs")	*Non-motor "offs"*	*Dyskinesias*
Slow "wearing-off"	Akathisia	Peak-dose chorea, ballism, and dystonia
Sudden "off"	Depression	Diphasic chorea and dystonia
Random "off"	Anxiety	"Off" dystonia
Yo-yo-ing	Dysphoria	Myoclonus
Episodic failure to respond	Panic	Simultaneous dyskinesias and parkinsonism
Delayed "on"		
Weak response at end of day		
Sudden transient freezing		
Variable response relative to meals		

an "off" phenomenon. Sensory or behavioral "offs" are the non-motor phenomena that may accompany a motor (parkinsonian) "off"; they may also present as an "off" in the absence of motor parkinsonian signs. Sensory "offs" can consist of pain, akathisia, depression, anxiety, dysphoria, or panic; usually more than one of these is present. Sensory "offs," like dystonic "offs," are extremely poorly tolerated. The presence of these sensory and behavioral phenomena – much more so than parkinsonian or dystonic "offs" – can drive patients to take more and more levodopa, turning them into "levodopa junkies."

A number of investigators have found that the major risk factors for motor complications are the duration[16,17] or dosage[18,19] of levodopa therapy. Several studies have also shown that using dopamine agonists rather than levodopa can delay the start of the "wearing off" effect, and reduce the risk that it will develop.[20–22] The CALM–PD trial also showed that levodopa was statistically more likely than pramipexole to induce both motor fluctuations and dyskinesias.[9]

Although early levodopa use has been associated with the development of motor complications, it is unclear whether this is due to putative toxic properties of levodopa. Increasing levodopa exposure is a marker for disease progression, which itself is a known risk factor for the development of dyskinesias and fluctuations in PD.[17,23–28] Thus, it is not known to what extent levodopa may be a causative factor in promoting motor complications.

Another possibility is that the association of levodopa with motor complications is a function of the higher potency and shorter half-life of levodopa as compared with dopamine agonists. Since the development of motor complications relates to the dose, it is probably best to use the lowest dose of levodopa possible to achieve adequate clinical benefit.[18,29] In light of concerns that pulsatile administration of levodopa may contribute to the development of motor complications,[30–32] there is some rationale for the initial use of extended-release levodopa preparations or catechol-O-methyltransferase (COMT) inhibitors to extend the half-life of levodopa. Unfortunately, clinical trials of early use of regular (Sinemet) versus long-acting (Sinemet CR) carbidopa/levodopa failed to show differences in the rate of development of motor fluctuations in the two treatment groups.[33–36] There are as yet no clinical trials to determine whether the early use of COMT inhibitors will delay motor complications.

IS LEVODOPA SAFE IN PATIENTS WITH A HISTORY OF MELANOMA?

Levodopa is an intermediary metabolite in the synthesis of melanin. For this reason, there has been longstanding concern that this medication might potentially promote the growth of melanoma. Melanoma obviously occurs in patients on levodopa therapy, and is more common in PD patients than in the general population.[37–40] In studies of patients with melanoma, levodopa exposure is rare.[41] Thus, although package inserts warn that levodopa should not be used by patients with melanoma or suspicious skin lesions,[42–45] there is no clinical evidence to support this admonition.[46–49] Nonetheless, in patients with PD and a history of melanoma, it would seem prudent both to defer levodopa therapy until other medications prove inadequate, and to monitor closely for recurrent melanoma.

WHEN SHOULD LEVODOPA THERAPY BE INITIATED?

When a patient is initially diagnosed with PD, the first question that must be addressed is whether treatment is needed. At the present time, there are no proven neuroprotective medications for PD; only symptomatic treatment is available. Given the cost, inconvenience, and potential complications of PD medications, it is usually preferable to defer therapy until a patient's symptoms begin to cause functional disability. The definition of "disability" is unique for each patient, but may include the decreased ability to maintain employment, perform activities of daily living, or handle a combination of domestic, financial, and social affairs.[50] Safety issues are also critical; appreciable worsening of gait or balance is also a common and important reason to begin treatment.

Once the decision has been made to begin symptomatic therapy, the next question is whether to use levodopa earlier or later in the course of disease. In light of the ongoing controversy about whether levodopa may hasten disease progression or promote the development of motor complications, there is as yet no "right answer" about how to manage PD. Instead, the treatment strategy should be tailored to the individualized needs of the patient, based on his/her age, medical history, social situation, and personal preferences.

As the most potent treatment for PD, levodopa is clearly the appropriate initial therapy for selected patients. In older patients (>70 years old), or those with dementia or other serious medical comorbidities, levodopa-sparing agents (such as dopamine agonists) are poorly tolerated due to cognitive and psychiatric side-effects. Long-term motor complications are also less of an issue in these patients, who have both a shorter future life expectancy and a lower propensity to develop these problems than younger patients.[24,51–53] In these patients, levodopa is the treatment of choice.

Early levodopa is also appropriate for younger patients who present with pronounced gait disturbance that puts them at risk of falling, or severe functional disability that threatens their independence or livelihood. In these patients, the lower potency and slower titration schedule of dopamine agonists makes them unacceptable as initial therapy. Once the patient's acute crisis has been addressed, then switching to (or supplementing with) a dopamine agonist should be considered.

The optimal initial treatment of PD in younger patients with mild disability is subject to greater debate. Younger patients (<60 years of age) are particularly prone to develop fluctuations and dyskinesias.[24,51–53] Moreover, the longer future life expectancy (and often greater financial obligations) of these patients magnifies any potential harm that might result from the occurrence of these motor complications. Given the mounting evidence that levodopa may hasten the development of motor complications as compared with dopamine agonists,[54–56] many physicians prefer to use levodopa-sparing strategies in young patients.[57–59] Others, however, still prefer to start with levodopa because of its greater potency.[7]

LEVODOPA DOSING AND ADMINISTRATION

At some point, all patients will require levodopa, because it is the only medication that is capable of controlling their symptoms. At that time, levodopa therapy must be initiated. In general, it is preferable to use the lowest dosage of medication that is adequate to control the patient's symptoms, since this may reduce the risk of early development of motor complications.

Combination with a Peripheral Dopa Decarboxylase Inhibitor

Levodopa is almost always administered in combination with a peripheral dopa decarboxylase inhibitor (DDI) such as carbidopa (available in the United States and other countries) or benserazide (available outside of the United States). These medications prevent the peripheral breakdown of levodopa into dopamine, thereby conferring three major advantages over levodopa monotherapy. First, by decreasing the availability of peripheral dopamine that can act at the area postrema (vomiting center, which is located outside of the blood–brain barrier), they block the development of anorexia, nausea, and vomiting. Second, by lowering the amount of dopamine that is available to peripheral catecholamine receptors, they reduce the risk of cardiac arrhythmias. Third, by decreasing the peripheral catabolism of levodopa, they increase the bioavailability of levodopa in the central nervous system (CNS). A comparable clinical benefit can therefore be attained with a four-fold reduction in the dosage of levodopa.

Although the mechanisms of action of carbidopa and benserazide are similar, their pharmacokinetics differ slightly. Benserazide is more potent, producing a stronger and faster but more fleeting benefit.[60,61] In clinical practice, however, there is little difference in the efficacy of the two DDIs, though some patients may report a preference for one or the other.[62,63]

Patients typically require at least 75–100 mg of carbidopa or benserazide per day (regardless of the total daily dose of levodopa) to maximally inhibit dopa decarboxylase and block peripheral side-effects.[64] Most of the time, this can be provided using standard preparations of carbidopa/levodopa or benserazide/levodopa. In some patients, however, higher doses of DDI are required early in the treatment course. In these patients, additional carbidopa (marketed in the United States as Lodosyn®) can be added.[65]

Available Preparations of Levodopa + DDI

Carbidopa/levodopa is available in standard-release (Sinemet®, Atamet®, Apo-Levocarb®, Nu-Levocarb®, Cronomet®, Sindopa®, Parcopa™, or generic) and controlled-release (Sinemet CR® or generic) formulations.[42] Levodopa/benserazide is also available in standard-release (e.g., Madopar® or Prolopa®) and controlled-release (Madopar CR®, Madopar HBS®, or Prolopa HBS®) forms. Standard-release preparations are characterized by a shorter half-life, more rapid onset of effect, and a more predictable pattern of absorption. In contrast, controlled-release preparations have a slightly longer plasma half-life, more delayed onset of benefit, and more irregular absorption (because a variable amount of medication is absorbed in the proximal small intestine before it passes to the distal small intestine and colon). Accordingly, the controlled-release preparations have a reduced bioavailability, equivalent to about two-thirds to three-quarters of that of standard formulations. All of these factors must be taken into consideration when switching patients from standard to controlled-release preparations.

Standard-release Carbidopa/Levodopa

Standard-release carbidopa/levodopa is available in 10/100 mg, 25/100 mg, and 25/250 mg tablets, with the first number denoting the dose of carbidopa, and the second the dose of levodopa. These formulations may be used as an initial treatment for PD, as add-on therapy, or as a substitute for other PD medications (e.g., in patients who are unable to tolerate dopamine agonists). The tablets can be broken in half when a slower titration schedule (or more precise dosing) is desired; they can also be crushed or dissolved when a more rapid onset of effect is necessary. Orally disintegrating tablets (10/100 mg, 25/100 mg, and 25/250 mg) became available in 2004 under the brand name Parcopa™; these can be taken without water, but are otherwise comparable to standard-release carbidopa/levodopa.[66]

When carbidopa/levodopa therapy is initiated, the 25/100 mg tablets should be used, in order to provide sufficient carbidopa to block peripheral side-effects. A typical starting dose is one tablet a day following a meal (with supplementary carbidopa if necessary), followed by a weekly increase by one tablet per day, to a goal of one tablet three times a day; this is often a therapeutic dose in patients with early PD. Taking the tablets with food reduces the risk of nausea or vomiting. Although this also has the potential to decrease and slow levodopa absorption, the effect is rarely of clinical significance (see below).

If symptoms of PD persist (or when they progress), then the dosage of carbidopa/levodopa 25/100 mg can be gradually increased to two tablets three times daily. After that, the addition of a dopamine agonist should be considered, before continuing to gradually increase the dose of levodopa as needed. When patients require more than 600 mg of levodopa a day, then the 25/250 mg tablets can be used. Of note, while most patients begin to improve with low-dose levodopa, a few may require as much as 2000 mg/day before they show a definite clinical response. Accordingly, patients should not be considered to be "levodopa-unresponsive" unless they have been tested on this dose.

Carbidopa/levodopa 10/100 mg tablets are used infrequently, because of the higher risk of peripheral side-effects and reduced CNS bioavailability of levodopa that occurs with lower levels of carbidopa. These tablets are occasionally helpful in patients with late-stage disease, in whom very low CNS doses of levodopa may be necessary to minimize dyskinesias or other motor complications. They can also substitute for 25/100 mg tablets when more than six tablets a day are taken. This substitution avoids excessively high dosages of carbidopa, which at such a level could conceivably cross the blood–brain barrier and reduce the conversion of levodopa to dopamine in the CNS.

Extended-release Carbidopa/Levodopa

Extended-release carbidopa/levodopa is available in two forms: 25/100 mg and 50/200 mg tablets. These preparations are consistently more expensive than standard-release forms. The 25/100 mg tablets are not scored; breaking them in half is not usually recommended, because this alters the time-release properties of the matrix. In contrast, the 50/200 mg tablets are scored, and can be broken in half as necessary for medication titration. Neither form of extended-release tablet should be crushed, since this destroys the time-release properties of the tablets, rendering them equivalent to standard-release preparations.

Extended-release carbidopa/levodopa can be used as initial therapy for PD, or as add-on therapy in patients taking other PD medications (e.g., dopamine agonists or standard-release carbidopa/levodopa). They are sometimes added in an attempt to "smooth out" symptoms in patients with prominent fluctuations, as discussed below. Because the extended-release tablets are more slowly absorbed, and result in lower peak plasma (and CNS) concentrations of levodopa, they are less likely to cause acute, peak-dose side-effects such as drowsiness, hallucinations, or confusion. For this reason, they are sometimes useful as initial therapy in patients over 70 years of age. In patients of all ages whose PD symptoms interrupt their sleep or nocturnal mobility, the use of extended-release carbidopa/levodopa at bedtime can also be helpful in alleviating these symptoms.

Unfortunately, the irregular absorption and unpredictable timing of response to these and other extended-release levodopa preparations make it more difficult to monitor their effectiveness and adjust the dosing appropriately. In some patients, for example, an unintended build-up of medication may also induce late-day dyskinesias. Thus, standard carbidopa/levodopa is the preferred initial treatment in younger patients (and often in older patients as well). When motor fluctuations develop, then the addition of extended-release carbidopa/levodopa is sometimes helpful in smoothing out the patient's symptoms (see below).

When treatment with extended-release carbidopa/levodopa is initiated, patients should be instructed to take one of the 25/100 mg tablets three times daily. This dose is often enough to provide symptomatic relief, particularly in patients who are already on dopamine agonist therapy. As with the standard-release tablets, taking the medication after meals is often helpful for reducing the risk of nausea and vomiting. Over time, the dose can be gradually increased as necessary to 50/200 mg three or four times daily. After that, the addition of a dopamine agonist should be strongly considered, if one is not already included in the medication regimen. The maximum daily dose of levodopa is determined empirically, based on clinical efficacy and adverse effects; this may exceed 2000 mg per day.

Liquefied Carbidopa/Levodopa

In patients with advanced PD, the maintenance of smooth serum levels of levodopa becomes increasingly important for reducing motor complications, as discussed in detail below. One way to accomplish this is to have patients sip small doses of liquefied carbidopa/levodopa at regular intervals throughout the day.[67] Although liquefied carbidopa/levodopa is not commercially available, it can be easily prepared. A standard recipe is to dissolve four 25/250 mg tablets in a liter of fluid. A milliliter of the solution will then provide one milligram of levodopa. The solution should be made up daily in an acidic fluid (e.g., diet soda, carbonated water, orange juice, or an ascorbic acid solution), and stored in the refrigerator in order to prolong the stability of the levodopa. Under those conditions, the solution is stable for up to one week.[68]

Standard-release Levodopa/Benserazide

Standard-release levodopa/benserazide is available in 50/12.5 mg, 100/25 mg, and 200/50 mg capsules or tablets; the dosage of levodopa is listed first (in contrast with the convention that is used for carbidopa/levodopa). Levodopa/benserazide is also available in dispersible tablets (50/12.5 mg and 100/25 mg), which can be used when a rapid onset of effect is desired.

Although the pharmacokinetics of benserazide differ slightly from those of carbidopa, the clinical differences between carbidopa/levodopa and levodopa/benserazide preparations are minimal (see above). Thus, the recommended dosage and administration of levodopa/benserazide are the same as for carbidopa/levodopa.

Extended-release Levodopa/Benserazide

Extended release levodopa/benserazide is available in 100/25 mg capsules (Madopar CR 125®, Madopar HBS®, Prolopa HBS®). The capsules must remain intact in order to retain their extended-release properties. The recommended dosing and administration of these capsules is similar to that of extended-release carbidopa/levodopa preparations, as detailed above. Once again, it is important to take into account the decreased bioavailability and more irregular absorption of extended-release levodopa preparations.

Short-term Adverse Effects of Levodopa Therapy

When starting levodopa therapy, physicians must be aware of a number of adverse effects that may occur. Gastrointestinal side-effects such as anorexia, nausea, and vomiting are especially common, particularly early in the treatment course. These symptoms result from the peripheral decarboxylation of levodopa, and as such can often be relieved by taking additional DDI, or taking the tablets with food, as discussed above. If these strategies fail, then premedication with domperidone (Motilium®), a peripherally acting dopamine D2 receptor antagonist (available outside of the United States), can be used. Constipation, which is frequently present in patients with PD, may also be exacerbated by levodopa therapy. This usually responds to standard treatments, including increased fluid and fiber intake.

Orthostatic hypotension is another common symptom in PD that may be potentiated by the peripheral decarboxylation of levodopa. As such, it may also respond to DDI supplementation. When orthostatic hypotension is severe at baseline, however, other established treatment strategies may be needed before patients are able to tolerate levodopa therapy.

Akathisia, or inner restlessness, occurs commonly in PD, usually as a side-effect of levodopa or other dopaminergic medications.[69] Less commonly, akathisia can be a manifestation of PD itself, which may acutely worsen when dopaminergic medications wear off. When a patient with PD develops akathisia, it is important to distinguish between these two possibilities, to determine whether a decrease or an increase in their dopaminergic medications is warranted.

Levodopa may also cause or exacerbate psychotic symptoms, including visual hallucinations, illusions, or delusions. These symptoms usually occur late in the course of the disease, and are most prominent in patients of advanced age or with baseline cognitive impairment. The dosage of levodopa is also important, because even young patients can develop drug-induced psychosis if the dosage is very high. Medication-induced psychosis often improves with lowering the dosage of levodopa (and other contributing agents), or the addition of atypical antipsychotic medications such as quetiapine or clozapine. Before attributing psychotic symptoms to levodopa, however, it is critical to exclude other treatable etiologies such as infection, stroke, intracranial mass lesions, endocrinopathies, or metabolic disturbances.

Excessive daytime sleepiness is a common and multifactorial problem in PD that may be caused or exacerbated by levodopa use, particularly in patients with advanced disease or dementia. Levodopa-related drowsiness typically occurs after each dose of levodopa. The symptom may improve with lowering the dose but at the risk of worsening the PD symptoms. Substitution of a long-acting levodopa preparation may be helpful, since these medications are associated with a slower rise in the CNS levels of levodopa.

Chronic Adverse Effects of Levodopa Usage

Wearing-off ("end of dose failure")

With time, the long-duration response to levodopa is lost,[16] and the clinical response persists only for as long as the plasma concentration of levodopa remains high.[2,70,71] Accordingly, the duration of effectiveness of a dose of levodopa becomes progressively shorter.[2,72] The term "short-duration response" is used when the effects of a dose of levodopa last for less than four hours. At that time, the patient begins to experience what is referred to as "wearing-off," or "end of dose failure," whereby the symptoms of PD gradually recur and increase until the next dose of medication takes effect. If the plasma level of levodopa can be maintained, however, then the clinical response persists.[30,70,73] Thus, "wearing-off" does not occur when levodopa is administered by a continuous intravenous[74] or intestinal[75–78] infusion. Because such infusions are both invasive and cumbersome, they have not proven to be a viable long-term treatment option for this problem. Fortunately, a number of other strategies have been moderately successful in treating "wearing-off."

Perhaps the most straightforward approach is to increase the dosing frequency of levodopa. While this strategy is effective for most patients with mild "wearing-off," it becomes less practical as the disease advances, and progressively shorter dosing intervals are required. As a result, it becomes increasingly inconvenient or impractical to administer levodopa as often as necessary to prevent "wearing-off." Another approach is to add (or substitute) long-acting levodopa preparations.[79–81] When a direct conversion is made, the reduced bioavailability of the longer-acting levodopa preparations must be taken into consideration. Even so, the inconsistent and delayed absorption of the long-acting preparations can sometimes precipitate other problems, such as delayed "ons" or unpredictable "offs," which can occur even with standard carbidopa/levodopa.

In many cases, the best way to treat "wearing-off" is to add a second medication. Selegiline, for example, can decrease "wearing-off" by potentiating the effects of levodopa, though the benefits are very mild.[82] Dopamine agonists, on the other hand, have both longer half-lives than levodopa and a higher potency than other available adjunctive therapies. As such, they are effective in decreasing the severity of the "off" state, and can also reduce the amount of "off" time per day. A third class of adjunctive agents, the catechol-O-methyltransferase (COMT) inhibitors, are also playing an increasingly important role in the treatment of "wearing-off." The use of these medications will be discussed in detail below, in the section on COMT inhibitors.

When "wearing-off" occurs, rescue doses of levodopa can be used as needed to abort or ameliorate the symptoms. Chewing or crushing levodopa, and administering with an acidic beverage such as carbonated water or orange juice, usually produces a response in about 10–15 minutes. Subcutaneous, intranasal, or sublingual apomorphine can also be used to achieve a rapid clinical response.[83–85] Unfortunately, levodopa ethyl ester (etilevodopa), a highly soluble prodrug of levodopa, was found to be no more effective than standard levodopa in a phase III clinical trial.[86,87]

"Off" Dystonia or Painful Cramps

In some patients, painful, sustained dystonic cramps may occur when the plasma level of levodopa is low, most often in the early morning.[88–90] Although the pathophysiological basis of this is unclear, the clinical management is the same as for other "off" phenomena. Extended-release levodopa preparations, in particular, may be helpful for patients with early-morning "off" dystonia.[81]

Sudden (Random) "On–Off"

The term "on–off" phenomenon was initially used to describe the sudden and unpredictable return of a patient's symptoms of PD, as if a light switch had suddenly been turned off.[91,92] More recently, the term has been broadened to denote any fluctuation of symptoms in parkinsonian patients. To avoid ambiguity, we refer to a rapid, random worsening of PD symptom as a "sudden off" or "sudden on–off." When "sudden offs" initially occur, they may be brief and mild. With time, however, the "offs" become longer and "deeper" (more severe); they may also be accompanied by increasingly debilitating non-motor symptoms, including depression, anxiety, or pain.[93–95]

In comparison with "wearing off," the "sudden off" phenomenon is typically a much more difficult problem to overcome. The addition of other medications, such as extended-release levodopa, selegiline, dopamine agonists, or amantadine, has proven to be ineffective. Minimizing the use of levodopa by supplementing with a dopamine agonist is sometimes moderately helpful. In most cases, however, it is not possible to prevent this phenomenon from occurring. Instead, rescue therapy with crushed levodopa preparations, liquefied levodopa preparations, or parenteral apomorphine[83–85] may be used to alleviate recurrent PD symptoms once they occur.

"Dose Failures" and "Delayed Ons"

Levodopa is absorbed only from the proximal small intestine; passage through the stomach is therefore necessary before it can enter the bloodstream and produce clinical benefit. In patients with advanced PD, if gastric emptying is delayed, "delayed ons" or "dose failures" can result[96] because levodopa is not absorbed from the small intestine in a timely fashion. "Dose failures" may occur at any time, even with the first dose in the morning;[97] when this occurs, patients may benefit from crushing their first daily dose of levodopa. When a "dose failure" or "delayed on" has already occurred, rescue therapy with crushed or liquefied levodopa, or parenteral apomorphine, can be used.[83–87]

In advanced disease, levodopa responsiveness may also begin to vary in relation to meals. Consumption of a large meal may further delay gastric emptying, resulting in impaired absorption of levodopa taken during or after a meal.[98] Thus, a dose of levodopa may prove to be inadequate when administered with food. In contrast, the same dose taken at least 20 minutes prior to eating may produce a good clinical benefit, or even an overdose. This variable response to levodopa can be a serious problem if it is unrecognized. Fortunately, once the problem has been identified, it can usually be ameliorated by adjusting the timing of medication doses in relation to meals.

Another potential factor influencing levodopa absorption is competition with amino acids derived from dietary protein. Levodopa is transported across the intestinal mucosa and blood–brain barrier by the large neutral amino acid carrier. The carrier at the blood–brain barrier, in particular, has been shown to be saturable under physiological conditions. For this reason, levodopa competes with large neutral amino acids for transport into the CNS[99,100] Thus, dietary protein has the potential to decrease levodopa absorption.[101]

Fortunately, this phenomenon is only rarely of clinical significance, even in advanced PD.[102]

For the few patients in whom dietary protein significantly impairs levodopa absorption, changes in the diet can often be made to overcome this problem. In particular, it can be helpful to minimize the consumption of protein at breakfast and lunch, when levodopa absorption is most critical.[103,104] Patients can compensate with a higher protein meal later in the day, since this is a time when an "off" is generally less problematic.

Dyskinesias

Dyskinesias are abnormal involuntary movements that can occur as a side-effect of levodopa use. They most commonly develop after several years of levodopa treatment,[105] but may appear much sooner in patients with advanced disease. The movements are usually choreic, although dystonic dyskinesias may also occur.[106] When mild, dyskinesias are often more bothersome to family members than to patients, who are sometimes unaware of them. When severe, however, dyskinesias may become distressing, painful, or functionally disabling.

Dyskinesias most commonly occur when levodopa levels in the blood and serum are maximal. These "peak-dose dyskinesias"[107] improve when the dose of levodopa is decreased, but at the cost of worsening the symptoms of PD. The goal for treating peak-dose dyskinesias is to maintain the levodopa at a constant level just below the threshold for dyskinesias but where the patient's symptoms are optimized – the PD symptoms are adequately treated, but dyskinesias are minimized. There are several different approaches for maintaining smooth serum levels of levodopa. One is to use smaller, more frequent dosing of levodopa. With time, however, the need for increasingly frequent and punctual administration of levodopa makes this increasingly impractical. In some cases, to achieve this effect, liquefied levodopa is required (see above).

Long-acting levodopa preparations can also be used in an attempt to smooth out the serum levels of levodopa. Unfortunately, the irregular absorption and delayed onset of effect of these medications often do not provide the desired effect of a stable serum level of levodopa. In particular, long-acting preparations often lead to accumulation of levodopa (and increased dyskinesias) at the end of the day. Another approach to maintaining steady medication levels is to gradually substitute a dopamine agonist for levodopa. Agonists have a lower potency and longer serum half-life than levodopa, and thereby provide smoother medication coverage, with an associated lower propensity to cause dyskinesias.

With time, the therapeutic window for levodopa becomes progressively narrower, making it increasingly difficult to control PD symptoms without precipitating dyskinesias. In some patients, peak-dose dyskinesias may even occur with subtherapeutic doses of levodopa, such that dyskinesias and "off" symptoms occur simultaneously. In these cases, the only effective treatment may be antidyskinetic agents such as amantadine[108–111] or clozapine.[112–115] In the future, adenosine α_{2A} receptor antagonists may also be useful in this setting.[116,117]

Dyskinesias are not always a peak-dose phenomenon. Sometimes they occur in a diphasic pattern, when the plasma level of levodopa is rising or falling, but not when it is at its peak.[107,118,119] A characteristic feature is that the dyskinesias may affect the legs either solely or predominantly. Affected patients often have dystonic as well as choreic dyskinesias; for this reason, diphasic dyskinesias were first described as occurring in a "DID" (dystonia–improvement–dystonia) pattern.[107] Diphasic dyskinesias are poorly understood, and very difficult to treat. Although the use of higher doses of levodopa has been advocated,[118] this tends to promote the development of peak-dose dyskinesias and other levodopa-induced adverse effects. Anti-dyskinetic agents are the most effective treatment for diphasic dyskinesias, though the benefit is usually suboptimal. It is sometimes also helpful to use a dopamine agonist, rather than levodopa, as the major therapeutic agent. When severe peak-dose or diphasic dyskinesias prove to be medically refractory, then deep-brain stimulator placement should be considered.[120]

Alternating "Offs" and Dyskinesias

In advanced PD, it is not uncommon for patients to experience both fluctuations ("wearing-off" or "on–offs") and dyskinesias. In most cases, patients prefer to have dyskinesias than to suffer with the disability (and discomfort) of the "off" state. For this reason, patients have a tendency to overdose themselves with levodopa in order to avert or alleviate their PD symptoms. As a result, they may spend the day alternating between "offs" and dyskinesias. In severe cases, there may be little or no time during which their PD symptoms are optimized; this has been described as "yo-yo-ing," in reference to the patient's constant "ups" and "downs."[71] The management is the same as for patients with concurrent dyskinesias and PD symptoms, as described above.

THE ADJUNCTIVE ROLE OF CATECHOL-O-METHYLTRANSFERASE INHIBITORS

Levodopa is metabolized through two different pathways. It is converted into dopamine by dopa decarboxylase, and to 3-O-methyldopa (an inactive metabolite) by catechol-O-methyltransferase (COMT). In patients receiving levodopa with a DDI such as carbidopa or benserazide, inhibition of COMT slows down the breakdown of levodopa. This increases the serum half-life of levodopa, thereby prolonging its duration of action. The net effect is to produce higher average serum levodopa levels, but with lower variability in these levels throughout the course of the day.[121]

Two COMT inhibitors are currently available for clinical use – tolcapone (marketed in the United States as Tasmar®) and entacapone (marketed in the United States as Comtan®). Tolcapone was the first of these to become available, and is the more potent of the two agents. It inhibits both central and peripheral 3-O-methylation of dopamine, though only the former effect is believed to be clinically significant.[122] Tolcapone has a longer half-life than entacapone, allowing for greater flexibility in the timing of each dose of medication. When administered three times daily to patients taking carbidopa/levodopa, it prolongs the half-life of levodopa by about 90 minutes.[123] It is available in 100 mg and 200 mg tablets. The starting dose is 100 mg a day, which can be gradually increased to 100 mg three times a day. At this dose, tolcapone decreases "wearing-off" by about two hours a day.[124] The maximum recommended daily dose of tolcapone is 200 mg three times daily. At this higher dose, it decreases "wearing-off" by about three hours a day.[124,125]

Unfortunately, tolcapone has been associated with two important side-effects that have limited its clinical usefulness. The first is diarrhea, which occurs in more than 15% of patients, and usually begins 6–12 weeks after treatment has been initiated. In 3–4% of patients, the diarrhea is severe, and may be explosive.[123] The second, and more serious, side-effect is hepatotoxicity. This resulted in three deaths from fulminant liver failure before routine monitoring of serum transaminase levels was mandated.[124,126,127] Fortunately, with close surveillance of serum transaminase levels (and discontinuation of the drug when these levels become elevated), no further deaths have occurred. Because of the risk of fatal hepatotoxicity, however, tolcapone should be reserved for patients with fluctuations who are refractory to other medical therapy. When tolcapone is used, physicians should discuss the potential risks with patients, and obtain written informed consent. If there is no substantial improvement in the patient's fluctuations after three weeks, then the medication should be discontinued.[123]

Entacapone is less likely to produce diarrhea than tolcapone, and does not appear to be hepatotoxic.[128] Because of this favorable side-effect profile, it is currently the COMT inhibitor of choice. It does not penetrate the blood–brain barrier, and therefore acts exclusively in extracerebral tissues.[129] It is available exclusively in 200 mg tablets; higher doses do not confer additional clinical benefit.[130,131] Entacapone has a relatively short half-life; for this reason, each tablet should be administered concurrently with a dose of levodopa + DDI. In some cases, it is preferable to use entacapone selectively, adding it to specific dose(s) of levodopa + DDI (e.g., the ones after which "wearing-off" usually occurs). In other cases, entacapone can be given with every dose of levodopa + DDI throughout the day, up to a maximum of eight tablets a day. When administered simultaneously with carbidopa/levodopa, 200 mg of entacapone prolongs the half-life of each dose of levodopa by about 30–60 minutes, and increases the total daily "on" time by one to two hours.[132–136]

In 2003, a single tablet containing carbidopa, levodopa, and entacapone also become available, marketed in the United States as Stalevo®.[45] Three different tablets of carbidopa/levodopa/entacapone are available: 12.5/50/200 mg (Stalevo 50®), 25/100/200 mg (Stalevo 100®), and 37.5/150/200 mg (Stalevo 150®). The major advantage of these combined preparations is that they can simplify the medication regimen, reducing the number of pills that a patient needs to take. The major disadvantage is that they do not allow for the doses of levodopa and entacapone to be individually titrated. For this reason, patients should initially be treated with separate tablets of carbidopa/levodopa and entacapone. When an effective dosing regimen has been established, then they can be switched to a comparable regimen using the combination tablets.[45] Even so, there are inherent limitations to these fixed-dose preparations; for example, it is not possible to administer more than 150 mg of levodopa at a time without providing excess entacapone.

One of the major advantages of COMT inhibitors is their rapid onset of benefit. Because they increase the average serum levels of levodopa, however, they can often precipitate or exacerbate levodopa side-effects such as dyskinesias, nausea, or hallucinations.[121,124] Accordingly, a reduction in the dose of levodopa is often necessary when COMT inhibitor therapy is initiated. Patients should also be warned that both tolcapone and entacapone can turn the urine a brownish orange color. This is a benign (but potentially alarming) side-effect.

OTHER ISSUES IN THE MANAGEMENT OF PD

The Withdrawal of Levodopa and Other PD Medications

The rapid withdrawal of levodopa has been associated with a rare but life-threatening "malignant withdrawal syndrome" that resembles neuroleptic malignant syndrome.[137–142] A similar phenomenon can also occur, though much less commonly, with the rapid discontinuation of other PD medications.[143,144] The syndrome is characterized by hyperthermia, rigidity, altered mental status, and autonomic instability. It can usually be avoided if levodopa and other PD medications are tapered off gradually, over a period of at least three days; in very rare cases, however, it may occur as an "off" phenomenon.[145,146] Since patients may not always report transient discontinuation of medications (for reasons such as intercurrent illness), physicians must have a high index of suspicion for this life-threatening syndrome. The management includes the administration of levodopa (or other dopaminergic medications) and supportive measures similar to those used in the treatment of neuroleptic malignant syndrome.[146]

The Management of PD when Oral Medications Cannot be Used

When patients require surgical procedures, there is often a period during which they need to remain "nothing per os" (NPO), and are not permitted to receive any food, liquids, or medications by mouth. Because this period is usually brief, the PD medications can be held before surgery, and restarted postoperatively. Even patients who are unable to take oral medications postoperatively (e.g., because of altered mental status, dysphagia, endotracheal intubation, or gastric surgery) can often be treated with liquefied levodopa via feeding tube, gastrostomy, or duodenostomy.[147]

There are some cases, however, in which patients may be unable to receive enteral medications on a long-term basis, rendering it much more difficult to manage their PD. If their PD remains untreated, however, then they may develop severe rigidity, akinesia, pain, impairment of gastrointestinal motility, decreased respiratory function, and contractures. These symptoms are not only distressing for the patient, but also potentially dangerous or life-threatening. In this setting, there are limited treatment options. Intravenous levodopa can be used[148] but is generally avoided because of the potential for serious complications such as arrhythmias or hypotension. Subcutaneous infusions of apomorphine[147,149] represent an effective and safer alternative, but premedication with antiemetics is necessary. In the future, other parenteral dopamine agonists may also be useful in this situation.[150,151]

REFERENCES

1. Marsden CD, Fahn S. Problems in Parkinson's Disease. In: Marsden CD, Fahn S (eds), Movement Disorders. London: Butterworth Scientific, 1982, pp. 1–7.
2. Muenter MD, Tyce GM. L-dopa therapy of Parkinson's disease: plasma L-dopa concentration, therapeutic response, and side effects. Mayo Clin Proc 1971;46:231–239.
3. Fahn S. Adverse effects of levodopa. In: Olanow CW (ed.), The Scientific Basis for the Treatment of Parkinson's Disease. Carnforth: Parthenon Publishing Group, 1992, pp. 89–112.
4. Jenner PG, Brin MF. Levodopa neurotoxicity: experimental studies versus clinical relevance. Neurology 1998;50(6 Suppl. 6):S39–43; discussion S44–48.
5. Melamed E, Offen D, Shirvan A et al. Levodopa: an exotoxin or a therapeutic drug? J Neurol 2000;247(Suppl. 2):II135–139.
6. Agid Y. Levodopa: is toxicity a myth? Neurology 1998;50:858–863.
7. Weiner WJ. The initial treatment of Parkinson's disease should begin with levodopa. Mov Disord 1999;14:716–724.
8. Factor SA. The initial treatment of Parkinson's disease. Mov Disord 2000;15:360–361.
9. Parkinson Study Group. Dopamine transporter brain imaging to assess the effects of pramipexole vs levodopa on Parkinson disease progression. J Am Med Assoc 2002;287:1653–1661.
10. Whone AL, Watts RL, Stoessl AJ et al. Slower progression of Parkinson's disease with ropinirole versus levodopa: the REAL–PET study. Ann Neurol 2003;54:93–101.
11. Marek K, Jennings D, Seibyl J. Do dopamine agonists or levodopa modify Parkinson's disease progression? Eur J Neurol 2002;9(Suppl. 3):15–22.
12. Morrish PK. Brain imaging to assess the effects of dopamine agonists on progression of Parkinson disease. J Am Med Assoc 2002;288:312; author reply 312–313.
13. Albin RL, Frey KA. Initial agonist treatment of Parkinson disease: a critique. Neurology 2003;60:390–394.
14. Fahn S. Parkinson disease, the effect of levodopa, and the ELLDOPA trial (earlier vs later L-dopa). Arch Neurol 1999;56:529–535.
15. Parkinson Study Group. Levodopa and progression of Parkinson disease: the ELLDOPA study. N Engl J Med 2004;351(24):2498–2508.
16. Horstink MW, Zijlmans JC, Pasman JW et al. Which risk factors predict the levodopa response in fluctuating Parkinson's disease? Ann Neurol 1990;27:537–543.
17. Roos RA, Vredevoogd CB, van der Velde EA. Response fluctuations in Parkinson's disease. Neurology 1990;40:1344–1346.
18. Poewe WH, Lees AJ, Stern GM. Low-dose L-dopa therapy in Parkinson's disease: a 6-year follow-up study. Neurology 1986;36:1528–1530.
19. Fabbrini G, Mouradian MM, Juncos JL et al. Motor fluctuations in Parkinson's disease: central pathophysiological mechanisms, part I. Ann Neurol 1988;24:366–371.
20. Montastruc JL, Rascol O, Senard JM et al. A randomised controlled study comparing bromocriptine to which levodopa was later added, with levodopa alone in previously untreated patients with Parkinson's disease: a five-year follow-up. J Neurol Neurosurg Psychiat 1994;57: 1034–1038.
21. Przuntek H, Welzel D, Gerlach M et al. Early institution of bromocriptine in Parkinson's disease inhibits the emergence of levodopa-associated motor side-effects: long-term results of the PRADO study. J Neural Transm Gen Sect 1996;103:699–715.
22. Rinne UK, Bracco F, Chouza C et al. Early treatment of Parkinson's disease with cabergoline delays the onset of motor complications: results of a double-blind levodopa controlled trial. The PKDS009 Study Group. Drugs 1998;55(Suppl. 1):23–30.
23. de Jong GJ, Meerwaldt JD, Schmitz PI. Factors that influence the occurrence of response variations in Parkinson's disease. Ann Neurol 1987;22(1):4–7.
24. Quinn N, Critchley P, Marsden CD. Young onset Parkinson's disease. Mov Disord 1987;2:73–91.
25. Blin J, Bonnet AM, Agid Y. Does levodopa aggravate Parkinson's disease? Neurology 1988;38: 1410–1416.
26. Horstink MW, Zijlmans JC, Pasman JW et al. Severity of Parkinson's disease is a risk factor for peak-dose dyskinesia. J Neurol Neurosurg Psychiatry 1990;53:224–226.
27. Caraceni T, Scigliano G, Musicco M. The occurrence of motor fluctuations in parkinsonian patients treated long term with levodopa: role of early treatment and disease progression. Neurology 1991;41:380–384.

28. Cedarbaum JM, Gandy SE, McDowell FH. "Early" initiation of levodopa treatment does not promote the development of motor response fluctuations, dyskinesias, or dementia in Parkinson's disease. Neurology 1991;41:622–629.
29. Lesser RP, Fahn S, Snider SR et al. Analysis of the clinical problems in parkinsonism and the complications of long-term levodopa therapy. Neurology 1979;29(9 Pt 1):1253–1260.
30. Mouradian MM, Heuser IJ, Baronti F et al. Modification of central dopaminergic mechanisms by continuous levodopa therapy for advanced Parkinson's disease. Ann Neurol 1990;27(1):18–23.
31. Chase TN. The significance of continuous dopaminergic stimulation in the treatment of Parkinson's disease. Drugs 1998;55(Suppl. 1):1–9.
32. Zappia M, Oliveri RL, Bosco D et al. The long-duration response to L-dopa in the treatment of early PD. Neurology 2000;54:1910–1915.
33. Block G, Liss C, Reines S et al. Comparison of immediate-release and controlled release carbidopa/levodopa in Parkinson's disease: a multicenter 5-year study. The CR First Study Group. Eur Neurol 1997;37(1):23–27.
34. Capildeo R. Implications of the 5-year CR FIRST trial. Sinemet CR Five-Year International Response Fluctuation Study. Neurology 1998;50(6 Suppl. 6):S15–17; discussion S44–48.
35. Wasielewski PG, Koller WC. Quality of life and Parkinson's disease: the CR FIRST Study. J Neurol 1998;245(Suppl. 1):S28–30.
36. Koller WC, Hutton JT, Tolosa E et al. Immediate-release and controlled-release carbidopa/levodopa in PD: a 5-year randomized multicenter study. Carbidopa/Levodopa Study Group. Neurology 1999;53(5):1012–1019.
37. Skibba JL, Pinckley J, Gilbert EF et al. Multiple primary melanoma following administration of levodopa. Arch Pathol 1972;93:556–561.
38. Olsen JH, Friis S, Frederiksen K et al. Atypical cancer pattern in patients with Parkinson's disease. Br J Cancer 2005;92(1):201–205.
39. Rampen FH. Levodopa and melanoma: three cases and review of literature. J Neurol Neurosurg Psychiatry 1985;48:585–588.
40. Fiala KH, Whetteckey J, Manyam BV. Malignant melanoma and levodopa in Parkinson's disease: causality or coincidence? Parkinsonism Relat Disord 2003;9:321–327.
41. Sober AJ, Wick MM. Levodopa therapy and malignant melanoma. J Am Med Assoc 1978;240: 554–555.
42. Sinemet CR [package insert]. Princeton, NJ: Bristol–Myers Squibb Co., 2002.
43. Madopar [summary of product characteristics]. Welwyn Garden City, Hertfordshire, UK: Roche Products Ltd, 2002.
44. Madopar CR [summary of product characteristics]. Wellwyn Garden City, Hertfordshire, UK: Roche Products Ltd, 2002.
45. Stalevo [package insert]. East Hanover, NJ: Novartis Pharmaceuticals Corp., 2003.
46. Weiner WJ, Singer C, Sanchez-Ramos JR et al. Levodopa, melanoma, and Parkinson's disease. Neurology 1993;43:674–677.
47. Woofter MJ, Manyam BV. Safety of long-term levodopa therapy in malignant melanoma. Clin Neuropharmacol 1994;17:315–319.
48. Pfutzner W, Przybilla B. Malignant melanoma and levodopa: is there a relationship? Two new cases and a review of the literature. J Am Acad Dermatol 1997;37(2 Pt 2):332–336.
49. Siple JF, Schneider DC, Wanlass WA et al. Levodopa therapy and the risk of malignant melanoma. Ann Pharmacother 2000;34:382–385.
50. Parkinson Study Group. DATATOP: a multicenter controlled clinical trial in early Parkinson's disease. Parkinson Study Group. Arch Neurol 1989;46:1052–1060.
51. Kostic V, Przedborski S, Flaster E et al. Early development of levodopa-induced dyskinesias and response fluctuations in young-onset Parkinson's disease. Neurology 1991;41(2 Pt 1):202–205.
52. Gershanik OS. Early-onset parkinsonism. In: Jankovic J, Tolosa E (eds), Parkinson's Disease and Movement Disorders, 2nd edn. Baltimore: Lippincott Williams & Wilkins, 1993, pp. 235–252.
53. Wagner ML, Fedak MN, Sage JI et al. Complications of disease and therapy: a comparison of younger and older patients with Parkinson's disease. Ann Clin Lab Sci 1996;26:389–395.
54. Oertel WH. Pergolide vs L-dopa (PELMOPET). Mov Disord 2000;15(Suppl. 3):5.
55. Parkinson Study Group. Pramipexole vs levodopa as initial treatment for Parkinson disease: a randomized controlled trial. Parkinson Study Group. J Am Med Assoc 2000;284:1931–1938.
56. Rascol O, Brooks DJ, Korczyn AD et al. A five-year study of the incidence of dyskinesia in patients with early Parkinson's disease who were treated with ropinirole or levodopa. 056 Study Group. N Engl J Med 2000;342:1484–1491.

57. Quinn NP. A case against early levodopa treatment of Parkinson's disease. Clin Neuropharmacol 1994;17:S43–49.
58. Fahn S. Parkinsonism. In: Rakel RE (ed.), Conn's Current Therapy. Philadelphia: WB Saunders, 1998, pp. 944–953.
59. Montastruc JL, Rascol O, Senard JM. Treatment of Parkinson's disease should begin with a dopamine agonist. Mov Disord 1999;14:725–730.
60. Lieberman A, Goldstein M, Gopinathan G et al. Combined use of benserazide and carbidopa in Parkinson's disease. Neurology 1984;34:227–229.
61. Da Prada M, Kettler R, Zurcher G et al. Inhibition of decarboxylase and levels of dopa and 3-O-methyldopa: a comparative study of benserazide versus carbidopa in rodents and of Madopar standard versus Madopar HBS in volunteers. Eur Neurol 1987;27(Suppl. 1):9–20.
62. Greenacre JK, Coxon A, Petrie A et al. Comparison of levodopa with carbidopa or benserazide in parkinsonism. Lancet 1976;ii(7982):381–384.
63. Lieberman A, Estey E, Gopinathan G et al. Comparative effectiveness of two extracerebral DOPA decarboxylase inhibitors in Parkinson disease. Neurology 1978;28(9 Pt 1):964–968.
64. Nutt JG, Woodward WR, Anderson JL. The effect of carbidopa on the pharmacokinetics of intravenously administered levodopa: the mechanism of action in the treatment of parkinsonism. Ann Neurol 1985;18:537–543.
65. Lodosyn [package insert]. Princeton, NJ: Bristol–Myers Squibb Co., 2002.
66. Parcopa [package insert]. Milwaukee, WI: Schwarz Pharma, 2003.
67. Djaldetti R, Melamed E. Management of response fluctuations: practical guidelines. Neurology 1998;51(2 Suppl. 2):S36–40.
68. Pappert EJ, Buhrfiend C, Lipton JW et al. Levodopa stability in solution: time course, environmental effects, and practical recommendations for clinical use. Mov Disord 1996;11:24–26.
69. Lang AE, Johnson K. Akathisia in idiopathic Parkinson's disease. Neurology 1987;37:477–481.
70. Shoulson I, Glaubiger GA, Chase TN. On–off response: clinical and biochemical correlations during oral and intravenous levodopa administration in parkinsonian patients. Neurology 1975;25:1144–1148.
71. Fahn S. Fluctuations of disability in Parkinson's disease: pathophysiological aspects. In: Marsden CD, Fahn S (ed.), Movement Disorders. London: Butterworth Scientific, 1982, pp. 123–145.
72. Contin M, Riva R, Martinelli P et al. A levodopa kinetic–dynamic study of the rate of progression in Parkinson's disease. Neurology 1998;51:1075–1080.
73. Hardie RJ, Lees AJ, Stern GM. On–off fluctuations in Parkinson's disease: a clinical and neuropharmacological study. Brain 1984;107(Pt 2):487–506.
74. Nutt JG. On–off phenomenon: relation to levodopa pharmacokinetics and pharmacodynamics. Ann Neurol 1987;22:535–540.
75. Sage JI, McHale DM, Sonsalla P et al. Continuous levodopa infusions to treat complex dystonia in Parkinson's disease. Neurology 1989;39:888–891.
76. Sage JI, Trooskin S, Sonsalla PK et al. Experience with continuous enteral levodopa infusions in the treatment of 9 patients with advanced Parkinson's disease. Neurology 1989;39(11 Suppl. 2):60–63; discussion 72–63.
77. Bredberg E, Nilsson D, Johansson K et al. Intraduodenal infusion of a water-based levodopa dispersion for optimisation of the therapeutic effect in severe Parkinson's disease. Eur J Clin Pharmacol 1993;45:117–122.
78. Kurth MC, Tetrud JW, Tanner CM et al. Double-blind, placebo-controlled, crossover study of duodenal infusion of levodopa/carbidopa in Parkinson's disease patients with "on–off" fluctuations. Neurology 1993;43:1698–1703.
79. Bush DF, Liss CL, Morton A. An open multicenter long-term treatment evaluation of Sinemet CR. Sinemet CR Multicenter Study Group. Neurology 1989;39(11 Suppl. 2):101–104; discussion 105.
80. Hutton JT, Morris JL. Long-acting carbidopa–levodopa in the management of moderate and advanced Parkinson's disease. Neurology 1992;42(1 Suppl. 1):51–56; discussion 57–60.
81. Pahwa R, Busenbark K, Huber SJ et al. Clinical experience with controlled-release carbidopa/levodopa in Parkinson's disease. Neurology 1993;43:677–681.
82. Golbe LI, Lieberman AN, Muenter MD et al. Deprenyl in the treatment of symptom fluctuations in advanced Parkinson's disease. Clin Neuropharmacol 1988;11:45–55.
83. Hughes AJ, Bishop S, Kleedorfer B et al. Subcutaneous apomorphine in Parkinson's disease: response to chronic administration for up to five years. Mov Disord 1993;8:165–170.
84. Ostergaard L, Werdelin L, Odin P et al. Pen injected apomorphine against off phenomena in late Parkinson's disease: a double-blind, placebo-controlled study. J Neurol Neurosurg Psychiatry 1995;58:681–687.

85. Dewey RB, Maraganore DM, Ahlskog JE et al. A double-blind, placebo-controlled study of intranasal apomorphine spray as a rescue agent for off-states in Parkinson's disease. Mov Disord 1998;13:782–787.
86. Djaldetti R, Melamed E. Levodopa ethylester: a novel rescue therapy for response fluctuations in Parkinson's disease. Ann Neurol 1996;39:400–404.
87. Djaldetti R, Inzelberg R, Giladi N et al. Oral solution of levodopa ethylester for treatment of response fluctuations in patients with advanced Parkinson's disease. Mov Disord 2002;17:297–302.
88. Melamed E. Early-morning dystonia: a late side-effect of long-term levodopa therapy in Parkinson's disease. Arch Neurol 1979;36:308–310.
89. Bravi D, Mouradian MM, Roberts JW et al. End-of-dose dystonia in Parkinson's disease. Neurology 1993;43:2130–2131.
90. Currie LJ, Harrison MB, Trugman JM et al. Early morning dystonia in Parkinson's disease. Neurology 1998;51:283–285.
91. Duvoisin RC. Variations in the "on–off" phenomenon. Adv Neurol 1974;5:339–340.
92. Fahn S. "On–off" phenomenon with levodopa therapy in parkinsonism: clinical and pharmacologic correlations and the effect of intramuscular pyridoxine. Neurology 1974;24:431–441.
93. Maricle RA, Nutt JG, Carter JH. Mood and anxiety fluctuation in Parkinson's disease associated with levodopa infusion: preliminary findings. Mov Disord 1995;10:329–332.
94. Ford B, Louis ED, Greene P et al. Oral and genital pain syndromes in Parkinson's disease. Mov Disord 1996;11:421–426.
95. Hillen ME, Sage JI. Nonmotor fluctuations in patients with Parkinson's disease. Neurology 1996;47:1180–1183.
96. Djaldetti R, Baron J, Ziv I et al. Gastric emptying in Parkinson's disease: patients with and without response fluctuations. Neurology 1996;46:1051–1054.
97. Melamed E, Bitton V, Zelig O. Delayed onset of responses to single doses of L-dopa in parkinsonian fluctuators on long-term L-dopa therapy. Clin Neuropharmacol 1986;9:182–188.
98. Contin M, Riva R, Martinelli P et al. Effect of meal timing on the kinetic–dynamic profile of levodopa/carbidopa controlled release [corrected] in parkinsonian patients. Eur J Clin Pharmacol 1998;54:303–308.
99. Frankel JP, Kempster PA, Bovingdon M et al. The effects of oral protein on the absorption of intraduodenal levodopa and motor performance. J Neurol Neurosurg Psychiatry 1989;52:1063–1067.
100. Tsui JK, Ross S, Poulin K et al. The effect of dietary protein on the efficacy of L-dopa: a double-blind study. Neurology 1989;39:549–552.
101. Nutt JG, Woodward WR, Hammerstad JP et al. The "on–off" phenomenon in Parkinson's disease: relation to levodopa absorption and transport. N Engl J Med 1984;310:483–488.
102. Juncos JL, Fabbrini G, Mouradian MM et al. Dietary influences on the antiparkinsonian response to levodopa. Arch Neurol 1987;44:1003–1005.
103. Pincus JH, Barry K. Influence of dietary protein on motor fluctuations in Parkinson's disease. Arch Neurol 1987;44(3):270–272.
104. Pincus JH, Barry K. Protein redistribution diet restores motor function in patients with dopa-resistant "off" periods. Neurology 1988;38:481–483.
105. Duvoisin RC. Hyperkinetic reactions with L-dopa. In Yahr MD (ed.), Current Concepts in the Treatment of Parkinsonism. New York: Raven Press, 1974, 203–210.
106. Fahn S. The spectrum of levodopa-induced dyskinesias. Ann Neurol 2000;47(4 Suppl. 1):S2–9; discussion S9–11.
107. Muenter MD, Sharpless NS, Tyce GM et al. Patterns of dystonia ("I-D-I" and "D-I-D") in response to L-dopa therapy for Parkinson's disease. Mayo Clin Proc 1977;52(3):163–174.
108. Verhagen Metman L, Del Dotto P, van den Munckhof P et al. Amantadine as treatment for dyskinesias and motor fluctuations in Parkinson's disease. Neurology 1998;50:1323–1326.
109. Metman LV, Del Dotto P, LePoole K et al. Amantadine for levodopa-induced dyskinesias: a 1-year follow-up study. Arch Neurol 1999;56:1383–1386.
110. Luginger E, Wenning GK, Bosch S et al. Beneficial effects of amantadine on L-dopa-induced dyskinesias in Parkinson's disease. Mov Disord 2000;15:873–878.
111. Snow BJ, Macdonald L, McAuley D et al. The effect of amantadine on levodopa-induced dyskinesias in Parkinson's disease: a double-blind, placebo-controlled study. Clin Neuropharmacol 2000;23(2):82–85.
112. Bennett JP, Landow ER, Schuh LA. Suppression of dyskinesias in advanced Parkinson's disease. II: Increasing daily clozapine doses suppress dyskinesias and improve parkinsonism symptoms. Neurology 1993;43:1551–1555.

113. Bennett JP, Landow ER, Dietrich S et al. Suppression of dyskinesias in advanced Parkinson's disease: moderate daily clozapine doses provide long-term dyskinesia reduction. Mov Disord 1994;9:409–414.
114. Durif F, Vidailhet M, Assal F et al. Low-dose clozapine improves dyskinesias in Parkinson's disease. Neurology 1997;48:658–662.
115. Pierelli F, Adipietro A, Soldati G et al. Low dosage clozapine effects on L-dopa induced dyskinesias in parkinsonian patients. Acta Neurol Scand 1998;97:295–299.
116. Bara-Jimenez W, Sherzai A, Dimitrova T et al. Adenosine A(2A) receptor antagonist treatment of Parkinson's disease. Neurology 2003;61:293–296.
117. Hauser RA, Hubble JP, Truong DD. Randomized trial of the adenosine A(2A) receptor antagonist istradefylline in advanced PD. Neurology 2003;61:297–303.
118. Lhermitte F, Agid Y, Signoret JL. Onset and end-of-dose levodopa-induced dyskinesias: possible treatment by increasing the daily doses of levodopa. Arch Neurol 1978;35:261–263.
119. Agid Y, Bonnet AM, Signoret JL et al. Clinical, pharmacological, and biochemical approach of "onset" and "end-of-dose" dyskinesias. In: Poirier LJ, Sourkes TL, Bedard PJ (eds), The Extrapyramidal System and its Disorders. New York: Raven Press, 1979, pp. 401–410.
120. Jankovic J. Complications and limitations of drug therapy for Parkinson's disease. Neurology 2000;55(12 Suppl. 6):S2–6.
121. Kieburtz K, Hubble J. Benefits of COMT inhibitors in levodopa-treated parkinsonian patients: results of clinical trials. Neurology 2000;55(11 Suppl. 4):S42–45; discussion S46–50.
122. Mercuri NB, Federici M, Bernardi G. Inhibition of catechol-O-methyltransferase (COMT) in the brain does not affect the action of dopamine and levodopa: in-vitro electrophysiological evidence from rat mesencephalic dopamine neurons. J Neural Transm 1999;106(11/12):1135–1140.
123. Tasmar [package insert]. Nutley, NJ: Roche Laboratories Inc., 1998.
124. Adler CH, Singer C, O'Brien C et al. Randomized, placebo-controlled study of tolcapone in patients with fluctuating Parkinson disease treated with levodopa–carbidopa. Tolcapone Fluctuator Study Group III. Arch Neurol 1998;55:1089–1095.
125. Rajput AH, Martin W, Saint-Hilaire MH et al. Tolcapone improves motor function in parkinsonian patients with the "wearing-off" phenomenon: a double-blind, placebo-controlled, multicenter trial. Neurology 1998;50(5 Suppl. 5):S54–59.
126. Assal F, Spahr L, Hadengue A et al. Tolcapone and fulminant hepatitis. Lancet 1998;352:958.
127. Watkins P. COMT inhibitors and liver toxicity. Neurology 2000;55(11 Suppl. 4):S51–52; discussion S53–56.
128. Comtan [package insert]. East Hanover, NJ: Novartis Pharmaceuticals Corp., 2000.
129. Goetz CG. Influence of COMT inhibition on levodopa pharmacology and therapy. Neurology 1998;50(5 Suppl. 5):S26–30.
130. Ruottinen HM, Rinne UK. A double-blind pharmacokinetic and clinical dose–response study of entacapone as an adjuvant to levodopa therapy in advanced Parkinson's disease. Clin Neuropharmacol 1996;19:283–296.
131. Heikkinen H, Varhe A, Laine T et al. Entacapone improves the availability of L-dopa in plasma by decreasing its peripheral metabolism independent of L-dopa/carbidopa dose. Br J Clin Pharmacol 2002;54:363–371.
132. Ruottinen HM, Rinne UK. Effect of one month's treatment with peripherally acting catechol-O-methyltransferase inhibitor, entacapone, on pharmacokinetics and motor response to levodopa in advanced parkinsonian patients. Clin Neuropharmacol 1996;19:222–233.
133. Ruottinen HM, Rinne UK. Entacapone prolongs levodopa response in a one-month double-blind study in parkinsonian patients with levodopa related fluctuations. J Neurol Neurosurg Psychiatry 1996;60:36–40.
134. Parkinson Study Group. Entacapone improves motor fluctuations in levodopa-treated Parkinson's disease patients. Ann Neurol 1997;42:747–755.
135. Rinne UK, Larsen JP, Siden A et al. Entacapone enhances the response to levodopa in parkinsonian patients with motor fluctuations. Nomecomt Study Group. Neurology 1998;51:1309–1314.
136. Larsen JP, Worm-Petersen J, Siden A et al. The tolerability and efficacy of entacapone over 3 years in patients with Parkinson's disease. Eur J Neurol 2003;10(2):137–146.
137. Toru M, Matsuda O, Makiguchi K et al. Neuroleptic malignant syndrome-like state following a withdrawal of antiparkinsonian drugs. J Nerv Ment Dis 1981;169:324–327.
138. Sechi GP, Tanda F, Mutani R. Fatal hyperpyrexia after withdrawal of levodopa. Neurology 1984;34:249–251.
139. Friedman JH, Feinberg SS, Feldman RG. A neuroleptic malignant-like syndrome due to levodopa therapy withdrawal. J Am Med Assoc 1985;254:2792–2795.

140. Gibb WR, Griffith DN. Levodopa withdrawal syndrome identical to neuroleptic malignant syndrome. Postgrad Med J 1986;62(723):59–60.
141. Hirschorn KA, Greenberg HS. Successful treatment of levodopa-induced myoclonus and levodopa withdrawal-induced neuroleptic malignant syndrome: a case report. Clin Neuropharmacol 1988;11:278–281.
142. Gordon PH, Frucht SJ. Neuroleptic malignant syndrome in advanced Parkinson's disease. Mov Disord 2001;16:960–962.
143. Simpson DM, Davis GC. Case report of neuroleptic malignant syndrome associated with withdrawal from amantadine. Am J Psychiatry 1984;141:796–797.
144. Takubo H, Harada T, Hashimoto T et al. A collaborative study on the malignant syndrome in Parkinson's disease and related disorders. Parkinsonism Relat Disord 2003;9(Suppl. 1):S31–41.
145. Pfeiffer RF, Sucha EL. "On/off"-induced lethal hyperthermia. Mov Disord 1989;4:338–341.
146. Ikebe S, Harada T, Hashimoto T et al. Prevention and treatment of malignant syndrome in Parkinson's disease: a consensus statement of the malignant syndrome research group. Parkinsonism Relat Disord 2003;9(Suppl. 1):S47–49.
147. Furuya R, Hirai A, Andoh T et al. Successful perioperative management of a patient with Parkinson's disease by enteral levodopa administration under propofol anesthesia. Anesthesiology 1998;89:261–263.
148. Rosin AJ, Devereux D, Eng N et al. Parkinsonism with "on-off" phenomena: intravenous treatment with levodopa after major abdominal surgery. Arch Neurol 1979;36:32–34.
149. Galvez-Jimenez N, Lang AE. Perioperative problems in Parkinson's disease and their management: apomorphine with rectal domperidone. Can J Neurol Sci 1996;23(3):198–203.
150. Fahn S, Parkinson Study Group. Rotigotine transdermal system (SPM-962) is safe and effective as monotherapy in early Parkinson's disease. Parkinsonism Relat Disord 2001;7(Suppl.):S55.
151. Metman LV, Gillespie M, Farmer C et al. Continuous transdermal dopaminergic stimulation in advanced Parkinson's disease. Clin Neuropharmacol 2001;24(3):163–169.

2

Drug Therapy: Dopamine Agonists

Werner Poewe

INTRODUCTION

Dopamine agonists were first introduced into clinical practice in the 1970s when Calne and coworkers reported on the beneficial effects of adjunctive treatment with bromocriptine in patients with a failing levodopa response.[1,2] Their development and clinical use in Parkinson's disease (PD) was based on the evolving understanding of the pharmacology of dopamine receptors. Since then, five human dopamine receptor subtypes have been identified and eventually cloned. They are divided into the D1-like (D1 and D5) and the D2-like (D2, D3, and D4) receptor families, based on their capability to stimulate or to inhibit adenylate cyclase, respectively. The presence or absence of stimulation of adenylate cyclase reflects their different interactions with the GTP-dependent regulatory G_i/G_o and G_s-proteins.[3] Dopamine receptors are encoded by genes localized on different chromosomes–the D1 receptor gene is localized on chromosome 5, both D2 and D4 receptor genes on chromosome 11, the D3 on chromosome 3, and the D5 on chromosome 4.[4–8] Dopamine receptors share some homologous amino acid sequences, probably reflecting common characteristics, while different sequences may reflect the different coupling of each subtype with one particular G protein (G_s or G_i/G_o), and their different drug specificities.

D1 and D2 receptors are mainly found in the striatum and in substantia nigra and they are thought to have a largely postsynaptic localization. D2 receptors can also function as autoreceptors, which have a feedback regulatory role at the presynaptic level, modulating dopamine synthesis and release and neuronal firing rate.[9] The nigrostriatal dopaminergic denervation which characterizes PD causes changes of these receptors at both the postsynaptic and presynaptic levels.

The antiparkinsonian effect of most dopamine agonists is related to stimulation of D2 receptors. Mixed D1/D2 agonism, however, may be important for a full reversal of parkinsonian motor deficits.[10]

Dopamine agonists act directly on postsynaptic dopamine receptors, thereby bypassing the need for metabolic conversion, storage, and release in degenerating nigrostriatal nerve terminals as required for the action of levodopa. Furthermore, dopamine agonists decrease endogenous dopamine turnover which is even enhanced by levodopa and may be one source of potentially neurotoxic free radical formation through auto-oxidation of accumulating dopamine. In addition, while all acting on D2-like dopamine receptors, dopamine agonists have selective subspecificities within the D2 family, offering the potential of specific clinical profiles and reduced risks for adverse reactions associated with specific types of receptor stimulation. Most of the currently marketed dopamine agonists for the treatment of PD have significantly longer half-lives than levodopa. In primate models of PD, exposure to long-acting dopamine agonists is not associated with the development of drug-induced dyskinesias, but exposure to levodopa or short-acting dopamine agonists is.[11] Such findings suggest that long-acting dopamine agonists will be associated with a decreased risk to develop motor complications in the long-term treatment of PD patients due to more continuous striatal dopamine receptor stimulation.

Finally, a number of in-vitro and in-vivo studies have produced findings suggestive of potential neuroprotective effects of dopamine agonists related to antioxidative, radical scavenging, and antiapoptotic properties.[12–14] Their pharmacological profile thus suggests potential advantages over levodopa (Table 2.1).

CLINICAL PHARMACOLOGY OF DOPAMINE AGONISTS

Currently used dopamine agonists in clinical practice include the ergot derivatives bromocriptine, cabergoline, dihydroergocriptine, lisuride, and pergolide, as well as the non-ergot compounds apomorphine, piribedil, pramipexole, and ropinirole. While most are available globally, dihydroergocriptine, apomorphine, and piribedil are currently marketed only in Europe. Their clinical pharmacological profile is summarized in Table 2.2. This section summarizes the clinical pharmacology of the different DA-agonists based on data generated in well-designed controlled clinical trials.

TABLE 2-1 Advantages of dopamine agonists in the treatment of Parkinson's disease

Direct DA-receptor-stimulation
D1/D2 subspecificity
No transport competition (GI-tract, BBB)
Longer half-life than levodopa (ropinirole, pramipexole, pergolide, cabergoline)
No oxidative metabolism
Neuroprotection in vitro
– radical scavenging
– antioxidative action
– antiapoptotic action

TABLE 2.2 Clinical pharmacology of dopamine agonists

Drug	*Dopamine receptor interaction*[a]	*Interaction with other receptors*		*Half-life (h)*
		NA	5-HT	
Bromocriptine	D2	+	+	3–6
Lisuride	D2	+	+	2–3
Pergolide	D2 > D1	+	+	15
Cabergoline	D2	+	+	65
Dihydroergocriptine[b]	D2 (± D1)	+	+	12–16
Apomorphine[b]	D2/D1	–	–	0.5
Piribedil[b]	D2	±	–	20
Pramipexole	D2	±	–	10
Ropinirole	D2	–	–	6

[a] Within D2 family, all agonists have D3/D2 affinity ratio of >1 except for lisuride, bromocriptine, and dihydroergocryptine.

[b] Not available in the United States.

Ergot Dopamine Agonists

Bromocriptine

Bromocriptine mesylate is a tetracyclic ergoline derivative and was the first DA-agonist marketed for the treatment of Parkinson's disease. Bromocriptine is not completely absorbed via the oral route and is extensively metabolized in the liver. Absolute oral bioavailability is less than 10%, maximum plasma levels are reached within 1–2 hours, and plasma half-life is 6–8 hours.

It acts as a D2 agonist with a D1 antagonist activity in nanomolar concentrations and as a partial D1 agonist in micromolar concentrations.

Like most ergot compounds, bromocriptine also has 5-HT_2 antagonistic and some adrenergic efficacy.

Clinical efficacy of bromocriptine as early monotherapy

While bromocriptine was initially introduced as adjunctive treatment to levodopa in advanced PD, later placebo-controlled studies have confirmed the efficacy of bromocriptine monotherapy in de-novo patients with Parkinson's disease.[15,16] Moreover, it was noted that sustained bromocriptine therapy in previously untreated patients with PD was associated with a very low rate of motor fluctuations or drug-induced dyskinesias in the long term.[17] This was later confirmed in several levodopa controlled randomized trials of early bromocriptine monotherapy where initial bromocriptine treatment produced significantly fewer motor complications than levodopa after 3 to 5 years.[18–20] In the 5-year randomized levodopa-controlled bromocriptine trial of Montrastuc and colleagues, later addition of levodopa to bromocriptine, when clinically needed, was still associated with significantly fewer drug-induced dyskinesias.

Clinical efficacy in terms of symptomatic control, however, was generally less with bromocriptine compared to levodopa in these studies, and the PDRG-UK trial found that only a third of patients could be satisfactorily controlled by bromocriptine monotherapy for more than 3 years and that virtually all patients eventually required levodopa by 10 years.[21]

Only a few randomized trials have compared efficacy of bromocriptine to that of other dopamine agonists as initial monotherapy. One short-term pergolide-controlled study found similar degrees of improvement with both drugs after 8 weeks of double-blind comparative treatment.[22] The only long-term data of bromocriptine monotherapy are from a ropinirole-controlled study.[23,24] At 6 months, ropinirole monotherapy (mean dose 8.3 mg/day) was slightly more efficacious in reducing UPDRS motor scores than bromocriptine monotherapy (mean dose 16.8 mg/day). After 3 years, patients completing the trial on ropinirole (12 mg/day) had significantly greater improvements in UPDRS ADL scores compared to patients receiving bromocriptine (24 mg/day) but the greater improvement in UPDRS motor scores for ropinirole was no longer statistically significant.[24]

This study found similarly low rates of motor complications, in particular dyskinesias, with both drugs regardless of levodopa supplementation. Dyskinesia rates after 3 years were 7.7% for ropinirole and 7.2% for bromocriptine.[24]

Doses of bromocriptine required for effective monotherapy are generally between 20 mg and 40 mg daily,[18] but individual patients may require higher doses of more than 60 mg/day.[19]

One randomized double-blind trial was performed to assess the effects of adjunctive treatment with deprenyl to either levodopa or bromocriptine on disease progression of early Parkinson's disease. This four-arm trial, which had a duration of 14 months (including a 2 months' washout of deprenyl), found similar declines of UPDRS scores versus baseline with either levodopa or bromocriptine monotherapy combined with placebo–indicating either no effect of bromocriptine on disease progression or effects which are similar to levodopa. There are no trials specifically designed to assess the disease-modifying potential of bromocriptine.[25]

Clinical efficacy of bromocriptine as adjunct to levodopa

Several placebo-controlled studies of adjunct therapy with bromocriptine in patients on chronic levodopa therapy experiencing motor fluctuations and/or dyskinesias have consistently shown significant improvements in "on" motor function as assessed by the UPDRS ADL and/or motor score with bromocriptine–generally dosed around 20 mg/day.[26–28]

Few controlled trials have compared bromocriptine with other ergot dopamine agonists as adjunctive treatment to levodopa. Inzelberg et al.[29] found similar effects of cabergoline (mean dose 3.2 mg/day) and bromocriptine (mean dose 22 mg/day) on UPDRS ADL and motor scores. In a comparative crossover study with pergolide, Pezzoli and colleagues[30] found significantly greater improvements in the New York University Parkinson's Disease Scale with pergolide (2.3 mg/day) versus 24.2 mg/day of bromocriptine. Similar findings using the UPDRS were reported by Boas et al.[31] in another, but open-label, crossover study.

All the above trials were primarily designed to assess efficacy of adjunctive treatment with bromocriptine with respect to the control of motor complications and found significant improvements in wearing-off motor fluctuations and/or reductions in total daily "off" time with bromocriptine versus placebo[26–28] (Figure 2.1). The active comparator trial versus cabergoline found significant greater "off"-time reductions with cabergoline compared to bromocriptine.[28]

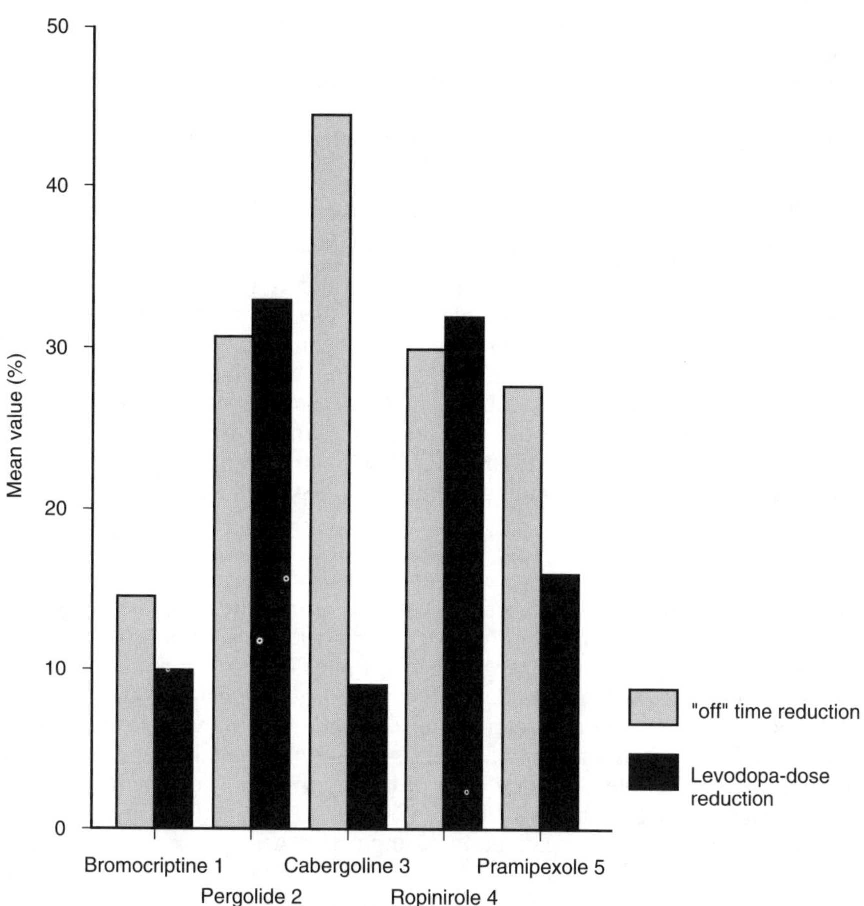

FIGURE 2.1 Results from double-blind controlled trials of add-on dopamine agonists in fluctuating Parkinson's disease. Sources of data–[1] Guttman et al., 1997; Inzelberg et al., 1996 (refs 28 and 29). [2] Olanow et al., 1994; Olanow et al., 1987; Jankovic et al., 1987; Diamond et al., 1985 (refs 55 and 86–88). [3] Inzelberg et al., 1996; Geminiani et al., 1996; Steiger et al., 1996 (refs 29, 89, and 90). [4] Lieberman et al., 1998 (ref. 83). [5] Guttmann, 1997; Lieberman et al., 1997; Pinter et al., 1999 (refs 28, 72, and 74).

Safety

Dopaminergic adverse reactions to bromocriptine include nausea, vomiting, dizziness and orthostatic hypotension as well as drug-induced hallucinosis and psychosis. Adjunctive bromocriptine in levodopa-treated patients with pre-existing dyskinesias can exacerbate these involuntary movements and necessitate concomitant dose reductions of levodopa. Like other dopamine agonists, and levodopa itself, bromocriptine has been associated with somnolence and daytime sleepiness, including occasional reports of "sleep attacks."[32] A rare and potentially serious adverse event reported in patients treated with bromocriptine and other ergot dopamine agonists is related to pleuropulmonary and/or peritoneal fibrosis.[33] Leg edema is not an uncommon side-effect of bromocriptine therapy–the mechanism of which is still poorly understood.

Peripheral dopaminergic side-effects of bromocriptine therapy can be prevented or controlled by adjunctive treatment with domperidone.[34]

Dihydroergocriptine (DHEC)

Dihydroergocriptine (DHEC) is a dihydroderivative of ergocriptine with a similar pharmacological profile to bromocriptine. It is marketed in several European countries but is not available in the United States. Efficacy regarding symptomatic control of parkinsonism has been established in placebo-controlled studies in de-novo patients[35] as well as an adjunct to levodopa[36] in stable responders, while there is limited trial data on its use to control motor complications. Therapeutic doses reported in clinical trials range between 30 mg/day to 60 mg/day. Safety of DHEC seems to be similar to that of other ergot dopamine agonists, including a small risk of pleural fibrosis.[37]

Cabergoline

Cabergoline is another orally active synthetic tetracyclic ergoline derivative with selective D2 receptor agonist properties, but with no significant affinity for D1 receptors. Its non-dopaminergic receptor profile (nor-adrenergic agonist, serotonergic antagonist) is similar to the other ergot dopamine agonists like bromocriptine. A unique characteristic of cabergoline is its very long elimination half-life of approximately 65 hours with an associated long duration of clinical effect. A single 1 mg oral dose of cabergoline has been shown to suppress prolactin levels for up to 21 days.[38] The pharmacokinetic profile of cabergoline therefore allows for once-daily dosing regimens.

Clinical efficacy of cabergoline as early monotherapy

There are no randomized placebo-controlled trials to assess the efficacy of cabergoline to control the motor symptoms of PD. However, a levodopa-controlled double-blind randomized trial has investigated efficacy and safety of cabergoline monotherapy in previously untreated patients with PD.[39] This study included 413 patients randomized to cabergoline or levodopa in a 1:1 ratio. Interim results were published after one year of study and subsequently final results covering a follow-up period between 3 and 5 years (mean 3.8 years) were also made available.[40] Cabergoline doses were 2.8 mg/day at year 1 and had increased to 3 mg/day by the end of long-term follow-up. After one year, 38% of patients in the cabergoline group received levodopa supplementation (mean dose 305 mg/day) but the decrease in UPDRS total scores was slightly larger in the levodopa group. This difference was, however, small (2.8 points) and percentages of patients with a 30% reduction in total UPDRS scores versus baseline were almost identical in both groups (81% versus 88%). The proportion of patients requiring levodopa supplementation, however, was significantly greater with cabergoline (38%) versus levodopa (18%) by year 1.

Patients receiving cabergoline had significantly fewer motor complications compared to those initially randomized to levodopa (22% versus 37% $p < 0.02$). Sixty-five percent of patients remaining in the trial on cabergoline required levodopa supplementation compared to 48% in the levodopa arm. "On"-period dyskinesias affected 14% of patients initially treated with levodopa compared to only 6% on cabergoline (Table 2.3). Cabergoline was somewhat less effective than levodopa in controlling motor symptoms as assessed by changes from baseline in UPDRS motor scores. Patients randomized to levodopa showed an average 30% improvement of UPDRS motor scores compared to 22–23% with cabergoline.

So far no study has investigated the effects of initial monotherapy with cabergoline on disease progression.

Cabergoline as adjunct to levodopa

A single placebo-controlled trial has investigated the efficacy of adjunctive treatment with cabergoline in 188 levodopa-treated patients with suboptimal motor control. Adjunctive cabergoline resulted in improvements of 15%–20% of the UPDRS ADL and motor part versus baseline, which was significantly superior to placebo. At the same time the levodopa dose was reduced by 175 mg/day in the cabergoline group (compared to 25.5 mg/day with placebo). In a small double-blind randomized comparative trial, Inzelberg et al.[29] had found 3.2 mg/day of cabergoline to be similarly effective in reducing UPDRS motor scores as bromocriptine (see above).

TABLE 2.3 Levodopa-controlled trials of early monotherapy with dopamine agonists: incidence of dyskinesias

Study	*Follow-up (years)*	*Agonist*	*Levodopa*	*Reference*
Cabergoline vs. levodopa[a]	3.8	6%	14%	40
Ropinirole vs. levodopa	5.0	5%/20%	36%/45%	79
Pergolide vs. levodopa	3.0	5%	14%	54
Pramipexole vs. levodopa	2.0	10%	31%	69
Pramipexole vs. levodopa	4.0	25%	54%	70

[a] "ON"-period dyskinesias only.

In their placebo-controlled add-on-study, Hutton et al.[41] also observed significantly greater reductions in "off" time with cabergoline and the drug was superior to bromocriptine in the study by Inzelberg et al.[29] – yielding 50% "off"-time reduction versus baseline compared to 20% with bromocriptine (see Figure 2.1).

Safety

Cabergoline treatment is associated with typical dopaminergic side-effects like nausea, vomiting, orthostatic hypotension and neuropsychiatric adverse events. Add-on-treatment in patients with levodopa-induced dyskinesias may exacerbate involuntary movements similarly to other dopaminergic agonists, and cabergoline has also been associated with daytime sleepiness and so-called "sleep attacks."[42] Also similar to other ergot-agonists, cabergoline has been associated with pleuropulmonary fibrosis[43] and the drug may also induce leg edema.

Lisuride

Lisuride is a semisynthetic α-aminoergoline with D2 dopaminergic activity and no apparent D1-receptor agonism. Lisuride has a relatively short half-life of about 2 hours and its absolute oral bioavailability is low due to extensive first-pass metabolism. As with most other ergot agonists, lisuride has also 5-HT_2 receptor activity.

Lisuride as early monotherapy

Lisuride improves motor symptoms of PD when given as initial monotherapy, but symptomatic efficacy is less than that seen with levodopa.[44] This is based on a single randomized open-label long-term comparative trial including 90 patients randomized to receive early lisuride monotherapy, levodopa monotherapy, or combined lisuride plus levodopa ("early combination"). After 3 months of treatment, patients randomized to lisuride had significantly less improvement on the Columbia University Rating Scale (CURS) compared to those receiving levodopa monotherapy (32% versus 56%, $p < 0.01$).

This study was designed as a 4-year prospective study, but only 17% of patients continued on lisuride monotherapy while all others had required levodopa supplementation. Combined treatment with lisuride (1.1 mg/day on average) and levodopa (mean 484 mg/day) produced similar improvements on the CURS compared to levodopa monotherapy (mean dose around 670 mg/day), but patients with early or late combination of lisuride plus levodopa had significantly fewer motor complications: 19% in the early combination arm had peak-dose dyskinesias compared to 64% in the levodopa monotherapy arm at final visit.[44] These data are insufficient, however, to assess the outcome of lisuride monotherapy in early Parkinson's disease since after 4 years of follow-up only five patients remained in this treatment group.

A second randomized open-label study comparing early combined lisuride plus levodopa versus levodopa treatment of early PD used UPDRS subsection

IV scores to assess motor complications after 5 years of treatment and failed to find significant differences between the two approaches.[45]

Lisuride as adjunct to levodopa

As stated above, early combined treatment with lisuride plus levodopa may be associated with fewer long-term motor complications compared to levodopa monotherapy. Both open-label randomized trials available[40,45] suggest similar symptomatic efficacy on the motor symptoms of PD as seen with higher doses of levodopa given as monotherapy. There are no properly randomized placebo-controlled studies to assess the efficacy of late adjunctive lisuride treatment in levodopa-treated patients with motor fluctuations. Active comparator studies with bromocriptine or dihydroergocriptine suggest similar efficacy regarding "on" motor function and reduction of motor fluctuations with lisuride as seen with the other ergot-agonists.[46–48]

Continuous subcutaneous infusions of lisuride via portable mini-pumps were introduced in the late 1980s by Obeso and collegues for PD patients with refractory response oscillations, and open-label studies have reported marked reductions in "off" time.[49] This approach, however, has been associated with an unacceptable incidence of drug-induced psychosis in the long term.[50] Some authors have reported evidence for pharmacodynamic dopamine receptor changes with increases of dyskinetic thresholds following subcutaneous lisuride infusions in patients with late levodopa failure, arguing for continuous dopaminergic stimulation as the optimal treatment modality in PD.[51] A recent prospective randomized clinical trial comparing standard oral levodopa based therapy with subcutaneous lisuride infusions in patients with advanced disease and motor complications has found significantly reduced dyskinesia scores with subcutaneous lisuride infusions.[52]

Safety

The safety profile of lisuride is identical to that of other ergot-dopamine agonists including gastrointestinal and cardiovascular side-effects as well as exacerbation of pre-existing dyskinesias. Neuropsychiatric reactions, in particular hallucinosis, have been common with lisuride subcutaneous infusions, and two comparative studies with bromocriptine and DHEC[46,48] have reported higher incidences of psychiatric adverse reactions with lisuride. Pleuro-pulmonary fibrosis has been reported in individual cases, as have been incidences of pathological daytime sleepiness with "sleep attacks."[32]

Pergolide

Pergolide mesylate is a semi-synthetic ergot derivative that acts at both D2 and D1 receptors. Pergolide reaches plasma peak concentrations in 1–3 hours and a single dose is completely cleared within 7 days, with a half-life of 15–42 hours. Molecular biological studies have shown that pergolide also has a high affinity for the D3 receptor. Studies using catecholamine synthesis inhibitors have shown that the dopaminergic action of pergolide is much less dependent on intact dopamine stores than that of bromocriptine, and this difference may be related to the mixed D1/D2 agonistic properties of pergolide.

Pergolide as early monotherapy

Efficacy of initial monotherapy with pergolide in de-novo patients with PD has been demonstrated in a double-blind placebo-controlled 3-month study in 105 patients.[53] At a mean dose of 2 mg/day, pergolide treatment resulted in significantly greater percentages of responders (defined as patients with 30% or greater improvement on the UPDRS motor scale) compared to placebo (57% versus 17%, $p < 0.001$). Pergolide was also superior on secondary endpoints like UPDRS ADL or Schwab and England scores as well as clinical global improvement.

A 3-year double-blind prospective levodopa-controlled study of pergolide in de-novo patients assessed the relative incidence of motor complications with either treatment as primary endpoint. Results have only been presented in abstract form and show significantly reduced frequencies of motor fluctuations and dyskinesias with pergolide monotherapy compared to levodopa (see Table 2.3). Symptomatic efficacy as judged by the UPDRS motor score, however, was also significantly less with pergolide at a mean dose of slightly more than 3 mg/day (compared to 500 mg/day of levodopa).[54]

Pergolide as adjunct to levodopa

Adjunctive treatment with pergolide in patients with advanced Parkinson's disease on levodopa was highly significantly superior to placebo in a large randomized study including 376 PD patients. At a mean dose of about 3 mg/day, pergolide was associated with significantly greater improvements in all parkinsonian scores including motor disability and activities of daily living, and was also associated with significantly greater decreases in levodopa daily dose compared to placebo (–25% versus –5%).

Two studies comparing adjunctive pergolide to bromocriptine in advanced PD also reported greater efficacy of adjunctive pergolide.[30,31]

The placebo-controlled study by Olanow et al.[55] demonstrated significant reductions of total daily "off" time by around 35% with pergolide (see Figure 2.1).

Safety

The side-effect profile of pergolide is typical for ergot dopamine agonists, including nausea, vomiting, orthostatic hypotension, and hallucinosis and psychosis. Pre-existing levodopa-induced dyskinesias can be exacerbated with adjunctive pergolide. Pleural or pulmonary fibrosis as well as cardiac valvular dysfunction have been rarely reported with pergolide. It has a similar propensity to induce daytime sleepiness as other ergot dopamine agonists.[56]

Non-ergot Dopamine Agonists

Apomorphine

Apomorphine is a potent mixed D1- and D2-type DA receptor agonist with powerful antiparkinsonian effects. Bioavailability is poor when administered orally due to extensive first-pass metabolism. The drug is readily absorbed via sublingual, intranasal, and rectal routes. With subcutaneous or intravenous injections, apomorphine has a half-life of about 30 minutes,[57] corresponding to a 45- to 60-minute duration of clinical effect. Following subcutaneous bolus injections, maximal plasma concentrations are reached in about 8 minutes and clinical effects have a latency of 10–20 minutes. Latencies are longer for the various transmucosal routes.[58–60]

Apomorphine as early monotherapy

While the so-called "apomorphine test" is used to test dopaminergic responsiveness in de-novo patients with PD as part of the diagnostic work-up in many centers, no data on subcutaneous apomorphine–or indeed any other apomorphine delivery route–as initial monotherapy in early PD are available.

Apomorphine as adjunct to levodopa

Apomorphine is currently marketed for subcutaneous therapy of levodopa-treated patients with motor fluctuations in several European countries. A number of open-label studies have consistently found reliable reversal of "off" periods with intermittent subcutaneous apomorphine injections and marked reductions in daily "off" time with continuous subcutaneous apomorphine infusions. Intermittent subcutaneous apomorphine injections are able to reverse "off" periods within 10–15 minutes ("rescue-injections") at single doses between 2 mg and 7 mg.[61] These effects have recently been confirmed in a double-blind placebo-controlled trial.[62] Special PEN-injection systems for subcutaneous apomorphine self-administration are currently marketed in several European countries (Figure 2.2).

Several groups have advocated the use of continuous subcutaneous apomorphine infusions via portable mini-pumps (see Figure 2.2) in patients suffering from complex unpredictable "on"/"off" oscillations refractory to conventional oral treatment[63] (see reference 61 for a review). Continuous subcutaneous apomorphine monotherapy may be associated with marked down-regulation of pre-existing levodopa-induced dyskinesias.[64,65]

Piribedil

Piribedil is a non-ergot, mixed D2/D3 agonist with some α_2 antagonistic effects. After oral administration, maximal plasma concentration (t_{max}) is reached within 1 hour. Piribedil has a long half-life of about 20 hours.

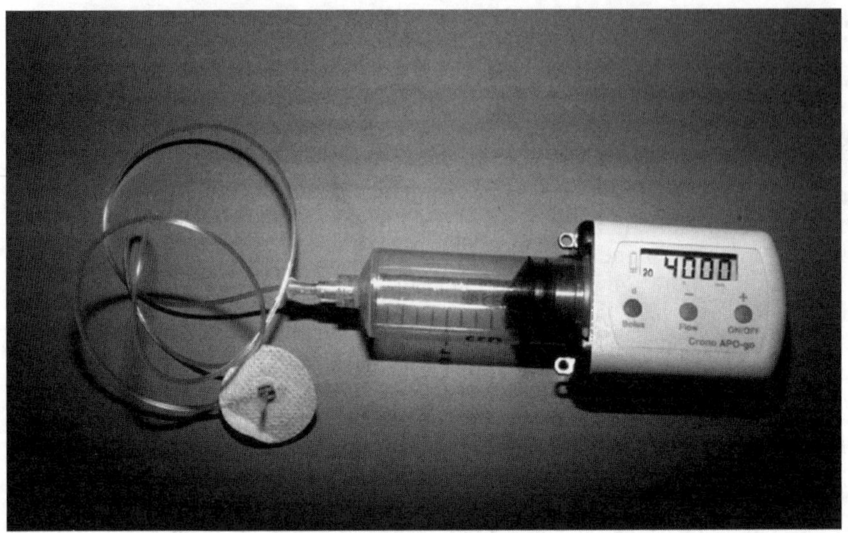

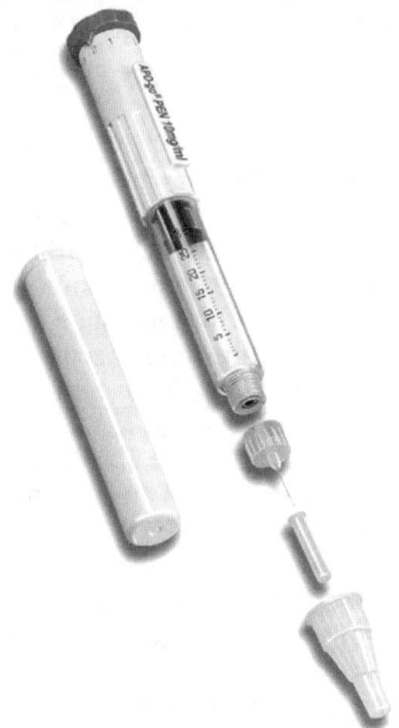

FIGURE 2.2 Commercially available infusion and injection systems for subcutaneous apomorphine therapy of PD (Crono-APO-GO pump; APO-GO pen).

Although there are no randomized controlled trials available regarding efficacy of piribedil given as monotherapy or adjunctively to levodopa in patients with PD, the drug is currently marketed as an antiparkinsonian agent in several European countries.

Pramipexole

Pramipexole is a benzothiazole derivative with full agonism at the D2-receptor family with preferential affinity for the D3-receptor subtype. It has no D1 affinity and very low affinity for non-DA receptors. It has been shown to improve parkinsonism in the 6-OHDA rat model as well as in MPTP-treated primates. Pramipexole is completely absorbed after oral administration with a bioavailability of more than 90%. Maximal plasma concentration (t_{max} is reached within 1–3 hours and the half-life is 9–12 hours).

Pramipexole as early monotherapy

Pramipexole monotherapy has been shown to be effective in the treatment of de-novo patients with PD in three double-blind placebo-controlled short-term trials.[66–68] Daily doses were between 1.5 and 6 mg, but a dose ranging trial has found no evidence for significant further improvement in total UPDRS scores beyond a daily dose of 1.5 mg compared to placebo. However, in the largest placebo-controlled study of pramipexole as early monotherapy, including 335 de-novo PD patients, mean effective doses associated with significant reductions of UPDRS ADL and motor scores were 3.8 mg/day.

A levodopa-controlled randomized double-blind prospective trial including 301 patients with early PD reported significantly less reductions in UPDRS total scores as well as motor and ADL subscores after 2 years with pramipexole–about half of whom had received supplemental open-label levodopa during the trial–compared to patients on levodopa monotherapy.[69] The primary endpoint of this CALM-PD trial was the occurrence of motor complications, and early monotherapy with pramipexole was associated with a significantly reduced risk of motor fluctuations and/or dyskinesias. After 2 years, 10% of patients in the pramipexole arm as compared to 30% in the levodopa arm had developed drug-induced dyskinesias. After 4 years, with ongoing levodopa supplementation in the pramipexole arm, this rose to 25% of patients versus 54% in the levodopa arm (see Table 2.3).

Recently, results of a dopamine-transporter (DAT) SPECT progression substudy to the CALM-PD trial have become available.[70] Eighty-one patients randomized to either pramipexole or levodopa monotherapy underwent sequential Beta-Cit SPECT scans to monitor progression of dopamine transporter dysfunction over a 4-year follow-up period. Similar to the main study, these patients received supplementary open-label levodopa as clinically required. Beta-Cit SPECT results at 22, 34, and 46 months showed significantly reduced declines in striatal Beta-Cit binding in the pramipexole- versus levodopa-treated patients. The exact interpretation of these results is difficult due to the lack of a placebo arm. Moreover, differential regulatory effects of pramipexole and levodopa on the expression and activity of the DAT-protein and ligand binding cannot be excluded.[71] Neuroprotective effects of pramipexole still are one possible explanation for the results of the CALM-CIT study. However, UPDRS motor scores assessed in the "off" condition were not statistically different between the two patient groups at years 3 and 2.

Pramipexole as adjunct to levodopa

Several well-designed randomized placebo-controlled double-blind studies have assessed efficacy and safety of adjunctive therapy with pramipexole in levodopa-treated patients with PD.[28,72–74] All found significant improvements of UPDRS ADL and motor scores with pramipexole as compared to placebo. UPDRS improvements versus baseline were between 20% and 40% in these different trials as compared to 4–13% with placebo. At the same time, several of these studies reported concomitant reductions in levodopa dose of around 30% when adjuncting pramipexole.[72,73]

Adjunctive pramipexole in patients with motor fluctuations has been shown to reduce "off" time by an average of 30% versus baseline[28,72–74] (see Figure 2.1).

One randomized double-blind trial has compared adjunctive pramipexole to placebo specifically in levodopa-treated patients with insufficient control of tremor. Many of these patients also had been receiving adjunctive therapy with other dopamine agonists without a satisfactory response. After appropriate washout, adjunctive treatment with pramipexole was significantly superior to placebo in reducing tremor in this trial.[75]

Safety

The profile of pramipexole regarding gastrointestinal, cardiovascular, and neuropsychiatric side-effects is similar to all other dopamine agonists. Also similar to other agonists, pramipexole has been reported to induce leg edema and excessive daytime sleepiness. The initial report stimulating the recent awareness of the potential of dopamine agonists (and levodopa) to induce pathological daytime sleepiness was based on a paper reporting sudden onset of sleep ("sleep attacks") in patients receiving pramipexole or ropinirole.[76] While this was initially interpreted as the new side-effect of the non-ergot dopamine agonists pramipexole and ropinirole, similar cases have since been reported with most other dopamine agonists.[32,42,56] Pleural or pulmonary fibrosis has so far not been reported with pramipexole treatment.

Ropinirole

Ropinirole is a selective non-ergoline DA-agonist at D2-like receptors with greatest affinity for the D3-subtype but no significant D1 activity. There is also no interaction with non-DA receptors. After oral administration, ropinirole is rapidly absorbed (slightly more than 1 hour after dosing). Its bioavailability is around 15% and its half-life around 6 hours.

Ropinirole as early monotherapy

Ropinirole monotherapy is effective in improving symptomatic control in de-novo patients with early PD as assessed in randomized double-blind placebo-controlled trials.[24,77–80] One trial found a trend towards greater improvement with ropinirole compared to bromocriptine monotherapy,[24] but efficacy is less than that seen with levodopa.[81] Effective doses for ropinirole monotherapy in early PD are generally above 9 mg/day and between 12 and 16 mg/day after 2–5 years of therapy.[79]

A 5-year levodopa-controlled double-blind randomized prospective trial in de-novo patients has demonstrated significantly reduced incidences of drug-induced dyskinesias with ropinirole monotherapy compared to levodopa. Even after open-label levodopa supplementation to initial ropinirole monotherapy, the reduction and dyskinesia incidence remains significant over levodopa[79] (see Table 2.3).

A 2-year randomized double-blind prospective trial of ropinirole versus levodopa has used 18-F-Dopa PET scanning as a surrogate marker to assess differential rates of progression of nigrostriatal dysfunction with either type of treatment in 186 de-novo patients not previously exposed to any dopaminergic therapy.[80] Ropinirole-treated patients had a significantly reduced rate of decline of putaminal 18-F-Dopa uptake compared to levodopa-treated patients, with a relative difference in favor of ropinirole of around 40%. As with the pramipexole versus levodopa Beta-Cit SPECT study, these results are difficult to interpret in the absence of a placebo control and without a clear clinical correlate.

Ropinirole as adjunct to levodopa

Adjunctive therapy with ropinirole in levodopa-treated patients with advanced PD and motor fluctuations has been less well studied compared to early ropinirole monotherapy in terms of controlled clinical trials. One 3-month, small, randomized placebo-controlled study in 46 patients used very low doses of ropinirole (3.3 mg/day) and found a decrease of total daily "off" time by 44%, which was statistically different from placebo only in the completor population of this study.[82] A larger randomized trial over 6 months included 149 levodopa-treated patients with motor fluctuations, and adjunctive ropinirole (maximum 24 mg/day) decreased daily "off" time and levodopa dose requirements compared to placebo; 35% of ropinirole-treated patients had both a 20% or greater decrease in levodopa dose plus a 20% or greater reduction in total daily "off" time compared to 13% of placebo-treated patients[83] (see Figure 2.1).

Safety

Ropinirole has a similar safety profile to other dopamine agonists. Specifically there were no significant differences in frequency and type of side-effects in a 3-year bromocriptine-controlled study of ropinirole in de-novo patients with PD.[24] Main side-effects include gastrointestinal, cardiovascular, and neuropsychiatric reactions. Adjunctive ropinirole may exacerbate pre-existing drug-induced dyskinesias and necessitate levodopa dose reductions. Concern about ropinirole-induced somnolence and "sleep attacks" have induced regulatory warnings for patients receiving ropinirole or pramipexole not to drive while taking these medications. Similar episodes have, however, also been reported with other agonists and even with levodopa monotherapy.

DOPAMINE AGONISTS IN CLINICAL PRACTICE

Dopamine agonists are first-line therapeutic agents in both early and advanced Parkinson's disease, where they are commonly used as initial monotherapy or adjunctively to levodopa, respectively. In spite of their different pharmacological profiles, there seem to be only minor differences between the various ergot and non-ergot compounds regarding efficacy and safety. The robustness of evidence from high-quality controlled clinical trials supporting their use, however, varies between different agents of this class.

Early Monotherapy

There is growing consensus that dopamine replacement therapy in early Parkinson's disease should generally be initiated with a dopamine agonist. Bromocriptine, dihydroergocriptine (DHEC), pergolide, pramipexole, and ropinirole have all been shown to be effective in placebo-controlled double-blind trials, while lisuride and cabergoline have only been compared to levodopa as initial monotherapy of de-novo PD patients[84] (Table 2.4). All dopamine agonists that have been tested in randomized controlled studies versus levodopa (bromocriptine, cabergoline, lisuride, pergolide, pramipexole, ropinirole) have been somewhat less effective than levodopa based on motor scores of different rating scales (most often UPDRS). Because of this difference in symptomatic efficacy, most patients started on dopamine agonist monotherapy will eventually require adjunctive levodopa. In recent levodopa-controlled clinical trials this percentage was close to 80% of the intent-to-treat population at 5 years and greater than 90% in the 10-year follow-up of the bromocriptine versus levodopa comparative trial conducted by the UK Parkinson's disease Research Group.

Initial monotherapy with dopamine agonists is effective in delaying the onset of motor complications, in particular drug-induced dyskinesias. This has been convincingly demonstrated for bromocriptine, cabergoline, pergolide, pramipexole, and ropinirole.

Doses of dopamine agonists required for sufficient symptomatic control in early monotherapy are summarized in Table 2.5.

There is experimental evidence for potential neuroprotective properties of dopamine agonists (see above), and two recent levodopa-controlled trials with pramipexole and ropinirole have used functional neuroimaging surrogate markers (Beta-Cit SPECT, 18-F-Dopa PET) to assess differential effects of these agonists versus levodopa on the rate of progression of nigrostriatal terminal function. Both trials have found similar reductions in the rate of decline of functional markers of nigrostriatal terminal activity in favor of the dopamine agonists. These findings do not, however, provide clear evidence for neuroprotective properties since both trials lacked placebo controls and there was no clinical evidence of different effects on progression of motor impairment between the agonists and levodopa. In addition, the issue of potential regulatory effects of dopamine agonists and/or levodopa on the imaging marker is not resolved.[71]

TABLE 2.4 Efficacy of dopamine agonists in the treatment of PD as assessed in randomized controlled trials (RCTs)

Drug	*Neuroprotection*	*Symptomatic control in early disease*	*Symptomatic control as adjunct*	*Prevent motor complications*	*Control motor complications*
Bromocriptine	?	+	+	+	+
Cabergoline	?	+	+	+	+
DHEC	?	+	?	?	?
Lisuride	?	+	+	?	?
Pergolide	?	+	+	?	+
Apomorphine	?	?	+	?	+
Piribedil	?	?	?	?	?
Pramipexole	?	+	+	+	+
Ropinirole	?	+	?	+	+

Based on [84].

+ = drugs assessed as "efficacious" or "likely efficacious" ? = drugs with insufficient evidence for efficacy from RCTs.

TABLE 2.5 Average daily dosage (mg) of dopamine agonists in the treatment of PD

Drug	*Monotherapy*	*Adjunct to levodopa*
Bromocriptine	25–45	15–25
Lisuride	0.8–1.6	0.6–1.2
Pergolide	1.5–5.0	0.75–5
Cabergoline	2–6	2–4
Dihydroergocryptine[a]	60–80	40
Apomorphine[a]	–	1.5–6 (s.c. bolus)
Piribedil[a]	150–250	150–250
Pramipexole	0.375–4.5	0.375–4.5
Ropinirole	6–18	6–12

[a] Not available in the United States.
s.c. = subcutaneous.

Dopamine Agonists as Adjunct to Levodopa

Dopamine agonists can effectively be added to levodopa to enhance symptomatic control, in patients with or without motor fluctuations. This has been convincingly shown in randomized controlled trials of bromocriptine, cabergoline, pergolide, and pramipexole, while there is less robust evidence for apomorphine, lisuride, and ropinirole. Doses required in this indication are generally similar to those required for initial monotherapy (see Table 2.5).

Apomorphine, bromocriptine, cabergoline, pergolide, pramipexole, and ropinirole have all been demonstrated to reduce motor fluctuations with an increase in "on" time and a reduction in "off" time in levodopa-treated patients with response oscillations, while lisuride, piribedil, and DHEC have been insufficiently tested in this regard (see Table 2.4). Adding dopamine agonists to levodopa in patients with advanced disease and motor complications generally allows for levodopa dose reductions and may thus help to reduce the duration and/or intensity of pre-existing levodopa-induced dyskinesias.

Long-acting dopamine agonists do not generally induce dyskinesias in primate models of PD, while levodopa or short-acting agonists do.[11] The ability of dopamine agonists to provide more continuous striatal dopamine receptor stimulation is believed to be the key factor explaining the reduced incidence of motor complications with initial agonist monotherapy consistently seen in levodopa-controlled studies of early PD. Several open-label clinical studies have reported significant decreases in duration and severity of pre-existing levodopa-induced dyskinesias when patients were switched to high-dose oral dopamine agonist monotherapy[85] or continuous subcutaneous infusions of apomorphine or lisuride.[52,64,65]

Side-effects

Currently available dopamine agonists share a wide range of side-effects with levodopa, due to peripheral and central dopaminergic stimulation. Nausea and vomiting, postural hypotension, dizziness, bradycardia, and other signs of autonomic peripheral stimulation are common peripheral dopaminergic side-effects of all dopamine agonists. In a small number of patients the first dopamine agonist dose can induce severe hypotensive reactions, so that small starting doses and slow titration schemes are recommended. Outside the United States, co-administration of the peripheral dopamine-receptor blocker *domperidone* can be used to counteract these peripherally induced dopaminergic side-effects if necessary. Both ergot and non-ergot dopamine agonists have been reported to induce leg edema.

In patients with levodopa-induced dyskinesias, adjunctive therapy with dopamine agonists can exacerbate these motor complications, but these can be counteracted by reducing the dose of levodopa. In individual patients with disabling levodopa-induced dyskinesias, switching to high-dose oral dopamine agonist monotherapy may significantly reduce pre-existing dyskinesias. Dopamine agonists appear to have a slightly greater potential than levodopa to induce central side-effects such as sedation, confusional states, and hallucinosis or paranoid psychosis. Elderly patients aged over 70, and those with concomitant cerebrovascular disease and cognitive decline, or antecedent history of psychiatric complications, are at particular risk.

Some case reports suggested that non-ergot dopamine agonists such as pramipexole and ropinirole may induce sleep attacks without warning, raising the question of safety of these medications for patients who drive. Subsequent reports described similar side-effects of excessive daytime sleepiness, including sleep episodes at the wheel, caused by ergot dopamine agonists that included bromocriptine, pergolide, cabergoline, and by levodopa monotherapy as well. Daytime sedation, therefore, must be regarded as a side-effect common to all dopaminergic agents and patients must be warned of this in particular with respect to driving.

Ergot-derivative dopamine agonists have been associated with the occurrence of pleuropulmonary and/or peritoneal fibrosis. So far, this has not been reported with non-ergot agonists such as pramipexole and ropinirole.

Subcutaneous injections frequently cause red itching nodules at injection sites, which are commonly well tolerated and transient. Problems of local tolerability with large areas of inflammation or subcutaneous abscesses or necrosis have been registered and are often related to noncompliance with hygiene rules for needle use. Sexual dysfunction (i.e. frequent erections and hypersexuality) have also been reported with subcutaneous apomorphine. Apomorphine-induced autoimmune hemolytic anemia is a rare complication, requiring monthly blood counts in patients on continuous subcutaneous infusions.

REFERENCES

1. Calne DB, Teychenne PF, Claveria LE et al. Bromocriptine in parkinsonism. Br Med J 1974;4:442–444.
2. Calne DB, Teychenne PF, Leigh PN, Bamji AN, Greenacre JK. Treatment of parkinsonism with bromocriptine. Lancet 1974;2:1355–1356.
3. Schwartz J-C, Giros B, Martres M-P, Sokoloff P. The dopamine receptor family: molecular biology and pharmacology. Sem Neurosci 1992;4:99–108.

4. Grandy DK, Marchionni MA, Makan H et al. Cloning of the cDNA and gene for a human D2 dopamine receptor. Proc Natl Acad Sci USA 1989;84:9762–9766.
5. Sunahara RK, Niznik HB, Weiner DM et al. Human dopamine D1 receptor encoded by an intronless gene on chromosome 5. Nature 1990;347:80–83.
6. Van Tol HHM, Bunzow JR, Guan HC et al. Cloning of the gene for a human dopamine D4 receptor with high affinity for the antipsychotic clozapine. Nature 1991;350:610–614.
7. Tiberi M, Jarvie KR, Silvia C et al. Cloning, molecular characterization, and chromosomal assignment of a gene encoding a second D1 dopamine receptor subtype: differential expression pattern in rat brain compared with the D1A receptor. Proc Natl Acad Sci USA 1991;88:7491–7495.
8. Le Coniat M, Sokoloff P, Hillion J et al. Chromosomal localization of the human D3 dopamine receptor gene. Hum Genet 1991;87:618–620.
9. Sokoloff P, Giros B, Martres M-P, Bouthenet M-L, Schwartz J-C. Molecular cloning and characterization of a novel dopamine receptor (D3) as a target for neuroleptics. Nature 1990;347:146–151.
10. Haverstick D, Rubestein A, Bannon M. Striatal tachykinin gene expression regulated by interaction of D-1 and D-2 dopamine receptors. J Pharmacol Exp Ther 1989;248:858–862.
11. Bedard PJ, Gomez-Mancilla B, Blanchette P et al. Role of selective D1 and D2 agonists in inducing dyskinesia in drug-naive MPTP monkeys. Adv Neurol 1993;60:113–118.
12. Olanow CW, Jenner P, Brooks D. Dopamine agonists and neuroprotection in Parkinson's disease. Ann Neurol 199844(suppl. 1):S167–174.
13. Yamamoto M. Do dopamine agonists provide neuroprotection? Neurology 1998;51(suppl. 2): S10–12.
14. Olanow CW, Schapira AHV, Agid Y. Neuroprotection for Parkinson's disease: prospects and promises. Ann Neurol 2003;53(suppl. 3)1–2.
15. Olanow CW. Single blind double observer-controlled study of carbidopa/levodopa vs bromocriptine in untreated Parkinson patients. Arch Neurol 1988;45:206.
16. Staal-Schreinemachers AL, Wesseling H, Kamphuis DJ, Burg WVD, Lakke JPWF. Low-dose bromocriptine therapy in Parkinson's disease: double-blind, placebo-controlled study. Neurology 1986;36:291–293.
17. Lees AJ, Stern GM. Sustained bromocriptine therapy in previously untreated patients with Parkinson's disease. J Neurol Neurosurg Psychiatry 1981;44:1020–1023.
18. Parkinson's Disease Research Group in the United Kingdom. Comparisons of therapeutic effects of levodopa, levodopa and selegiline, and bromocriptine in patients with early, mild Parkinson's disease: three year interim report. Br Med J 1993;307:469–472.
19. Montastruc JL, Rascol O, Senard JM, Rascol A. A randomised controlled study comparing bromocriptine to which levodopa was later added, with levodopa alone in previously untreated patients with Parkinson's disease: a five year follow-up. J Neurol Neurosurg Psychiatry 1994;57:1034–1038.
20. Hely MA, Morris JGL, Reid WGJ. The Sydney multicentre study of Parkinson's disease: a randomized, prospective five year study comparing low dose bromocriptine with low dose levodopa–carbidopa. J Neurol Neurosurg Psychiatry 1994;57:903–910.
21. Lees AJ, Katzenschlager R, Head J, Ben-Shlomo Y. Ten-year follow-up of three different initial treatments in de-novo PD: a randomised trial. Neurology 2001;57:1687–1694.
22. Mizuno Y, Kondo T, Narabayashi H. Pergolide in the treatment of Parkinson's disease. Neurology 1995;45(suppl. 31):S13–21.
23. Korczyn AD, Brooks DJ, Brunt ER et al. Ropinirole versus bromocriptine in the treatment of early Parkinson's disease: a 6-month interim report of a 3-year study. The 053 Study Group. Mov Disord 1998:13:46–51.
24. Korczyn AD, Brunt ER, Larsen JP et al. A 3-year randomized trial of ropinirole and bromocriptine in early Parkinson's disease. The 053 Study Group. Neurology 1999;53:364–370.
25. Olanow CW, Hauser RA, Gauger L et al. The effect of deprenyl and levodopa on the progression of Parkinson's disease. Ann Neurol 1995;38:771–777.
26. Hoehn MMM, Elton RL. Low dosages of bromocriptine added to levodopa in Parkinson's disease. Neurology 1985;35:199–206.
27. Toyokura Y, Mizuno Y, Kase M et al. Effects of bromocriptine on parkinsonism: a nationwide collaborative double-blind study. Acta Neurol Scand 985;72:157–170.
28. Guttman M, International Pramipexole-Bromocriptine Study Group. Double-blind randomized, placebo controlled study to compare safety, tolerance and efficacy of pramipexole and bromocriptine in advanced Parkinson's disease. Neurology 1997;49:1060–1065.

29. Inzelberg R, Nisipeaunu P, Rabey JM et al. Double-blind comparison of cabergoline and bromocriptine in Parkinson's disease patients with motor fluctuations. Neurology 1996;47:785–788.
30. Pezzoli G, Martignoni E, Pacchetti C et al. Pergolide compared with bromocriptine in Parkinson's disease: a multicenter, cross-over, controlled study. Mov Disord 1994; 9:431–436.
31. Boas J, Worm-Petersen J, Dupont E, Mikkelsen B, Wermuth L. The levodopa dose-sparing of pergolide compared with that of bromocriptine in an open-label, cross-over study. Eur J Neurol 1996;3:44–49.
32. Ferreira J J, Galitzky M, Montastruc JL, Rascol O. Sleep attacks and Parkinson's disease treatment. Lancet 2000;355:1333–1334.
33. Ben-Noun L. Drug-induced respiratory disorders: incidence, prevention and management. Drug Saf 2000;23:143–164.
34. Quinn N, Illas A, Lhermitte F, Agid Y. Bromocriptine and domperidone in the treatment of Parkinson's disease. Neurology 1981;31:662–667.
35. Bergamasco B, Frattola L, Muratorio A et al. Alpha-dihydroergocryptine in the treatment of de novo parkinsonian patients: results of a multicentre, randomized, double-blind, placebo-controlled study. Acta Neurol Scand 2000;101:372–380.
36. Martignoni E, Pacchetti C, Sibilla L et al. Dihydroergocryptine in the treatment of Parkinson's disease: a six month's double-blind clinical trial. Clin Neuropharmacol 1991;14:78–83.
37. Oechsner M, Groenke L, Mueller D. Pleural fibrosis associated with dihydroergocryptine treatment. Acta Neurol Scand 2000;101:283–285.
38. Fariello RG. Pharmacodynamic and pharmacokinetic features of cabergoline: rationale for use in Parkinson's disease. Drugs 1998;55(suppl. 1):10–16.
39. Rinne UK, Bracco F, Chouza C et al. Cabergoline in the treatment of early Parkinson's disease: results of the first year of treatment in a double-blind comparison of cabergoline and levodopa. The PKDS009 Collaborative Study Group. Neurology 1997;48:363–368.
40. Rinne UK, Bracco F, Chouza C et al., and the PKDS009 Study Group. Early treatment of Parkinson's disease with cabergoline delays the onset of motor complications. Drugs 1998;55 (suppl. 1):23–30.
41. Hutton JT, Koller WC, Ahlskog JE et al. Multicenter, placebo-controlled trial of cabergoline taken once daily in the treatment of Parkinson's disease. Neurology 1996;46:1062–1065.
42. Ebersbach G, Norden J, Tracik F. Sleep attacks in Parkinson's disease: polysomnographic recordings. Mov Disord 2000;15(suppl. 3):89.
43. Ling LH, Ahlskog JE, Munger TM, Limper AH, Oh JK. Constrictive pericarditis and pleuropulmonary disease linked to ergot dopamine agonist therapy (cabergoline) for Parkinson's disease. Mayo Clin Proc 1999;74:371–375.
44. Rinne UK. Lisuride, a dopamine agonist in the treatment of early Parkinson's disease. Neurology 1989;39:336–339.
45. Allain H, Destée A, Petit H et al. Five-year follow-up of early lisuride and levodopa combination therapy versus levodopa monotherapy in de-novo Parkinson's disease. The French Lisuride Study Group. Eur Neurol 2000;44:22–30.
46. LeWitt PA, Gopinathan G, Ward CD et al. Lisuride versus bromocriptine treatment in Parkinson disease: a double-blind study. Neurology 1982;32:69–72.
47. Laihinen A, Rinne UK, Suchy I. Comparison of lisuride and bromocriptine in the treatment of advanced Parkinson's disease. Acta Neurol Scand 1992;86:593–595.
48. Battistin L, Bardin PG, Ferro-Milone F et al. Alpha-dihydroergocryptine in Parkinson's disease: a multicentre randomized double blind parallel group study. Acta Neurol Scand 1999;99:36–42.
49. Obeso JA, Luquin MR, Martinez-Lage JM. Lisuride infusion pump: a device for the treatment of motor fluctuations in Parkinson's disease. Lancet 1986;1(8479):467–470.
50. Vaamonde J, Luquin MR, Obeso JA. Subcutaneous lisuride infusion in Parkinson's disease. Response to chronic administration in 34 patients. Brain 1991;114:601–617.
51. Chase TN, Engber TM, Mouradian MM. Striatal dopaminoceptive system changes and motor response complications in levodopa-treated patients with advanced Parkinson's disease. Adv Neurol 1993;60:181–185.
52. Stocchi F, Ruggieri S, Vacca L, Olanow CW. Prospective randomised trial of lisuride infusion versus oral levodopa in patients with Parkinson's disease. Brain 2002;125:2058–2066.
53. Barone P, Bravi D, Bermejo-Pareja F et al., and the Pergolide Monotherapy Study Group. Pergolide monotherapy in the treatment of early PD. A randomized controlled study. Neurology 1999;53:573–579.

54. Oertel WH. Pergolide versus levodopa (PELMOPET). Mov Dis 2000;15(suppl. 3):4.
55. Olanow CW, Fahn S, Muenter M et al. A multicenter double-blind placebo-controlled trial of pergolide as an adjunct to Sinemet in Parkinson's disease. Mov Disord 1994;9:40–47.
56. Schapira AH. Sleep attack (sleep episodes) with pergolide. Lancet 2000;355:1332–1333.
57. Gancher ST, Woodward WR, Boucher B, Nutt JG. Peripheral pharmacokinetics of apomorphine in humans. Ann Neurol 1989;26:232–238.
58. Durif F, Deffond D, Tournilhac M et al. Efficacy of sublingual apomorphine in Parkinson's disease. J Neurol Neurosurg Psychiatry 1990;53:1105.
59. Kapoor R, Turjanski N, Frankel J et al. Intranasal apomorphine: a new treatment in Parkinson's disease. J Neurol Neurosurg Psychiatry 1990;53:1015.
60. van Laar T, Jansen EN, Neef C, Danhof M, Roos RA. Pharmacokinetics and clinical efficacy of rectal apomorphine in patients with Parkinson's disease: a study of five different suppositories. Mov Dis 1995;10:433–439.
61. Poewe W, Wenning GK. Apomorphine: an underutilized therapy for Parkinson's disease [review]. Mov Dis 2000;15:789–94.
62. Dewey RB, Hutton JT, LeWitt PA, Factor SA. A randomized, double-blind, placebo-controlled trial of subcutaneously injected apomorphine for parkinsonian off-state events. Arch Neurol 2001;58:1385–1392.
63. Frankel JP, Lees AJ, Kempster PA, Stern GM. Subcutaneous apomorphine in the treatment of Parkinson's disease. J Neurol Neurosurg Psychiatry 1990;53:96–101.
64. Colzi A, Turner K, Lees AJ. Continuous subcutaneous waking day apomorphine in the long-term treatment of levodopa induced interdose dyskinesias in Parkinson's disease. J Neurol Neurosurg Psychiatry 1998;64:573–576.
65. Poewe W, Kleedorfer B, Wagner M, Bosch S, Schelosky L: Continuous subcutaneous apomorphine infusions for fluctuating Parkinson's disease: long-term follow-up in 18 patients. Adv Neurol 1993;60:656–659.
66. Hubble JP, Koller WC, Cutler NR et al. Pramipexole in patients with early Parkinson's disease. Clin Neuropharmacol 1995;18:338–347.
67. Parkinson Study Group. Safety and efficacy of pramipexole in early Parkinson disease: a randomized dose-ranging study. JAMA 1997;278:125–130.
68. Shannon KM, Bennett JP, Friedman JH, for the Pramipexole Study Group. Efficacy of pramipexole, a novel dopamine agonist, as monotherapy in mild to moderate Parkinson's disease. Neurology 1997;49:724–728.
69. Parkinson Study Group. Pramipexole vs levodopa as initial treatment for Parkinson's disease: a randomized controlled trial. JAMA 2000;284:1931–1938.
70. Parkinson Study Group. Dopamine transporter brain imaging to assess the effects of pramipexole vs levodopa on Parkinson disease progression. JAMA 2002;287:1653–1661.
71. Ahlskog JE. Slowing Parkinson's disease progression: recent dopamine agonist trials. Neurology 2003;60:381–389.
72. Lieberman A, Ranhosky A, Korts D. Clinical evaluation of pramipexole in advanced Parkinson's disease: results of a double-blind, placebo-controlled, parallel-group study. Neurology 1997;49:162–168.
73. Wermuth L, and the Danish Pramipexole Study Group. A double-blind, placebo-controlled, randomized, multi-center study of pramipexole in advanced Parkinson's disease. Eur J Neurol 1998;5:235–242.
74. Pinter MM, Pogarell O, Oertel WH. Efficacy, safety, and tolerance of the non-ergoline dopamine agonist pramipexole in the treatment of advanced Parkinson's disease: a double-blind, placebo controlled, randomised, multicentre study. J Neurol Neurosurg Psychiatry 1999;66:436–441.
75. Pogarell O, Gasser T, van Hilten JJ et al. Pramipexole in patients with Parkinson's disease and marked drug resistant tremor: a randomised, double-blind, placebo-controlled multicentre study. J Neurol Neurosurg Psychiatry 2002;72:713–720.
76. Frucht S, Rogers JD, Greene PE, Gordon MS, Fahn S. Falling asleep at the wheel: motor vehible mishaps in persons taking pramipexole and ropinirole. Neurology 1999;52:1908–1910.
77. Adler CH, Sethi KD, Hauser RA et al., for the Ropinirole Study Group. Ropinirole for the treatment of early Parkinson's disease. Neurology 1997;49:393–399.
78. Brooks DJ, Abbott RJ, Lees AJ et al. A placebo-controlled evaluation of ropinirole, a novel D2 agonist, as sole dopaminergic therapy in Parkinson's disease. Clin Neuropharmacol 1998;21:101–107.
79. Rascol O, Brooks DJ, Korczyn AD et al., for the 056 Study Group. A five-year study of the incidence of dyskinesia in patients with early Parkinson's disease who were treated with ropinirole or levodopa. N Engl J Med 2000;342:1484–1491.

80. Whone AL, Watts RL, Stoessl AJ et al. REAL-PET Study Group. Slower progression of Parkinson's disease with ropinirole versus levodopa. Ann Neurol 2003;54:93–101.
81. Rascol O, Brooks DJ, Brunt ER et al., on behalf of the 056 Study Group. Ropinirole in the treatment of early Parkinson's disease: a 6-month interim report of a 5-year levodopa-controlled study. Mov Disord 1998;13:39–45.
82. Rascol O, Lees AJ, Senard JM et al. Ropinirole in the treatment of levodopa-induced motor fluctuations in patients with Parkinson's disease. Clin Neuropharmacol 1996;19:234–245.
83. Lieberman A, Olanow CW, Sethi K et al., and the Ropinirole Study Group. A multicenter trial of ropinirole as adjunct treatment for Parkinson's disease. Neurology 1998;51:1057–1062.
84. Rascol O, Goetz C, Koller W, Poewe W, Sampaio C. Treatment interventions for Parkinson's disease: an evidence based assessment. Lancet 2002;359:1589–1598.
85. Facca A, Sanchez-Ramos J. High-dose pergolide monotherapy in the treatment of severe levodopa-induced dyskinesias. Mov Disord 1996;11:327–329.
86. Olanow CW, Alberts MJ. Double-blind controlled study of pergolide mesylate in the treatment of Parkinson's disease. Clin Neuropharmacol 987;10:178–185.
87. Jankovic J, Orman J. Parallel double-blind study of pergolide in Parkinson's disease. Adv Neurol 1987;45:551–554.
88. Diamond SG, Markham CH, Treciokas LJ. Double-blind trial of pergolide for Parkinson's disease. Neurology 1985;35:291–295.
89. Geminiani G, Fetoni V, Genitrini S et al. Cabergoline in Parkinson's disease complicated by motor fluctuations. Mov Disord 1996;11:495–500.
90. Steiger MJ, El-Debas T, Anderson T, Findley LJ, Marsden CD. Double-blind study of the activity and tolerability of cabergoline versus placebo in parkinsonians with motor fluctuations. J Neurol 1996;243:68–72.

3

Other Drug Therapies for Parkinson's Disease

Maria Graciela Cersosimo and William C. Koller

ANTICHOLINERGICS

Introduction

The clinical efficacy of the belladonna alkaloids–such as atropine, scopolamine, and stramonium – was first reported by Charcot and his student Ordenstein in 1867.[1] Since that time, and for almost a century, anticholinergics were the only possible treatment for parkinsonian syndromes and were widely used. The utility of anticholinergic drugs, based only on clinical observations, was well established long before their mechanism of action was understood.[2] In fact it was thought that anticholinergic's effects were the result of a peripheral action. Feldberg in 1945 first proposed that the clinical efficacy of atropine and scopolamine in parkinsonism might be due to a central acetylcholine antagonism.[3] Duvoisin and colleagues in 1967 tested the hypothesis that the therapeutic efficacy of scopolamine and benztropine in parkinsonism was due to a central action. They administrated 1 mg intravenous of physostigmine in 20 patients with Parkinson's disease (PD) and observed a prompt exacerbation of parkinsonian symptoms in 17 patients. Subsequently these effects were reversed by the injection of scopolamine hydrobromide 0.5–1 mg or benztropine mesylate 2 mg. Interestingly, the quaternary anticholinesterase compound edrophonlam, which does not penetrate into the CNS, failed to accentuate parkinsonian symptoms. The authors concluded that the aggravation of parkinsonism by physostigmine is due to the inhibition of acetylcholinesterase in the CNS, and that the therapeutic effect of scopolamine and benztropine is also due to a central anticholinergic action.[2]

More recently, natural compounds have been largely displaced by synthetic agents such as benztropine (Cogentin), trihexyphenidyl (Artane), cycrimine (Pagitane), procyclidine (Kemadrin), biperiden (Akineton), ethopropazine

(Parsidol), orphenadrine (Disipal), and diethazine (Diparcol). Although less potent than the natural alkaloids, these drugs possess similar pharmacological properties and a strong anticholinergic activity.

Basic Pharmacology

In Parkinson's disease, dopamine depletion results in a state of relative cholinergic sensitivity, so cholinergic drugs exacerbate and anticholinergic drugs improve parkinsonian symptoms. Although the exact mechanism of action of the anticholinergic agents remains unclear, it is generally accepted that they exert their action by correcting the disequilibrium between striatal dopaminergic and cholinergic neurotransmitter systems.[2]

Some anticholinergics such as benztropine also have a dopaminergic action by inhibiting striatal presynaptic reuptake of dopamine. However, it is uncertain whether this contributes to their mechanism of action. The acetylcholine receptors may be muscarinic (G-protein-linked receptors) or nicotinic (ligand gated ion channels), but the anticholinergics used in the treatment of PD are specific for muscarinic receptors. Some of these compounds – such as diphenhydramine or benztropine – are also antihistaminic agents, but that does not contribute to their antiparkinsonian action.

Trihexyphenidyl (Artane) is a synthetic product introduced in 1948 as an antispasmodic and antiparkinsonian drug. Its structural formula is 3-(1-piperidyl)-1-phenyl-cyclohexyl-1-propanol hydrochloride and it is the more widely used anticholinergic agent. Nonetheless, there is no evidence that any of these compounds are superior to another in terms of efficacy or side-effects.[4] Trihexyphenidyl is well absorbed after oral administration, reaches peak plasma concentration in 2–3 hours, and is able to penetrate into the CNS. The duration of action varies from 1 to 12 hours.

Trihexyphenidyl therapy is usually initiated at 0.5–1 mg twice a day (b.i.d.) and increased gradually to a dosage of 2 mg b.i.d. or three times a day (t.i.d.). Benztropine (Cogentin) has a recommended initial dose of 0.5–1 mg at bedtime and can be increased to 4–6 mg/day. Procyclidine (Kemadrin) is initiated with 2.5 mg t.i.d. after meals and may be increased to 5 mg b.i.d. or t.i.d.[5]

Symptomatic Treatment

Anticholinergics are typically used in younger PD patients when tremor is the more relevant clinical feature and cognitive function is preserved. These agents appear to be more useful for the treatment of resting tremor and less effective for akinesia and postural problems. However, the data available are insufficient to be sure about this issue.[6,7]

Cantello and colleagues performed a randomized, double-blind crossover study of bornaprine versus placebo. Thirty patients with Parkinson's disease were included, aged between 50 and 70 years. Disease severity on the Hoehn–Yahr scale ranged from 2 (14 patients) to 5 (1 patient). All patients were treated with stable dosages of levodopa and/or bromocriptine, without adequate control of their symptoms, especially tremor. Bornaprine (mean dose 8.25 mg/day) or placebo were added in randomized sequence, with 30 days on each treatment arm.

Patients were assessed using the Webster Rating Scale before, during, and after each stage of the treatment.

Statistical analysis of the results showed the superiority of bornaprine over placebo in reducing tremor and, in a lesser degree, other parkinsonian symptoms such as bradykinesia, rigidity, posture, and facial expression. No relevant side-effects were found apart from dryness of the mouth, which was more frequent with bornaprine.[8]

Martin et al.[9] investigated the clinical utility of trihexyphenidyl in association with levodopa. The authors performed a 6-month randomized double-blind study in which 30 PD patients were treated either with levodopa plus trihexyphenidyl hydrochloride or levodopa with placebo. All patients were receiving anticholinergic drugs at the time to entry to the study. This medication was withdrawn for a period of seven to ten days and then treatment was begun with levodopa plus trihexyphenidyl or placebo. The levodopa dosage was initially 500 mg/day and was increased by 500 mg every three days until the patient had maximal improvement, intolerable side-effects occurred, or a dose of 6.5 g/day was achieved. At the same time, the patients started with tablets of 2 mg of trihexyphenidyl hydrochloride or placebo t.i.d. Assessments were obtained first while the patient was receiving the usual medication (time 0), 10 days after withdrawn medication (time 1), 5 weeks after treatment was initiated (time 2), and 6 months later (time 3). Although this was a controlled study, the two groups were not entirely comparable: patients in the placebo group were older, had more disability, and their mean disease duration was 16.9 years versus 7.9 years in the active treatment group.

The authors reported no difference between groups with regard to tremor and rigidity, although in the control group less improvement in speech was found. The average dosage of levodopa required to sustain optimal control of symptoms was similar in the two groups.

The results of the study indicated that the addition of trihexyphenidyl hydrochloride to levodopa was not associated with a greater improvement in function when compared with levodopa alone. Nonetheless, the large differences between the two groups diminishes the validity of the conclusions.

Cooper et al.[10] compared the effects of anticholinergics, levodopa, and bromocriptine monotherapies on cognition and motor control in a randomized, controlled, single-blind trial during a 4-month period. The study included 82 de-novo PD patients and 22 healthy controls. Fifteen patients elected not to take medication; the remaining 67 patients were randomized to one of three monotherapy regimens: levodopa (mean dose 415 mg/day), bromocriptine (mean dose 13.5 mg/day), or anticholinergics (21 patients on benzhexol, mean dose 5.9 mg/day, and one on orphenadrine, 150 mg/day).

The assessments were performed before the treatment was started and after 4 months of therapy. Motor function was evaluated with King's College Rating Scale and Fine Finger Movements Test, Wechsler Memory Scale, Brown–Peterson Distractor Paradigm, Wisconsin Card Sorting Test, Digit Ordering Test; and other neuropsychological tests were used for the assessment of cognitive function.

The authors concluded: (1) levodopa and anticholinergic groups (but not bromocriptine-treated patients) showed improvement in motor control; (2) dopaminergic, but not anticholinergic, therapy produced a specific improvement in the performance on the Digit Ordering Test for working memory; and (3) anticholinergic therapy, but not dopaminergic therapy, was associated with a detrimental effect on several aspects of memory function. A selective deficit of short-term memory was found in the anticholinergic group, in addition with an exacerbation of pre-existing deficits on memory aquisition and immediate memory without accelerating the rate of forgetting.

Friedman et al.[11] investigated the effects of benztropine (mean dose 3 mg/day) compared with the atypical neuroleptic clozapine (mean dose 39 mg/day) for the treatment of tremor in Parkinson's disease. It was a non-randomized, double-blind crossover study. Twenty-two patients were enrolled of whom 19 completed the study. Inclusion criteria were diagnosis of PD and a minimum score of 2 on the tremor of the Unified Parkinson's Disease Rating Scale (UPDRS). The duration of the study was 14 weeks, with 6 weeks in each treatment arm (benztropine or clozapine) and a 2-week washout period. Tremor was measured using the UPDRS tremor question and the Fahn Tolosa–Marin tremor scale. Fourteen patients were better on clozapine than at baseline and 18 were better on benztropine than at baseline. The reduction of tremor was around 30% in both groups. The authors conclude that benztropine and clozapine were equally effective in improving tremor in patients with Parkinson's disease.

Treatment of Motor Complications

There are no data supporting anticholinergic efficacy in the treatment of motor complications in Parkinson's disease.

Prevention of Disease Progression

There are no data supporting anticholinergic efficacy for the prevention of Parkinson's disease progression.

Adverse Reactions

Adverse effects of anticholinergic drugs are common and often limit their clinical use. Elderly patients with cognitive impairment are particularly sensitive to these agents. Younger patients appear to tolerate these drugs better, although neuropsychiatric tests have shown impairment of executive function. Even in patients without obvious cognitive impairment, improvement of short- and long-term memory has been demonstrated after withdrawal from anticholinergics.[5] The most important CNS side-effects are memory impairment, acute confusion, hallucinations, sedation, and dysphoria. Anticholinergics may interfere with normal mental function, this representing one of the most important limiting factors to their use.

Dyskinesias have been reported in a small number of patients receiving anticholinergic drugs either as monotherapy or in combination with levodopa. Hauser et al.[12] reported the occurrence of dyskinesias in a 60-year-old PD patient after the introduction of trihexyphenidyl 2 mg b.i.d. in addition to his levodopa regimen. Dyskinesias were orobuccal and persisted for 5 days until trihexyphenidyl was discontinued. A few more cases of anticholinergic-induced dyskinesias in PD patients have been mentioned in the literature. They are described in association with ethopropazine, trihexyphenidyl, procyclidine, biperiden, or phenadrine and prophenamine. All cases presented as orobuccal dyskinesias, with the exception of two patients who developed generalized chorea. Dyskinesias appeared with a mean latency of 16.6 days following the introduction of anticholinergics, and resolved after a mean latency of 20.9 days following their withdrawal. While levodopa-induced dyskinesias typically involve the limbs and trunk, dyskinesias secondary to anticholinergics are predominantly orobuccal, similar in appearance to tardive dyskinesias. Anticholinergic-induced dyskinesias have also been observed in patients with focal dystonias such as blepharospasm, torticollis, writer's cramp, oromandibular dystonia, and essential tremor. The mechanism by which anticholinergics induce chorea is not known.[12,13]

Peripheral antimuscaric side-effects include dry mouth, constipation, blurred vision due to accommodation impairment, nausea, urinary retention, impaired sweating, and tachycardia.

Anticholinergic drugs are contraindicated in patients with prostate hypertrophy, closed-angle glaucoma, tachycardia, gastrointestinal obstruction, or megacolon.

Anticholinergics should be discontinued gradually and with caution because abrupt withdrawal may be associated with a marked deterioration of the parkinsonian syndrome even in patients who did not appear to have a clinical benefit.[14,15]

Anticholinergics: Conclusions

Anticholinergic drugs have a limited efficacy in the treatment of Parkinson's disease. They may be useful in younger patients when resting tremor is the dominant symptom. Anticholinergics should be used with caution in the elderly. The occurrence of adverse reactions is common and this often limits their use. Anticholinergics should be discontinued gradually to avoid withdrawal effects.

AMANTADINE

Introduction

Amantadine hydrocloride has long been known for its modest antiparkinsonian activity and recently because of its antidyskinetic properties. The drug was initially introduced as an antiviral agent effective against A2 influenza.[16] Its antiparkinsonian effect was first published by Schwab and colleagues in 1969. It was discovered fortuitously in a 58-year-old woman with PD who experienced a remission of her symptoms while taking amantadine to prevent influenza. After this single case, the authors conducted a trial with 163 patients with PD and observed improvement in 66% of them. Since that time a peculiar property of amantadine has been observed, namely its transient clinical benefit.[17]

Over the years, the introduction of a number of different agents – including dopamine agonists – resulted in more limited use of amantadine. This was in part due to its modest antiparkinsonian action, but also because of the short duration of the clinical benefit.[18] Many clinical trials have investigated the efficacy of amantadine, and recent reviews on PD treatment placed amantadine as a secondary therapy for PD.

Interest in this agent has recently reappeared since Shanon et al.[19] found that amantadine decreased motor fluctuations, and Stoof et al.[20] demonstrated amantadine's activity at glutamate receptors suggesting that its antiparkinsonian effect might be related to blockade of *N*-methyl-D-aspartic (NMDA) receptors.[20]

Amantadine has many controversial and not completely resolved features, such as its mechanism of action, the transient benefit reported in the literature, and the clinical observation that amantadine withdrawal in patients treated for longer than one year may result in a substantial increase of motor disability or delirium.[21]

Basic Pharmacology

Amantadine interacts with several different neurotransmitter systems, but its exact mechanism of action is not established. It is classically described that the drug has dopaminergic and anticholinergic properties, and more recently reported is its antagonist activity at NMDA glutamatergic receptors.[20] Amantadine exerts its dopaminergic effects by acting at presynaptic and postsynaptic levels. Presynaptically, the drug interacts with dopaminergic neurotransmission in two ways, first by enhancing the release of dopamine and other catecholamines from dopaminergic terminals, and second by inhibiting the reuptake processes at the presynaptic terminal. Postsynaptically, a direct action of the drug on dopamine receptors results in changes in dopamine receptor affinity. Additionally, studies on the chronic effect of amantadine have shown an increase in striatal spiroperidol binding, suggesting D2 dopamine receptor blockade.[22–24]

Stoof et al.[20] and colleagues reported amantadine's antiglutamatergic properties via blockade of NMDA receptors from rat neostriatum at therapeutic doses. It has been demonstrated that amantadine acts as a non-competitive NMDA antagonist, producing a concentration-, time-, and voltage-dependent blockade of open NMDA channels.[25,26] Recently it has been established that amantadine belongs to a type of blocker manifesting the so-called "trapping block" of NMDA channels. These drugs can enter an open NMDA channel and bind to its blocking site located deep in the pore. The blocking molecules can remain in the pore for a relatively long time, being trapped behind the closed activation gate. Agonist reapplication opens the gate and allows the blocker to leave the channel. The molecular mechanisms of the trapping of blockers are at present unclear.[26,27]

Interestingly, despite the many different pharmacological properties attributed to this drug, it is not clear how they contribute to its clinical effect. The classical idea that the antiparkinsonian effect of amantadine is the result of its dopaminergic or anticholinergic activities is not supported by more recent studies. In fact, therapeutic doses of amantadine *in vitro* are not associated with increased extracellular brain levels of dopamine. Similarly, the presumed anticholinergic effect is also unlikely as amantadine binds to acetylcholine receptors only at very high concentrations.[28,29]

Regarding the antidyskinetic effect of amantadine, compelling data support the hypothesis that it is related to the anti-NMDA properties of the drug. Furthermore, some authors propose NMDA antagonism as the mechanism for its antiparkinsonian effect. Amantadine hydrocloride is l-amino-adamantamine, the salt of a symmetric 10-carbon primary amine. It is a compound that is stable, white, crystalline, and freely soluble in water.[17] In humans, it is well absorbed after oral administration. Blood levels peak at 1–4 hours after an oral dose of 2.5 mg/kg. The drug has a plasma half-life of 10–28.5 hours and is excreted largely unmetabolized in the urine. Amantadine hydrocloride is used clinically as 100 mg capsules, and recommended doses for PD disease treatment are 100 mg b.i.d. or t.i.d.[30,31]

Symptomatic Treatment of Parkinsonism

Amantadine has a mild antiparkinsonian effect and appears to be more effective in the control of bradykinesia and rigidity and less effective with regard to tremor. Schwab et al. conducted the first clinical experiments to assess efficacy of amantadine in 163 patients with Parkinson's disease. However, this was a not controlled study. Patients received a maximum daily dose of 200 mg of amantadine in addition to their usual antiparkinsonian medication. The authors found improvement of akinesia, rigidity, and tremor in 66% of the patients and noted that in 58% the benefit was sustained for a period of 3–8 months.[17]

Since that first report many trials have been performed to investigate amantadine's effectiveness in the treatment of PD as monotherapy or in association to other antiparkinsonian drugs. A double-blind, placebo-controlled crossover study was performed on 30 PD patients; all patients were on monotherapy with amantadine, with the exception of three who also received anticholinergic or antihistaminic therapy.[32] Clinical assessments consisted on evaluations of tremor, rigidity, all physical signs, daily activities, repetitive motions, and an overall average. Amantadine resulted in a statistically significant 12% overall improvement over placebo. Ten patients continued treatment for 10–12 months. Improvements in tremor and rigidity remained relatively constant, while there was some apparent loss of efficacy in timed tests and quality of timed tests.

Fahn et al.[33] conducted a randomized, double-blind, crossover, placebo-controlled trial in 23 PD patients. During the first crossover period the patients were randomized to placebo or amantadine 200 mg/day. The authors reported a favorable response in 16 of 23 patients (70%). The most common adverse reactions were insomnia, anorexia, dizziness, nervousness, irritability, depression, and sleepiness.

Parkes et al.[34] investigated the efficacy of amantadine compared with anticholinergics in 17 PD patients in a randomized, double-blind crossover trial. Patients were randomized to amantadine 200 mg/day, benzhexol 8 mg/day, or amantadine plus benzhexol. The improvement observed with amantadine or benzhexol as monotherapy was a reduction of 15% in functional disability without significant differences between the two drugs, while both drugs in combination resulted in a reduction of 40% of total disability.

Amantadine is superior to placebo when administered in patients receiving anticholinergics. Walker et al.,[35] in a double-blind crossover trial in which

42 PD patients were evaluated, found amantadine superior to placebo in 74% of cases.

As adjunctive therapy to levodopa, amantadine is somewhat efficacious in the symptomatic treatment of Parkinson's disease. In a randomized, double-blind crossover study, Sarvey et al.[36] added amantadine to the regimen of 42 PD patients treated with levodopa/carbidopa. The clinical picture after a period of 9 weeks was a significant improvement of symptoms. Similarly, Fehling et al.,[37] in a randomized, double-blind crossover study, compared the effect of amantadine or placebo in 21 patients receiving levodopa/carbidopa, and found amantadine significantly more effective than placebo in improving PD symptoms. Nonetheless, these findings were not confirmed by other authors who found no differences in the evaluation of patients treated with levodopa/carbidopa with and without amantadine.[38,39]

It is generally described that amantadine produces a transient clinical benefit with a loss of efficacy after 6–12 months probably due to a tachyphylaxis phenomenon. Nonetheless, some authors have questioned the validity of this notion. Stewart and colleagues, in a critical review of 22 studies of amantadine, found that many of them included patients with post-encephalitic parkinsonism, multiple system atrophy, or progressive supranuclear palsy. The range of duration of amantadine therapy was 4 days to 12 months, and in 13 studies the decline of efficacy was not mentioned, suggesting there are not enough reliable data to support this notion.[18,40] Zeldowicz et al.[41] performed a clinical trial with 77 PD patients to evaluate whether there was a decline in efficacy. Nineteen patients with good to excellent response to amantadine monotherapy maintained that improvement for an average of 21 months, with the longest duration being 30 months. In addition, a marked deterioration took place when amantadine was switched in a random fashion to placebo.

Treatment of Motor Complications

Amantadine was found to be effective in the treatment of levodopa-induced dyskinesias in patients with Parkinson's disease. Preclinical studies suggest that the development of levodopa-induced motor complications is associated with an increased phosphorylation state of NMDA receptors in striatal medium spiny neurons, as a result of which synaptic efficacy is enhanced and corticostriatal glutamatergic input is amplified affecting striatal GABAergic output and probably leading to motor response complications. Therefore, it is conceivable that amantadine exerts its antidyskinetic effect by normalizing striatal NMDA receptor hyperfunction.[42,43]

Verhagen Metman et al.[29] conducted the first controlled clinical trial to evaluate the effects of amantadine on levodopa-associated dyskinesias and motor fluctuations in 18 advanced PD patients (average age 60 years, Hoehn–Yahrs stage 2 to 5) in a double-blind, crossover, placebo-controlled study during a 6-week period. All patients received amantadine or placebo for 3 weeks each. Amantadine doses were 100–400 mg/day depending on age, renal function, and tolerance. At the end of each study period patients received an intravenous levodopa infusion for 7 hours at an individually determined optimal rate defined as the lowest rate producing the maximal antiparkinsonian effect. The evaluations were performed during the last 2 hours of the levodopa infusion; choreiform dyskinesias and parkinsonian symptoms were scored every 10 minutes. Dyskinesias were also videotaped and subsequently scored by a second blinded neurologist. Parkinsonian symptoms and dyskinesias were assessed using the Unified Parkinson's Disease Rating Scale (UPDRS) part III, items 20, 22, 23, 26, and 31 and a modified Abnormal Involuntary Movement Scale (AIMS). Motor fluctuations were assessed with the UPDRS part IV, items 32 (duration of dyskinesias), 33 (severity of dyskinesias), and 39 (proportion of the day in the "off" state), as well as patient diaries on the last 2 or 3 days of each study arm. The statistical analysis of measures showed a significant ($p < 0.001$) reduction on dyskinesia severity which was 60% lower with amantadine compared with placebo. In this study, amantadine substantially ameliorated levodopa-induced peak-dose dyskinesias without worsening parkinsonian symptoms. Diphasic dyskinesias could not be evaluated as they did not occur during the optimal rate of levodopa infusion. Only four patients withdrew from the study because of adverse reactions (confusion 1, hallucinations 1, palpitations 1, nausea 1).[29]

One year later, Metman et al.[44] reported the results of a one-year follow-up of the previous study. Seventeen of the original 18 patients participated in this study with a non-randomized, double-blind, placebo-controlled design. Ten days prior to the follow-up assessment, amantadine was replaced with capsules containing either amantadine or placebo. On the test day, patients received an intravenous infusion of levodopa followed by the motor assessment. The results showed that one year after initiation of amantadine co-therapy its antidyskinetic effect was similar in magnitude. The reduction of dyskinesia severity was 56% compared with 60% one year earlier. The authors conclude that the beneficial effects of amantadine on levodopa-induced dyskinesias are maintained for at least one year after treatment initiation.

In the two previous studies, amantadine was administrated orally and the benefit was observed days or weeks after treatment initiation. Del Dotto et al.[45] investigated the possible occurrence of an acute effect of amantadine after an intravenous infusion. They conducted a randomized, double-blind, placebo-controlled study including nine PD patients with peak-dose levodopa-induced choreiform dyskinesias. Their mean age was 59.7 years, disease duration 8.4 years, Hoehn–Yahr stage in "off" condition 3, and the daily dose of levodopa immediately prior to the study was 860 mg. All patients were evaluated on two different days for 5 hours while taking their usual antiparkinsonian medications. The nine patients received their first morning levodopa dose, followed by 2 hours of intravenous amantadine (200 mg) or placebo infusion. The parkinsonian symptoms and dyskinesias were assessed every 15 minutes during the infusion and 3 hours thereafter using the UPDRS scale part III, tapping test, and the AIMS. The average of dyskinesia scores during amantadine infusion was 50% lower compared with placebo ($p<0.01$). These results indicate that the antidyskinetic effect of amantadine occurs acutely, not requiring days or weeks to develop.

The antidyskinetic effect of amantadine has been confirmed by other authors. Snow et al.[46] performed a double-blind, placebo-controlled, crossover study to assess the effect of amantadine (200 mg/day orally) versus placebo on levodopa-induced dyskinesia in 24 PD patients. There was a significant reduction ($p < 0.004$) of 24% in the total dyskinesia score after amantadine administration.

Prevention of Disease Progression

Several recent studies indicate that amantadine could have neuroprotective properties in addition to its symptomatic effects. It has been suggested that the enhancement of excitatory amino acid neurotransmission might play a role in the pathogenesis of several chronic neurodegenerative diseases, including Parkinson's.[47,48] Studies in monkeys indicate that excitatory amino acids such as glutamate are involved in the pathophysiological cascade of neuronal cell death due to MPTP (1-methyl-4-phenyl-1,2,3,6-tetrahydropyridine). This observation supports the hypothesis that glutamate antagonists such as amantadine may be able to retard progression of the disease.[49] In addition, several in-vitro studies have recently shown neuroprotective properties of amantadine and its congener compound memantine at therapeutically used doses (KOR-2).

Uitti et al.[50] studied survival in patients with Parkinson's disease and other parkinsonian syndromes. They employed standard survival curves and a Cox regression model to identify independent predictive variables for survival. Patients treated or not treated with amantadine were similar in terms of age, gender, type of parkinsonism, Hoehn–Yahr stage, and cognitive status. The authors found that the use of amantadine is an independent predictor of improved survival.

Glutamate-receptor antagonist agents appear to be promising for the neuroprotective therapy of Parkinson's disease.[51] Several compounds with antiparkinsonian effects–such as amantadine, memantine, and budipine–have been shown to be non-competitive NMDA-receptor antagonist and are candidates for clinical trials searching for their possible neuroprotective effect in PD patients.[49]

Adverse Events

The most frequent adverse reactions associated with the use of amantadine include: insomnia, anxiety, dizziness, impaired coordination, nervousness, nausea, and vomiting. These side-effects are usually mild although they can be severe in elderly patients. In fewer than 5% of patients, irritability, headaches, depression, ataxia, confusion, hallucinations, nightmares, somnolence, agitation, diarrhea, constipation, livedo reticularis, and xerostomia are reported. Dry mouth and blurred vision are considered peripheral anticholinergic side-effects. Livedo reticularis is more often seen in women and is frequently associated with persistent ankle edema.[52] Exceptionally, some patients can present with hyperkinesias, urinary retention, rash, or decreased libido. Toxic manifestations of amantadine include acute psychosis, coma, cardiovascular toxicity, and death. Amantadine toxicity may be associated with overdose or renal insufficiency as 90% of an oral dose is excreted unchanged in the urine.[53] These toxic effects may be exacerbated by the concomitant use of anticholinergic agents.

More rare adverse reactions are reported as isolated cases, such as vocal myoclonus, heart failure, or peripheral neuropathy.[54,55] Shulman et al.[56] reported a case of sensory motor peripheral neuropathy secondary to chronic administration of amantadine in a 48-year-old woman in whom the discontinuation of the drug resulted in resolution of trophic skin ulcers, paresthesias, and distal weakness.

Withdrawal effects of amantadine are not frequent but may be serious. Factor et al.[21] reported three PD patients who, after gradual tapering of amantadine, experienced acute delirium, paranoid reaction, and agitation in addition to worsening of their motor symptoms. In all patients the syndrome rapidly resolved after amantadine restitution. Some characteristics were common among these patients. They were elderly and had had hallucinations in the past, dementia, advanced PD, and a long duration of amantadine therapy – representing possible risk factors for this complication.

Amantadine: Conclusions

Amantadine has mild antiparkinsonian and antidyskinetic effects. It may be used as monotherapy in the early stages of Parkinson's disease in patients with mild to moderate rigidity or bradykinesia when tremor is not the major problem. In advanced disease, amantadine is useful for the control of levodopa-induced dyskinesias in patients with motor complications. The duration of the drug's benefit is not established. Amantadine is relatively safe and well tolerated. Further studies are warranted with regard to its potential neuroprotective properties.

SELEGILINE

Basic Pharmacology

Selegiline causes irreversible inhibition of monoamine oxidase (MAO) type B, which catalyzes the oxidative deamination of neuroactive amines such as dopamine.[57,58] The drug is an irreversible or suicide inhibitor forming a covalent bond with the flavin adenine dinucleotide cofactor of MAO. Selegiline is a relatively selective MAO-B inhibitor, but this selectively is lost at higher doses of the drug. Selegiline may enhance the activity of catecholaminergic neurons by other mechanisms besides MAO-B inhibition. Furthermore, selegiline possesses other pharmacologic activity that could be important for its putative neuroprotective mechanism of action, such as an effect on mitochondrial membrane potential activity, an antiapoptosis effect, and reduction of oxidative stress.

Selegiline is rapidly absorbed from the gastrointestinal tract. Its main metabolites are desmethylselegiline, methamphetamine, and amphetamine. These compounds are less pharmacologically active L-isomers. Selegiline is metabolized mainly in the liver and disappears rapidly from the serum with a half-life of 0.15 hours. Peak metabolite levels are seen 0.5–2 hours after an oral dose. The majority of the drug is bound to plasma protein. Selegiline is an irreversible inhibitor, so the effect on MAO-B is significantly longer than the drug elimination half-life. It depends on the resynthesis of enzyme protein, and is likely to be longer than one month.

Symptomatic Treatment of Parkinsonism

Selegiline appears to have a mild symptomatic effect in some patients as demonstrated by several studies. In the DATATOP study,[59] a small but statistically significant clinical effect was observed with selegiline monotherapy in de-novo PD patients at doses of 10 mg/day. At 1 and 3 months after treatment ("wash-in"), selegiline was significantly better than placebo in all components of the UPDRS. The authors considered these changes not to be clinically relevant. However, statistically significant deterioration was noted upon selegiline withdrawal at 1 and 2 months ("wash-out").

In a randomized, double-blind, placebo-controlled crossover study of 20 de-novo PD patients, Teravainen evaluated doses of selegiline between 5 and 30 mg/day.[60] Clinically significant changes were not observed in any patient, nor was subjective benefit reported. The mean scores on the 30 mg/day dose were approximately 10% less than placebo (not statistically significant). The study was problematic because of the crossover design where there was no washout period between treatment phases.

Myllyla et al.[61] reported that 27 PD patients treated with selegiline improved compared to 25 placebo controls. Scores for rating scales were significantly lower for selegiline. This effect was observed for up to one year. The sum of scores for tremor, rigidity, and bradykinesia also were significantly better at one year in the selegiline group compared to the placebo group. The most pronounced differences were found in rigidity and bradykinesia. However, the mean scores in the selegiline group reached the baseline score after four months. The initial improvement time was about 3 months.

Allain et al.[62] tested selegiline (10 mg/day) for treatment in 93 PD patients (average age 64.9 years) who were from 13 centers in France. Patients were followed for 3 months and evaluated by the UPDRS, Hoehn–Yahr, Schwab–England, and Hamilton Depression Scale. In 48 patients, selegiline was significantly better than placebo (47 patients) for the motor UPDRS score and for the depression scores. There was no difference between selegiline and placebo in global scores, scores of activities of daily living, and Hoehn–Yahr stage.

Mally et al.[63] evaluated 20 de-novo PD patients (Hoehn–Yahr 1 to 3, average age 62.5 years, average disease duration 2.1 years), in a randomized, placebo-controlled, parallel study design. Significant changes were observed in motor behavior and daily activity (UPDRS) after 3 weeks of treatment with selegiline at 10 mg/day. The total scores of the UPDRS and Northwestern University Disability Scale (NUDS) were significantly changed after 4 weeks. Hypokinesia and walking improved the most. Rigidity was not changed. The authors conclude that hypokinesias can be significantly improved with selegiline treatment.

Treatment of Motor Complications

Selegiline appears to have some efficacy in the treatment of motor fluctuations. Lees et al.[64] evaluated 41 PD patients (average age 62.5 years, average disease duration 8.0 years) in a double-blind, placebo-controlled study of selegiline

(10 mg/day) added to levodopa in both mild and severe fluctuating patients. Selegiline improved "wearing-off" disabilities in approximately 65% of patients. No statistically significant improvement occurred in diurnal akinesia, and there was no improvement in patients with severe "on/off" disabilities with freezing and rapid oscillation.

Lieberman et al.[65] investigated 33 PD patients (average age 63.3 years) in a randomized, double-blind, placebo-controlled parallel study of selegiline (10 mg/day) added to levodopa for 8 weeks. Seventeen patients were randomly assigned to the selegiline group and 16 to the placebo group. All patients completed the 8-week trial. The patients who were randomly assigned to the selegiline group experienced a significant 22% decrease in their parkinsonian symptoms, a significant 17.4% decrease in their parkinsonian signs, and a significant 21% decrease in their levodopa dose. The patients did not, as a group, experience an improvement in the number of hours that they were "on". Overall, the conditions of 12 of the 17 patients (71%) were judged to have improved. Although there was no increase in number of hours "on," patients reported that their dose of levodopa lasted longer, that the transitions between their "on" and "off" periods were less abrupt, that the "on" periods were better, and that the "off" periods were less severe.

Golbe et al.[66] investigated selegiline (10 mg/day) and placebo added to levodopa in 99 PD patients (average age 62.4 years, Hoehn–Yahr stage 2 to 4) in a randomized, double-blind, placebo-controlled, multicenter, parallel study (6-week study period). Using diary forms, patients recorded disability hourly at home, three days a week, during a 2-week baseline, and during a 6-week treatment period. Mean hourly overall symptom control significantly improved in 29 patients (58%) taking selegiline and in 12 patients (26.1%) taking placebo. Patients' mean pretreatment baseline hourly self-assessment scores for "drug working" in selegiline and placebo groups were 1.29 and 1.28, respectively. Mean scores (measured hourly) over the 6 weeks of treatment were 1.41 and 1.11 for selegiline versus placebo, respectively. No significant improvement occurred in the objective quality of the "on" state with selegiline. Mean daily levodopa dosage decreases were 17% in the selegiline group and 7% in the placebo group.

Prevention of Disease Progression

Selegiline has been suggested to be neuroprotective in Parkinson's disease but conclusive clinical data are lacking. Tetrud and Langston[67] were the first to study the effect of selegiline (10 mg/day) as putative neuroprotective therapy. They evaluated 54 patients (average age 61.0 years). Forty-four completed the trial for the duration of 36 months. The authors reported that, for the primary outcome, selegiline significantly delayed the need for levodopa therapy. Analysis of Kaplan–Meier survival curves for each group showed that selegiline delayed the need for levodopa therapy; the average time until levodopa was needed was 312.1 days for patients in the placebo group and 548.9 days for patients in the selegiline group. Disease progression, as monitored by assessment scales (e.g. UPDRS, Hoehn–Yahr, Schwab–England) was slowed by selegiline as compared to placebo. The authors suggested the drug may have neuroprotective properties but they did not directly consider potential confounding symptomatic effects of selegiline.

In a DATATOP study, both selegiline (10 mg/day) and tocopherol were studied in 800 patients (average age 61.1 years) with mild disease in a 2×2 factorial study design.[59] The authors found that selegiline significantly delayed the development of disability requiring levodopa therapy (the primary endpoint). Only 97 subjects who received selegiline reached the endpoint during an average 12-month follow-up, compared with 176 subjects who did not receive selegiline. The risk of reaching the endpoint was significantly reduced by 57% for the subjects who received selegiline. The subjects who received selegiline also had a significant reduction in their risk of having to give up full-time employment. However, there was improvement in motor scores after initiation of selegiline and worsening after drug withdrawal, suggesting that the beneficial effects of selegiline may be related, in part, to a symptomatic amelioration of Parkinson's disease. However, there was a statistically significant reduction in disability as compared to placebo even among selegiline-treated subjects who initially had no improvement in motor scores. This suggests that the results may not be entirely explained by the symptomatic effects of selegiline. Symptomatic deterioration may have been observed in all patients if a washout period was preformed prior to reaching the endpoint. Symptomatic deterioration also may have been observed over a longer period of time.

An additional study done by the Parkinson Study Group[68] reported the results of 310 patients who did not reach the endpoint. These patients all received selegiline, but the blindness of the original assessment was maintained. If selegiline had a neuroprotective effect, the subjects who had originally received selegiline would have shown superior and sustained benefits after reinitiation of selegiline treatment compared with subjects not previously treated with selegiline. However, during the extended trial, 108 subjects assigned previously to selegiline reached the endpoint of disability faster than 121 subjects not assigned selegiline. This suggests that the initial advantages of selegiline were not sustained. Firm conclusions from this study are difficult because the selegiline patients had more severe impairment at baseline, there was a 2-month interruption of therapy, and there were variations in interpretations of open-label assignments.

In a Finnish trial,[61] the authors reported long-term effects of selegiline (10 mg/day) in previously untreated patients with early disease. They followed 47 selegiline-treated patients for 2 years. The median duration of time before initiation of levodopa was 545 ± 90 days with selegiline and 372 ± 28 days with placebo ($p = 0.03$). Disability was significantly less in the selegiline group than in the placebo group for up to 12 months. A reduction in the need for long-term levodopa therapy was noted. The authors concluded that the drug may have neuroprotective properties and that it may slow down the rate or progression of Parkinson's disease. However, this study includes the same confounding issues as reviewed in the DATATOP study.

Olanow et al.[69] used a different study design to address the issue of neuroprotection with selegiline (10 mg/day). This 14-month trial was aimed at minimizing confounding symptomatic effects by including a 2-month washout of selegiline before assessing the final outcome. One-hundred and one patients (average age 66.2 years) were evaluated at baseline (untreated) and again after the final visit following withdrawal of antiparkinsonian medication. Deterioration of parkinsonian scores (motor UPDRS) between the two visits – baseline and 14 months – were used as the index of disease progression. Selegiline was withdrawn 2 months prior and levodopa 7–14 days prior to the final visit. Placebo-treated patients deteriorated by 5.8 ± 1.4 points on the UPDRS, while selegiline-treated patients changed only 0.4 ± 1.3 points ($p < 0.001$). This investigation shows that selegiline prevents deterioration of clinical scores in patients with early Parkinson's disease. The observed effects are more readily explained by a neuroprotective rather than a symptomatic action of the drug. However, in spite of the 2-month washout, this time period still may not have been long enough to eliminate all symptomatic effects of the drug.

In a similar design to the DATATOP clinical trial, Palhagen et al.[70] studied 157 PD patients (average age 63.8 years) over a 12-month period with a 2-month washout prior to the initiation of levodopa therapy. The primary endpoint was "time to disability sufficient to require levodopa therapy." Analysis of Kaplan–Meier survival curves for each group showed that selegiline significantly delayed the need for levodopa therapy. The semiannual rate of disability progression was slowed significantly in the selegiline group as analyzed with the UPDRS (total and motor scores). Selegiline had a wash-in effect (i.e. an initial symptomatic amelioration of PD at 6 weeks and 3 months). However, after the 8-week washout period, no significant differences in the deterioration of disability between the groups was revealed in any of the scales. Similarly, the progression of symptoms from baseline to the end of the washout period was significantly slower in the selegiline group when the progression was adjusted by the time to reach the endpoint. Selegiline significantly delayed the need to start levodopa in early Parkinson's disease. Additionally, after a 2-month washout period, there was no significant symptomatic effect of selegiline. The authors concluded that their data supported the concept of a neuroprotective property of the drug.

Adverse Events

Selegiline, in general, is a well-tolerated drug. When used as monotherapy, infrequently reported side-effects include insomnia (especially if the drug is given late in the day), headache, nausea, loss of balance, dry mouth, and gastrointestinal symptoms (flatulence, discomfort, and constipation). No significant changes in blood pressure have been reported. Many studies find no difference in the incidence of reported adverse reactions between selegiline and placebo. Dopaminergic adverse reactions (such as hallucinations and dyskinesia) can occur when selegiline is added to levodopa therapy. These adverse reactions usually subside when the dose of levodopa is reduced.

Lees et al.[71] reported that the mortality in previously untreated PD patients (520 patients in 93 British hospitals) was higher for those treated with levodopa plus selegiline than for those treated with levodopa alone (28% vs 18%; adjusted for age, sex, and other baseline factors; hazard ratio = 1.57). In a follow-up to this study, whereby the patient number was increased to 624, an increased mortality for the combined treatment group was still detected, but the hazard ratio was lower than in the previous report, and no longer statistically significant (adjusted hazard ratio = 1.30). The increased mortality appeared to be associated with the second to fourth years of treatment. The authors could not explain the increased mortality, but suggested that the combined therapy be avoided in patients with postural hypotension, frequent falls, confusion, or dementia.

These studies showing increased mortality have been extensively discussed and criticized and a number of objections have been raised, including problems with design and statistics.[72] Furthermore, other long-term studies of selegiline have not found an increased mortality with selegiline.

Selegiline: Conclusions

Selegiline is used less frequently in Parkinson's disease because its neuroprotective action remains unproven, it provides only minimal symptomatic control, and it is also not a particularly effective drug for treating motor fluctuations. Clearly there are more potent symptomatic drugs and more effective agents to treat motor complications. Nonetheless, it is a relatively safe drug and may be helpful in the treatment of some PD patients.

REFERENCES

1. Ordestein L. Sur la paralyse agitante et lasclérose en plaques generalisee. Paris: E Martinet, 1867, p. 32.
2. Duvoisin RC. Cholinergic–anticholinergic antagonism in parkinsonism. Arch Neurol 1967;17:124–136.
3. Feldberg W. Present views on the mode of action of acetylcholine in the central nervous system. Physiol Rev 1945;25:596.
4. Doshay LJ, Constable K. Artane therapy for parkinsonism: a preliminary study of results in one hundred and seventeen cases. JAMA 1949;140:1317–1322.
5. Lang AE. Treatment of Parkinson's disease agents others than levodopa and dopamine agonists: controversies and new approaches. Can J Neurol Sci 1984;11(suppl.):210–220.
6. Weiner WJ, Lang AE. Movement Disorders: a Comprehensive Survey. Mount Kisco, NY: Futura Publishing, 1989.
7. Koller WC. Pharmacological treatment of parkinsonian tremor. Arch Neurol 1986;43:126–127.
8. Cantello R, Riccio A, Gilli M et al. Bornaprine vs placebo in Parkinson disease: double-blind controlled cross-over trial in 30 patients. Ital J Neurol Sci 1986;7(1):139–143.
9. Martin WE, Loewenson RB, Resch JA, Baker AB. A controlled study comparing trihexyphenidyl hydrochloride plus levodopa with placebo plus levodopa in patients with Parkinson's disease. Neurology 1974;24:912–919.
10. Cooper JA, Sagar HJ, Doherty SM et al. Different effects of dopaminergic and anticholinergic therapies on cognitive and motor function in Parkinson's disease: a follow-up study of untreated patients. Brain 1992;115:1701–1725.
11. Friedman JH, Koller WC, Lannon MC et al. Benztropine versus clozapine for the treatment of tremor in Parkinson's disease. Neurology 1997;48:1077–1081.
12. Hauser RA, Ollanow CW. Orobuccal dyskinesia associated with trihexyphenidyl therapy in a patient with Parkinson's disease. Mov Disord 1993;8:512–514.
13. Birket-Smith E. Abnormal involuntary movements induced by anticholinergic therapy. Acta Neurol Scand 1974;50:801–811.
14. Hughes RC, Polgar JG, Weightman D, Walton JN. Levodopa in parkinsonism: the effects of withdrawal of anticholinergic drugs. Brit Med J 1971;2:487–491.
15. Goetz CG, Nausieda PA, Weines PH, Klawans HL. Practical guidelines for drug holidays in parkinsonian patients. Neurology1981;31:641–642.
16. Jackson GG, Muldoon RL, Akers LW. Serological evidence for prevention of influenza infection in volunteers by an anti-influenza drug, amantadine hydrochloride. Antimicrob Agents Chemother 1963;3:703–707.

17. Schwab RS, England AC, Poskanzer DC. Young RR. Amantadine in the treatment of Parkinson's disease. JAMA 1969;208:1168–1170.
18. Factor SA, Molho ES. Transient benefit of amantadine in Parkinson's disease: the facts about the myth. Mov Disord 1999;14:515–517.
19. Shannon KM, Goetz CG, Carroll VS, Tanner CM, Klawans HL. Amantadine and motor fluctuations in chronic Parkinson's disease. Clin Neuropharmacol 1987;10:522–526.
20. Stoof JC, Booij J, Drukarch B. Amantadine as *N*-methyl-D-aspartic acid receptor antagonist: new possibilities for therapeutic applications. Clin Neurol Neurosurg 1992;94:s4–6.
21. Factor SA, Molho ES, Brown DL. Acute delirium after withdrawal of amantadine in Parkinson's disease. Neurology 1998;50:1456–1458.
22. Von Voigtlander PF, Moore KE. Dopamine release from the brain *in vivo* by amantadine. Science 1971;174:408–410.
23. Bailey EV, Stone TW. The mechanism of action of amantadine in parkinsonism: a review. Arch Int Pharmacodyn Ther 1975;216:246–262.
24. Gianutsos G, Chute S, Dunn JP. Pharmacological changes in dopaminergic systems induced by long term administration of amantadine. Eur J Pharmacol 1985;110:357–361.
25. Kornhuber J, Bormann J, Hubers M, Rusche K, Riederer P. Effects of l-amino adamantanes at the MK-801 binding site of the NMDA receptor-gated ion channel: a human postmortem brain study. Eur J Pharmacol 1991;206:297–300.
26. Sobolevski AI, Koshelev SG, Khodorov BI. Interaction of memantine and amantadine with agonist inbound NMDA-receptor channels in acutely isolated rat hippocampal neurons. J Physiol 1998;512(1):47–60.
27. Banplied TA, Boeckman FA, Aizenman E, Johnson JW. Trapping channel block of NMDA receptors activated responses by amantadine and memantine. J Neurophysiol 1997;77:309–323.
28. Brown F, Redfern PH. Studies on mechanism of action of amantadine. Br J Pharmacol 1976;58:561–567.
29. Metman LV, Del Dotto P, van den Munckhof P et al. Amantadine as treatment for dyskinesias and motor fluctuations in Parkinson's disease. Neurology 1998;50:1323–1326.
30. Goetz C. New lessons from old drugs: amantadine and Parkinson's disease. Neurology 1998;50:1211–1212.
31. Aoki FY, Sitar DS. Clinical pharmacokinetics of amantadine hydrochloride. Clin Pharmacokinet 1988;14:35–51.
32. Butzer JF, Silver DE, Sahs AL. Amantadine in Parkinson's disease: a double-blind, placebo-controlled, crossover study with long-term follow-up. Neurology 1975;25:603.
33. Fahn S, Isgreen WP. Long term evaluation of amantadine and levodopa combination in parkinsonism by double-blind crossover analyses. Neurology 1975;25:695–700.
34. Parkes JD, Baxter RC, Marsden CD, Rees JE. Comparative trial of benzhexol, amantadine and levodopa in the treatment of Parkinson's disease. J Neurol Neurosurg Psychiatry 1974;37:422–426.
35. Walker JE, Albers JW, Tourtellotte WW et al. A qualitative and quantitative evaluation of amantadine in the treatment of Parkinson's disease. J Chronic Dis 1972;25:149–182.
36. Savery F. Amantadine and a fixed combination of levodopa and carbidopa in the treatment of Parkinson's disease. Dis Nerv Sys 1977;38:605–608.
37. Fehling C. The effect of adding amantadine to optimum levodopa dosage in Parkinson's syndrome. Acta Neurol Scand 1973;49:245–251.
38. Millac P, Hasan I, Espir ML, Slyfield DG. Treatment of parkinsonism with levodopa and amantadine. Lancet 1970;2:720.
39. Callagham N, McIlroy M, O'Connor M. Treatment of Parkinson's disease with levodopa and amantadine used as a single drugs and in combined therapy. Ir J Med Sci 1974;143:67–78.
40. Marsden CD. The drug therapy of early Parkinson's disease. In: Stern MB, Hurtig HH (eds), The Comprehensive Management of Parkinson's disease. New York: PMA Publishing, 1988, pp. 79–88.
41. Zeldowicz LR, Huberman J. Long term therapy of Parkinson's disease with amantadine alone and combined with levodopa. Can Assoc J 1973;109:588–593.
42. Chase TN, Engber TM, Mouradian MM. Contribution of dopaminergic and glutamatergic mechanisms to the pathogenesis of motor response complications in Parkinson's disease. Adv Neurol 1996;69:497–501.
43. Dunah AW, Wang Y, Yasuda RP et al. Alteration in subunit expression, composition, and phosphorylation of striatal *N*-methyl-D-aspartate glutamate receptors in a rat 6-hydroxidopamine model of Parkinson's disease. Mol Pharmacol 2000;57:342–352.
44. Metman LV, Del Dotto P, LePoole K et al. Amantadine for levodopa induced dyskinesias: a 1-year follow-up study. Arch Neurol 1999;56:1383–1386.

45. Del Dotto P, Pavese N, Gambaccini G et al. Intravenous amantadine improves levodopa-induced dyskinesias: an acute double-blind placebo-controlled study. Mov Disord 2001;16:515–520.
46. Snow BJ, Macdonald L, Mcauley D, Wallis W. The effect of amantadine in levodopa induced dyskinesias in Parkinson's disease: a double-blind, placebo-controlled study. Clin Neuropharmacol 2000;23(2):82–85.
47. Kornhuber J, Weller M, Schoppmeyer K, Riederer P. Amantadine and memantine are NMDA receptor antagonists with neuroprotective properties. J Neural Transm 1994;43(suppl.):91–104.
48. Danysz W, Parsons CG, Kornhuber J, Schmidt WJ, Quack G. Amino adamantanes as NMDA receptor antagonists and antiparkinsonian agents: preclinical studies. Neurosci Biobehav Rev 1997;21:455–468.
49. Lange KW, Kornhuber J, Riederer P. Dopamine/glutamate interactions in Parkinson's disease. Neurosci Biobehav Rev 1997;21:393–400.
50. Uitti RJ, Rajput AH, Ahlskog JE et al. Amantadine treatment is an independent predictor of improved survival in Parkinson's disease. Neurology 1996;46:1551–1552.
51. Kornhuber J, Weller M. New therapeutic possibilities with low-affinity MNDA receptor antagonists. Nervenarzt 1996;67(1):77–82.
52. Loffler H, Habermann B, Effendy I. Amantadine induced livedo reticularis. Hautarzt 1998;49:224–227.
53. Macchio GJ, Ito V, Sahgal V. Amantadine-induced coma. Arch Phys Med Rehabil 1993;74:1119–1120.
54. Vale JA, Maclean KS. Amantadine-induced heart failure. Lancet 1977;1(8010):548.
55. Pfeiffer RF. Amantadine-induced vocal myoclonus. Mov Disord 1996;11:104–106.
56. Shulman LM, Minagar A, Sharma K, Weiner WJ. Amantadine-induced peripheral neuropathy. Neurology 1999;53:1862–1865.
57. Knoll J. Deprenyl [selegiline]: the history of its development and pharmacological action. Acta Neurol Scan 1983;95:57–80.
58. Riederer P, Youdim MB, Rausch WD et al. On the mode of action of L-deprenyl in the human central nervous system. J Neural Transm 1978;43:217–226.
59. Parkinson's Study Group. Effect of deprenyl on the progression of disability in early Parkinson's disease. N Engl J Med 1989;321:1364–1371.
60. Teravainen H. Selegiline in Parkinson's disease. Acta Neurol Scand 1990;81:333–336.
61. Myllyla VV, Sotaniemic KA, Vuorinen JA, Heinonen EA. Selegiline as initial treatment in de-novo parkinsonian patients. Neurology 1992;42:339–343.
62. Allain H, Pollak P, Neukirch HC. Symptomatic effect of selegiline in de-novo parkinsonian patients: the French Selegiline Multicenter Trial. Mov Disord 1993;8(suppl. 1):s36–40.
63. Mally J, Kovacs AB, Slone TW. Delayed development of symptomatic improvement by L-deprenyl in Parkinson's disease. J Neurol Sci 1995;134:143–145.
64. Lees AJ, Shaw KM, Kohout LJ et al. Deprenyl in Parkinson's disease. Lancet 1977;2:791–795.
65. Lieberman AN, Gopinathan G, Neophytides A, Foo SH. Deprenyl versus placebo in Parkinson's disease: a double-blind study. NY State J Med 1987;87:646–649.
66. Golbe LI, Lieberman AN, Muenter MD et al. Deprenyl in the treatment of symptom fluctuations in advanced Parkinson's disease. Clin Neuropharmacol 1988;11:45–55.
67. Tetrud JW, Langston JW. The effect of deprenyl (selegiline) in the natural history of Parkinson's disease. Science 1989;245:519–522.
68. Parkinson Study Group. Impact of deprenyl and tocopherol treatment on Parkinson's disease in DATATOP subjects not requiring levodopa. Ann Neurol 1996;39:29–36.
69. Olanow CW, Hauser RA, Gauger L et al. The effect of deprenyl and levodopa on the progression of Parkinson's disease. Ann Neurol 1995;38:771–777.
70. Palhagen S, Heinonan EH, Hagglund J et al. Selegiline delays the onset of disability in de-novo parkinsonian patients: Swedish Parkinsons Study Group. Neurology 1998;51:520–525.
71. Lees A, for the Parkinson's Disease Research Group of the UK. Comparison of therapeutic effects and mortality data of levodopa and levodopa combined with selegiline in patients with early, mild Parkinson's disease. Br Med J 1995;311:1602–1607.
72. Olanow CW, Myllyla VV, Sotaniemi KA et al. Effects of selegiline on mortality in patients with Parkinson's disease: a meta-analysis. Neurology 1998;51:825–830.

4
Pathogenesis of Motor Complications

Thomas N. Chase

INTRODUCTION

The pharmacological treatment of Parkinson's disease (PD) has changed little over the past three decades or so.[1,2] Core motor dysfunction, notably tremor, rigidity and bradykinesia, have long been known to arise as a consequence of nigrostriatal dopamine (DA) system degeneration.[3,4] Clinical disability begins when denervation of striatal DA receptors becomes sufficient to overwhelm compensatory mechanisms, and striatal levels of the transmitter amine fall below the physiological range.[5,6] During early-stage disease, the restoration of dopaminergic transmission by administering either levodopa, the immediate precursor of DA, or a direct-acting DA agonist generally affords adequate relief of cardinal parkinsonian signs. But eventually dopaminomimetic therapy becomes increasingly unsatisfactory, due largely to the appearance of adverse events, especially characteristic alterations in the motor response to treatment. For many late-stage patients, motor disabilities associated with these iatrogenic complications ultimately rival those produced by the basic disease itself.

CLINICAL CHARACTERISTICS OF EARLY WEARING-OFF FLUCTUATIONS

Parkinsonian patients can manifest a variety of alterations in their motor response to dopaminergic therapy. These changes may be broadly divided into involuntary movements and response fluctuations. While retrospective studies generally find that patients report onset of either complication type at about the same time,[7–9] objective measurements in parkinsonian animals and patients suggest the shortening in motor response to dopaminomimetic therapy underlying fluctuations of the wearing-off type begins well before symptom severity rises to the level of patient reportability;[10–12] wearing-off fluctuations thus appear to presage other motor complications. They occur predictably after each dose of levodopa or a DA agonist and become a source of increasing disability as the duration of the antiparkinsonian effect becomes progressively shorter. In patients treated only with levodopa, administration just two or three times a day can provide a stable antiparkinsonian response. But eventually, parkinsonian signs re-emerge within a few hours of each dose. While early on the increasing severity of this end of dose deterioration can be ameliorated by simply reducing the interdose interval, eventually the response shortening becomes so pronounced that even dosing every 1.5 or 2 hours fails to stablize the response adequately. Events with DA agonist monotherapy are similar, although wearing-off fluctuations usually present later, occur less frequently, and cause less clinical disability.

The reported frequency of wearing-off fluctuations varies widely, reflecting differences in patient characteristics, therapeutic regimens, and study methodology.[13] There does, however, appear to be some general agreement that patients treated with levodopa have about an additional 10% risk of developing these fluctuations with each year of therapy and disease progression.[9,14–18] Typically, parkinsonian patients may go for 1–2 years after diagnosis before starting dopaminergic therapy; from then until onset of the first motor complication may take another 2–5 years with levodopa monotherapy and several more years with DA agonist treatment.[19–21]

PATHOGENESIS OF INITIAL WEARING-OFF FLUCTUATIONS

The pathogenesis of early wearing-off phenomena has been inferred from results of both animal model studies and clinical investigations. While early research focused on mechanisms affecting the bioavailability and pharmacokinetics of levodopa, subsequent investigations showed that these factors cannot fully account for wearing-off fluctuations.[10,22–26] For example, the antiparkinsonian efficacy of levodopa diminishes following ingestion of large protein-containing meals, due to competition for uptake from the gut and especially through the blood–brain barrier by other large neutral amino acids; but these dietary effects are generally small and hardly explain wearing-off phenomena that occur in the absence of food ingestion.[27–30] Thus it now appears that the functional changes underlying early wearing-off fluctuations, like the onset of parkinsonian signs, reflect the loss of DA neurons; wearing-off fluctuations do not manifest clinically until PD is moderately advanced and subsequent progression parallels that of the underlying disorder.[10,11,17,22,31,32]

The neuronal basis for these clinical events has become increasingly well understood. In early-stage PD, exogenous levodopa is taken up by striatal dopaminergic terminals where it is rapidly decarboxyated to DA.[33] These terminals act to protect the newly synthesized amine against enzymatic degradation through storage in synaptic vesicules as well as to regulate its extracellular release. As a result, levodopa's initial duration of action (averaging about 280 minutes) far exceeds its plasma half-life (about 90 minutes), and the antiparkinsonian response to levodopa remains clinically stable despite relatively infrequent dosing.[11] But, as nigrostriatal system degeneration progresses, the proportion of exogenous levodopa entering residual dopaminergic terminals steadily declines. More is taken up and converted to DA in other striatal amino acid decarboxylase-containing cells, especially serotoninergic neurons.[34,35] The rapid escape of newly synthesized DA from serotoninergic terminals suggests that it involves neither vesicular mechanisms nor neuronal regulation. On the other hand, recent evidence indicates that it may be affected by nerve impulse activity under the control of the serotonin 5-HT_{1A} autoreceptor.[36–38] Indeed, initial findings in parkinsonian patients also suggest that DA synthesized from exogenous levodopa may to some extent be released from serotoninergic terminals by vesicular mechanisms and that suppressing impulse activity in these terminals by 5-HT_{1A} autoreceptor stimulation can smooth out the fluctuations in DA release characteristically attending periodic levodopa dosing.[39]

Wearing-off phenomena begin when the number of surviving DA terminals is no longer sufficient to buffer the swings in striatal levodopa produced by the periodic administration of this short half-life amino acid.[10,11,31,40–43] Indirect evidence that wearing-off fluctuations are associated with a decline in DA storage is provided by the results of levodopa infusion studies showing that the half-time of the antiparkinsonian response averages 108 minutes in patients who have just begun to manifest wearing-off phenomena, compared to 146 minutes in those who still maintain a stable response to levodopa.[11] Moreover, initial wearing-off fluctuations virtually disappear upon switching levodopa treatment from intermittent oral administration to continuous intravenous infusion.[31,40,41] Finally, cerebral imaging study results are generally consistent with the view that early wearing-off fluctuations reflect the diminished capacity of residual striatal dopaminergic terminals to smooth out the oscillations in precursor availability associated with standard levodopa treatment. For instance, a positron emission tomography (PET) evaluation found that striatal [^{18}F]6-fluorodopa uptake into presynaptic dopaminergic terminals was reduced more in PD patients with fluctuations than in those with a steady response to levodopa.[44] A subsequent PET study using [^{11}C]raclopride observed that stable responders maintain increased levels of intrasynaptic DA longer after oral levodopa administration than those with fluctuations.[45]

In patients receiving DA agonist monotherapy, onset of wearing-off phenomena also relates to the loss of dopaminergic neurons. But DA agonists do not depend on surviving dopaminergic terminals for biotransformation to the active molecule, for vesicular storage, or for extraneuronal release. Thus the degeneration of DA neurons has no direct effect on the duration of their antiparkinsonian action. Nevertheless, wearing-off fluctuations present clinically as ambient striatal DA levels decline to the degree that the restoration of normal dopaminergic transmission relies on agonist stimulation. Accordingly, with DA agonists as well as with levodopa, the latency to onset and subsequent course of early wearing-off fluctuations tend to more closely reflect the rate of natural disease progression than treatment-related factors.[11,31,32] On the other hand, since DA agonists have a longer half-life than levodopa (4 hours or more compared with approximately 90 minutes), wearing-off fluctuations associated with agonist monotherapy occur less frequently throughout the day and thus are less disabling for the patient. Later wearing-off fluctuations occurring with DA agonists or levodopa reflect additional pathogenic mechanisms, as discussed below.

CLINICAL DESCRIPTION OF LATE MOTOR FLUCTUATIONS AND DYSKINESIAS

As PD advances, the duration of benefit from dopaminergic treatment continues to diminish and other motor complications become clinically evident. Thus with levodopa treatment, wearing-off periods occur more frequently; with either levodopa or DA agonists, "off" periods become more disabling. In addition to wearing-off phenomena, other response fluctuations begin to appear that are characteristically unpredictable and bear no temporal relation to dosing. Most common are fluctuations of the "on"/"off" type. Occurring in about 20% of levodopa-treated PD patients, these response variations are characterized by sudden, random switches between periods when parkinsonian signs disappear ("on" or hyperkinetic state) and periods when they re-emerge ("off" or hypokinetic state).[11,14,31,42,46,47] Unlike early wearing-off fluctuations, "on"/"off" responses are not rapidly alleviated by switching from intermittent oral to continuous intravenous levodopa administration.[31,40,41] Onset is associated with a substantially increased slope of the levodopa dose – the antiparkinsonian response relation.[42] As a result of this dose–response modification, relatively small fluctuations in circulating levodopa, and thus in striatal DA, induce large shifts in dopaminergic transmission, and thus in motor function. In addition, various other unpredictable, complex response variations, including dose failures and delayed "on"s, can also appear in those with relatively advanced disease.[48–50]

Dyskinesias that complicate dopaminomimetic therapy of mid- and late-stage PD most commonly manifest clinically while brain DA concentrations peak following each levodopa dose. Less commonly, diphasic, "off"-period and other types of choreiform and dystonic involuntary movements may also appear.[48–52] Peak-dose dyskinesias comprise a mixture of chorea and mobile dystonia that is usually painless.[17,53] Clinically, they reflect the progressive reduction in the threshold for inducing these abnormal movements that also accompanies advancing disease.[42,54] Since there is no associated change in the threshold dose for ameliorating parkinsonian signs, the therapeutic window for levodopa essentially vanishes. At this point, the dose of levodopa necessary to alleviate PD symptoms becomes sufficient to produce dyskinesias.

The more common motor complications, including peak-dose dyskinesias and wearing-off and "on"/"off" fluctuations, behave like a syndrome: most patients eventually develop several types of response change, suggesting they may reflect a common pathogenic mechanism. The reported frequency of the major motor complications varies considerably between studies.[13] On average, dyskinesias occur rarely during the first year of levodopa therapy, but rise in frequency to about 30% by the second year and to nearly 40% by 4–6 years of treatment; motor fluctuations already approach 50% in those given levodopa for 1–2 years, and nearly all PD patients manifest both types of motor complication after some 10 years of dopaminomimetic drug treatment.[9,15–18,20,55–57]

The most prominent factors suggested as predictors of the time to onset of late-onset motor complications are discussed below.

Treatment Dosage

Increasing the intensity of DA receptor stimulation increases the risk of motor complications in animal models of PD[58] and in parkinsonian patients.[21,55,59,60] Indeed, even normal monkeys can develop dyskinesias upon exposure to a sufficiently high levodopa dose.[61]

Treatment Intermittency

In parkinsonian rats, motor response alterations as well as associated striatal biochemical changes (see below) occur with intermittent (such as twice daily) but not continuous (24 hours per day) dopaminomimetic treatment.[62–68] Specifically, chronic intermittent levodopa treatment of parkinsonian rats alters motor responses in ways that mimic human motor fluctuations: the response duration is shortened as occurs in those with wearing-off fluctuations; the slope of the levodopa dose/motor response relation becomes steeper as with "on"/"off" fluctuations; and the frequency with which an ordinarily effective dose of levodopa does not benefit motor function increases as happens with "dose failures." In parkinsonian monkeys, motor complications appear after 1 or 2 weeks of once- or twice-daily DA agonist administration, but not in animals given many months of agonist treatment by continuous infusion.[69,70] Dyskinesias begin sooner in parkinsonian monkeys and in parkinsonian patients treated with levodopa, which has a half-life of about 90 minutes, than in those given DA agonists, which have half-lives exceeding 4 hours and thus provide more continuous dopaminergic replacement.[51,71–77] Conversely, motor complications tend to remit when intermittent dopaminergic therapy is replaced by relatively continuous modes of administration.[22,40,41,52,78–80]

Treatment Duration and Disease Severity

The time to onset of motor complications following initiation of dopaminomimetic treatment is highly dependent on the degree of DA neuron loss.[32,57,68,69,81–83] Response modifications of this type have not been reported in normal individuals mistakenly given levodopa for long periods.[84,85] Patients with mild PD (Hoehn and Yahr stage 1.5) rarely if ever manifest motor complications, while 60–70% of those with advanced disease (stage 4) have fluctuations and dyskinesias.[17] Parkinsonian patients in whom levodopa is introduced at stage 3 develop dyskinesias and fluctuations more rapidly than those begun in stage 1 or 2.[57] Indeed, when DA neuron destruction is very severe, onset can be quite rapid. For example, in rodent and nonhuman primates rendered parkinsonian by more than 95% neurotoxin-induced DA depletion, just a few days or weeks of intermittent treatment is sufficient to induce the characteristic alterations in motor response.[81,86–89] Similarly, in parkinsonian patients markedly damaged by MPTP,[90] or those in whom dopaminomimetic therapy was delayed until relatively late-stage disease, motor complications can appear within a few weeks.[91,92] But in the more typical situation, when dopaminomimetic medications are introduced at a milder stage of DA neuron loss, it generally takes several years for the characteristic response changes to make their clinical appearance.[9,16–18,59,60,93,94] Since patients with more advanced disease ordinarily have been treated longer, studies of complex motor fluctuations and dyskinesias also generally find that onset correlates with the duration of levodopa therapy.[16,17,59,60,93,94] Nevertheless, the delay to motor complication onset is not primarily attributable to the time needed for dopaminergic treatment to induce the adverse response, but rather to the rate of DA system degeneration: latency to onset of these complications mainly reflects the time for natural disease progression to advance sufficiently so that the buffering provided by residual dopaminergic terminals no longer protects postsynaptic DA receptors against the detrimental effects of intermittent stimulation.[11,31,42,78,95]

PATHOGENESIS OF LATE MOTOR FLUCTUATIONS AND DYSKINESIAS

The weight of current evidence suggests that the progression of wearing-off fluctuations as well as the appearance of dyskinesias and other motor response complications reflect changes downstream from the nigrostriatal DA system. While peripheral pharmacokinetic factors have the potential to affect levodopa responses, none alone accounts for the totality of the motor complication syndrome. Moreover, levodopa or DA agonist treatment rapidly shortens the motor response duration of parkinsonian rodents and primates even though their complement of DA neurons remains unchanged.[68,88] Thus wearing-off phenomena in parkinsonian models and patients must reflect not only the loss of DA neurons but also changes occurring postsynaptic to their striatal terminals.[10,22,41,42,78] Indeed, clinical studies with apomorphine[96,97] confirm what had been inferred from observations in animal models[62,64,98] as well as in parkinsonian patients given levodopa infusions.[11,22,31,42,43,96] The acute parenteral administration of this DA agonist replicates the shortened response duration, steeper dose/response slope, and diminished dyskinesia threshold observed with acute levodopa challenge.[22,97] Since the motoric effects of parenterally administered apomorphine depend on its ability to directly stimulate postsynaptic dopaminergic receptors, the observed response modifications must reflect changes downstream from the DA system, at the striatal level or beyond. Thus while DA terminal degeneration alone and the resultant loss of buffering contributes to the initial appearance of the wearing-off phenomenon, it now appears that secondary alterations postsynaptic to the nigrostriatal system ultimately make a substantial contribution to the underlying shortening in motor response duration[22,31,96] as well as to the associated pharmacodynamic changes underlying unpredictable "on"/"off" fluctuations and peak dose dyskinesias.[10,31,42,54,95]

Clinical studies have suggested that over 80% of the motor response variance in advanced levodopa-treated parkinsonian patients reflects alterations occurring beyond the level of the striatal dopaminergic projections.[31]

Medium Spiny Neurons

Dopaminergic projections from the pars compacta of substantia nigra make synaptic contact with receptors expressed on the dendrites of striatal medium-sized spiny neurons. These GABAergic neurons account for more than 90% of striatal nerve cells.[99] They not only receive dopaminergic axons ascending from the substantia nigra but also are richly invested by glutamatergic axons descending from all areas of cerebral cortex. In addition, spiny neurons receive terminals from numerous other transmitter systems both intrinsic and extrinsic to the striatum.[100,101] In turn, they project both directly and indirectly to the major output nuclei of the basal ganglia, the internal segment of globus pallidus and pars reticulata of substantia nigra.[102,103] Medium spiny neurons are thus critically situated to integrate cortical input with the complex signal processing occurring within the basal ganglia.

Not unexpectedly, primary spiny neuron damage, such as occurs in Huntington's disease and progressive supranuclear palsy, or secondary dysfunction such as now appears to contribute to symptom production in both untreated and treated PD, can seriously compromise motor performance.

Non-physiological DA Receptor Stimulation

The nigrostriatal dopaminergic system mainly operates tonically. Nerve impulse activity in this pathway thus generally occurs at a modal rate of about 4 Hz, except when interrupted by higher-frequency phasic bursts triggered by novel sensory stimuli.[104,105] Since the amount of transmitter release is a function of the rate of neuronal firing, striatal DA concentrations at both intrasynaptic and extrasynaptic dopaminergic receptors normally remain within a narrow physiological range.[106–108] But this situation changes dramatically in PD when striatal dopaminergic receptors become exposed to non-physiological levels and patterns of stimulation.[22,31,40,43,54,62,63,75] Initially, it changes as dopaminergic neurons degenerate and transmitter levels progressively decline. The abnormally low-intensity stimulation endured by striatal dopaminergic receptors in untreated PD gives rise to the cardinal signs of this disorder.[33,109] Later, it changes even further upon initiation of dopaminomimetic therapy.

With few residual DA neurons, standard treatment regimens subject postsynaptic DA receptors to intermittent high-intensity stimulation. As already noted, intermittency is the inevitable consequence of DA neuron loss. High intensity is suggested by the results of DA and DA metabolite assays in lumbar CSF and striatal tissue, showing that levels during levodopa treatment of parkinsonian patients far exceeds those found in normal individuals.[110–114] Episodic, high-intensity stimulation is no more physiological than the subthreshold stimulation caused by the loss of dopaminergic innervation.[115] Accordingly, striatal DA-mediated transmission remains abnormal in those with advanced PD whether left untreated or given standard therapy. Current evidence suggests that either type of non-physiological dopaminergic receptor stimulation may be able to alter spiny neuron function in ways that contribute to the increasing severity of wearing-off fluctuations as well as to the onset of unpredictable fluctuations and peak-dose dyskinesias.[10,11,31,42,52,54,78,116]

Medium Spiny Neuron Alterations

Chronic exposure of DA receptors on striatal spiny neurons to non-physiological stimulation has profound functional consequences. Although early attention focused on possible effects on the responsivity of the DA receptors themselves in relation to the pathogenesis of motor complications, subsequent investigations failed to confirm consistent alterations in the number or affinity of these receptors.[82,117–120]

Later studies began an examination of both the structure[121,122] and function of the host spiny neurons. Observations in rodent and primate models of PD revealed changes in their neurotransmitters, intraneuronal signaling cascades, and the synaptic efficacy of their ionotropic glutamatergic receptors. For example, activity of the GABA synthesizing enzyme, glutamic acid decarboxylase, increases with denervation and to an even greater extent with intermittent dopaminergic therapy.[62,123] mRNA and protein levels of several spiny neuron peptide cotransmitters also undergo characteristic alterations in both these conditions. Unilateral injection of the catecholamine neuron specific toxin 6-hydroxydopamine (6-OHDA) into rat substantia nigra permanently destroys DA neurons projecting to the ipsilateral striatum and produces contralateral hypokinesia mimicking what occurs in human PD.[124,125] Concomitantly, striatal enkephalin and neurotensin levels increase.[123,126] Subsequent levodopa treatment, when administered intermittently to simulate dosing schedules in parkinsonian patients, causes alterations in motor response within a few weeks that closely resemble human wearing-off and "on"/"off" fluctuations.[62,68] Animals given the same daily dose of levodopa by continuous round-the-clock infusion do not develop these response changes. Intermittently treated rats, but not those given levodopa continuously, manifest additional neuropeptide alterations. Most conspicuous is a large rise in both dynorphin and neurotensin.[123,124,127–130] Similar changes in the genes encoding these striatal neuropeptides and in their cellular expression occur in parkinsonian monkeys given intermittent levodopa or DA agonists.[118,131–133] Pharmacological studies suggest that these peptide modifications affect spiny neuron function in ways that contribute to the associated changes in motor behavior.[134–138]

Neurophysiological evaluations of striatal function in the parkinsonian state are consistent with this view. Single-unit recordings in intact, freely moving rats indicate that only a few dorsal striatal neurons fire spontaneously, usually at rates in the 1–4 Hz range.[139] With a unilateral 6-OHDA lesion, more ipsilateral cells become active (firing rates increase over 4-fold) and more burst firing occurs (by nearly 10-fold), rate changes that tend to be normalized by the acute administration of the DA agonist apomorphine.[139,140]

Glutamate Receptor Phosphorylation

Plastic responses to continuous low-intensity or intermittent high-intensity receptor stimulation, of the type occurring in parkinsonian striatum, have been extensively studied in various brain areas, especially in relation to long-term depression and long-term potentiation in the hippocampus.[141–143] More recently, extensions of this research to the striatum have begun to show how activity patterns of mesencephalic dopaminergic systems can affect the regulation of synaptic function at certain stages of learning and memory.[144,145] In this regard, particular attention has focused on how DA receptor-mediated mechanisms modulate the synaptic efficacy of ionotropic glutamatergic receptors.[115,122,146,147]

Since dopaminergic receptors are located in close proximity to both *N*-methyl-D-aspartate (NMDA) and alpha-amino-3-hydroxy-5-methyl-4-isoxazole proprionic acid (AMPA) receptors on the dendritic spines of striatal medium-sized neurons, these mechanisms could be crucial to understanding the persisting changes in motor behavior associated with the non-physiological stimulation of these DA receptors.[148–150]

Ionotropic glutamatergic receptors of the NMDA type function as ligand-gated ion channels, especially for calcium, while those of the AMPA type serve as channels for sodium and other monovalent ions.[151] The NMDA receptor complex is a tetramer, assembled from NR1 subunits (occurring in any of eight splice variants) and NR2 subunits (composed of four homologous isoforms, with the NR2B and less frequently the NR2A occurring in striatum).[152–154] AMPA receptors are composed of tetrameric combinations of GluR1–4 subunits; all but the GluR-4 subunits appear to be expressed by medium spiny neurons.[155–157] NMDA and AMPA receptor subunits are critically regulated by protein phosphorylation, especially at sites along their intracellular carboxy tails.[158–160] Phosphorylation of serine/threonine residues has been most closely related to the regulation of receptor anchoring to plasma membranes, while tyrosine phosphorylation has been primarily linked to the modulation of channel characteristics, including open-state probability.[161–163]A number of phosphorylation sites as well as protein kinases mediating phosphorylation at these sites have now been identified in mammalian brain.

Tyrosine Residue Phosphorylation

The phosphorylation state of tyrosine residues on striatal ionotropic glutamatergic receptors undergoes characteristic alterations as a result of dopaminergic denervation and later as a consequence of intermittent dopaminomimetic drug treatment. NMDA NR2A and NR2B subunits, but not NR1 subunits, can be directly phosphorylated by Src family protein tyrosine kinases, including Fyn.[164–168] At least seven specific tyrosine residues have been identified on the carboxy-termini of NR2B subunits that are phosphorylated by Fyn,[169] while three tyrosine residues within the NR2A carboxy-terminal domain are known to mediate src-induced changes in NMDA receptor function.[170] In rats, the 6-OHDA induced destruction of the nigrostriatal pathway increases NR2B tyrosine phosphorylation in striatal homogenates, without altering receptor protein expression.[171,172] On the other hand, for NMDA receptors located on striatal membranes, NR2B subunit tyrosine phosphorylation and the abundance of NR1-NR2B protein are reduced by 6-OHDA, without altering striatal NR1 gene expression, suggesting a redistribution of these receptors from the membrane to the cytoplasmic compartment.[173,174] Following intermittent levodopa treatment sufficient to induce motor response alterations, there is a substantial rise in tyrosine phosphorylation of both total and membrane associated NR2A and especially NR2B subunits, while the protein changes are normalized.[172,173]

Alterations in striatal NMDA receptor phosphorylation associated with dopaminergic denervation and subsequent intermittent stimulation reflect the activity of intracellular signal transduction cascades linking coexpressed dopaminergic and glutamatergic receptors. DA receptors are located relatively proximally along the necks of spiny neuron spines, while ionotropic glutamate receptors are situated within the postsynaptic density at the distal spine tips.[175,176] The distance between these receptors is relatively small, thus facilitating bidirectional signaling between these and multiple other neurotransmitter receptors.[177] The pattern and degree of NMDA subunit phosphorylation can change quickly, reflecting the countervailing actions of relevant kinases and phosphatases.[168]

Tyrosine Kinase Effects

An association between dopaminergic regulation of motor function and tyrosine phosphorylation of NMDA receptors has been explored using compounds that selectively inhibit tyrosine kinases. The unilateral injection of genestein, an antagonist of both soluble and membrane bound forms of protein tyrosine kinase, into the striatum of rats whose ipsilateral nigrostriatal system has been interrupted by 6-OHDA has modest antiparkinsonian efficacy as evidenced by the induction of contralateral rotation.[172] The intrastriatal administration of genistein to parkinsonian rats given intermittent levodopa treatment normalizes the motor response shortening and attenuates the enhanced tyrosine phosphorylation of both the NR2A and NR2B subunits.[172] These results support the possibility that hyperphosphorylation of tyrosine residues on NMDA receptor subunits, due to the aberrant activation of the appropriate kinases, contributes to the motor dysfunction induced by dopaminergic denervation as well as by subsequent levodopa treatment.

The phosphorylation state of tyrosine residues on AMPA receptors has received relatively little investigative attention and striatal changes have not been reported in parkinsonian animals.[157,158,178] DA system destruction has, however, been found to reduce AMPA GluR1 subunit expression in rat striatum.[174,179]

Serine Residue Phosphorylation

The phosphorylation state of serine/threonine residues is also an important contributor to the regulation of ionotropic glutamatergic receptors.[115,144,153] A number of serine phosphorylation sites have now been identified on NMDA receptor NR1 subunits where, for example, cyclic AMP-protein kinase A (PKA), can phosphorylate Ser897 and protein kinase C (PKC) phosphorylates Ser890 and Ser896,[180,181] and on NR2B subunits where PKC directly phosphorylates Ser1303 and Ser1323 and calcium/calmodulin-dependent protein kinase II (CaMKII) phosphorylates Ser1303 and/or the cognate site on the NR2A subunit.[182–184] Altered serine phosphorylation of striatal NMDA receptors occurs in association with dopaminergic denervation, where NR2A increases modestly (along with NR2A protein) as well as with levodopa treatment, which further elevates serine phosphorylation of NR2A but not of NR2B subunits (due to opposite D1 and D2 DA receptor mediated effects) without associated changes in subunit protein levels.[185] A 6-OHDA lesion decreases serine phosphorylation of membrane-associated NR1 subunits at residues 890 and 896; intermittent levodopa treatment markedly increases NR1 phosphorylation at Ser890, Ser896, and Ser897.[173] The abundance of NR1 protein in striatal membranes decreases in lesioned animals but normalizes with levodopa treatment.[173,174,179]

Thus while the precise role of the observed serine phosphorylation changes in modulating channel conductance and subcellular localization of NMDA receptors remains unclear, current evidence suggests that they could contribute to the alterations in motor function associated with DA system degeneration as well as the ability of dopaminomimetics to reverse the effects of denervation but ultimately induce motor response complications.

The serine phosphorylation of AMPA receptors also serves a crucial regulatory role. PKA, PKC, and CaMKII PKC contribute to the regulation of AMPA channel function, in part, through phosphorylation of GluR1 subunits (mediated for example at Ser831 by PKC and CaMKII and at Ser845 by PKA) and GluR2 subunits (mediated by PKC at Ser863 and Ser880.[182,186–190] In cultured nucleus accumbens cells, GluR1 phosphorylation at Ser845 increases with D1 DA agonist stimulation, a response that is attenuated by D2 agonist stimulation.[191] In rats, a 6-OHDA lesion of the DA system reduces AMPA GluR1 mRNA expression in striatal tissues,[174] but has no effect on serine phosphorylation at the GluR1 Ser831 PKC site; levodopa treatment sufficient to induce motor response changes in parkinsonian rats, on the other hand, increases Ser831 phosphorylation.[192] Similarly, striatal GluR1 Ser845 phosphorylation is unaffected by dopaminergic denervation, but rises with levodopa-induced motor response changes.[89]

Serine Kinase Effects

Recent studies have also begun to identify signaling pathways within striatal neurons that mediate the ability of DA receptors to modulate the phosphorylation state of serine residues on coexpressed glutamatergic receptors.[149,159,193] All three of the major second-messenger-regulated protein kinases – PKA, PKC, and CaMKII – have now been implicated in the altered serine phosphorylation of NMDA and AMPA receptors associated with the non-physiological stimulation of rat striatal dopaminergic receptors. PKA inhibition in medium spiny neurons by the intrastriatal injection of Rp-cAMPS has rather limited motoric activity in parkinsonian rats but potently reverses the motor response changes produced by intermittent levodopa therapy.[194] Since Rp-cAMPS normalizes the shortened response duration to D1 but not to D2 DA receptor agonist challenge, the participation of PKA in the pathogenesis of these response modifications may be limited to striatal spiny neurons expressing functioning D1 DA receptors and projecting via the direct striatonigral pathway. Inhibition of CaMKII by intrastriatally injected KN-93 has no antiparkinsonian activity but ameliorates levodopa-induced response alterations.[185] In contrast to results with PKA inhibition, selective CaMKII inhibition affects D2 as well as D1 DA receptor-mediated mechanisms. Chronic levodopa treatment elevates serine phosphorylation of striatal NR2A subunits, but not that of NR2B subunits, without associated changes in subunit protein levels. Chronic D1 agonist treatment increases NR2A but decreases NR2B serine phosphorylation, while chronic D2 agonist treatment has no effect on NR2A but increases NR2B phosphorylation. The acute intrastriatal injection of the CaMKII inhibitor KN93 not only appears to reverse levodopa-induced motor response alterations but also to attenuatethe D1 and D2 receptor-mediated changes in serine phosphorylation of NR2A and NR2B subunits, respectively. Conversely the protein phosphatase 1/2A inhibitor, okadaic acid, potentiates these response alterations.

PKC augmentation as a consequence of the direct intrastriatal transfer of the catalytic domain of constitutively active PKC by herpes simplex virus type 1 elevates Ser831 phosphorylation of GluR1 receptor subunits and hastens onset of the shortened motor response duration produced by levodopa therapy.[192] In pCMVpkc? transfected animals, intrastriatal injection of the PKC inhibitor NPC-15437 attenuated both the increased GluR1 phosphorylation and the accelerated onset of the levodopa-induced response modifications. The effects of PKC augmentation evidently occur in both D1 and D2 expressing medium spiny neurons, since pCMVpkc? gene transfer influences the motor response to both SKF 38393 and quinpirole challenge after levodopa therapy. While PKC also phosphorylates NMDA subunits, either directly[183,195] or by promoting tyrosine phosphorylation of NR2 subunits,[196,197] these results are consistent with the view that PKC-mediated phosphorylation of AMPA GluR1 subunits contributes to the initial appearance of the altered motor response.

Denervation or intermittent stimulation of rat striatal dopaminergic receptors activate kinases capable of directly phosphorylating ionotropic glutamatergic receptor subunits. Conceivably, sensitization of NMDA and AMPA receptors on striatal spiny neurons as a result of altered subunit phosphorylation contributes to the appearance of parkinsonian signs and levodopa-associated response alterations. In either case, changes in glutamatergic input to striatum from cerebral cortex may modify striatal output in ways that affect motor function.

Glutamate Receptor Sensitization

If the synaptic efficacy of ionotropic glutamatergic receptors on striatal spiny neurons increases as a result of changes in their phosphorylation state due to the non-physiological stimulation of coexpressed dopaminergic receptors, then pharmacological manipulation of these glutamate receptors might be expected to influence the associated motor dysfunction. Mounting evidence from studies in parkinsonian models and patients now indicates that alterations in the sensitivity of both NMDA and AMPA receptors do indeed occur with denervation-associated parkinsonism as well as with treatment-associated response complications.

NMDA Receptor Antagonists

NMDA receptor antagonists can augment the antiparkinsonian actions of dopaminomimetics and suppress levodopa-induced response alterations in parkinsonian rodents.[198–201] Direct injection studies indicate that the effects of systemically administered NMDA antagonists are mediated in the striatum, presumably at receptors expressed on the dendrites of medium spiny neurons.[199] The motoric responses to both competitive and non-competitive NMDA antagonists may reflect a preferential activity on the D2 DA receptor-mediated indirect striatopallidal pathway.[201–204] In MPTP lesioned monkeys, the non-competitive NMDA antagonist amantadine evidences mild antiparkinsonian activity, but strongly suppresses levodopa-induced dyskinesias in animals given levodopa treatment.[205] While other NMDA antagonists reduce levodopa-induced fluctuations and dyskinesias in parkinsonian primates, not all non-competitive or competitive antagonists share this ability despite a generally similar subunit non-selective profile.[206,207] Nevertheless, animal model studies strongly support the view that dopaminergic denervation, and especially intermittent DA receptor stimulation, can induce striatal NMDA receptor sensitization.

In parkinsonian patients, the ability of the NMDA receptor antagonist, amantadine, to palliate symptoms in those with early-stage disease is well established.[208] Recently, this and other non-competitive NMDA receptor antagonists, including dextrorphan and dextromethorphan, have been found to diminish levodopa-induced motor response fluctuations and peak-dose dyskinesias.[55,209,210] Subsequent studies have corroborated the safety and enduring efficacy of amantadine in treating motor complications.[211–215] They further suggest that mechanisms underlying motor dysfunction in PD patients resemble those occurring in animal models of this disorder.

The motoric effects of drugs that primarily block NMDA receptor NR2B subunits differ from those that mainly block NR2A subunits in parkinsonian animals. In 6-OHDA lesioned rats, selective antagonism of NR2B subunits with Co 101244/PD 174494 or CP101,606, but not of NR2A subunits with the competitive antagonist MDL 100,453, reverses levodopa-induced response alterations.[172,216] In parkinsonian monkeys, NR2B blockade with ifenprodil or CP101,606 exhibits antiparkinsonian activity when given *de novo*[217] or with levodopa,[218] while NR2B blockade with Co 101244/PD 174494 reduces levodopa-induced dyskinesias.[218,219] Selective NR2A antagonism with MDL 100,453, on the other hand, potentiates antiparkinsonian responses but at the same time exacerbates dyskinesias.[219]

Taken together, these results support the possibility that the previously noted increase in tyrosine phosphorylation of NR2B subunits (possibly together with increased serine phosphorylation of NR2B subunits in D2 DA containing spiny neurons) may be particularly crucial to the NMDA receptor sensitization that favors the appearance of parkinsonism and especially to the altered dopaminergic responses produced by levodopa treatment. Since NR2B subunits predominate in mammalian striatum, while NR2A subunits are more highly expressed in other brain regions, the foregoing possibilities may explain the relatively weak antiparkinsonian action of subunit non-selective NMDA antagonists. Furthermore, they suggest that NR2B subunit selective antagonists may have a better therapeutic index than non-subunit selective NMDA antagonists in PD patients.

AMPA Receptor Antagonists

The contribution of striatal AMPA receptor sensitization to motor dysfunction in parkinsonian animals has also received increasing investigative attention. Studies in 6-OHDA lesioned rats, for example, suggest that some AMPA antagonists can reduce parkinsonian signs when administered alone or with levodopa as well as prevent or reverse levodopa-induced motor response alterations.[201,204,220–222] Interestingly, the competitive AMPA antagonist NBQX has no effect on D2 DA agonist-induced rotations, but potentiates the antiparkinsonian response to a D1 agonist.[201] On the other hand, the competitive AMPA antagonist LY293558 reverses the response alterations elicited by a D2 agonist but not those occurring with a D1 agonist in levodopa-treated rats.[223] Thus in rodents the ability of AMPA antagonists to diminish denervation-induced parkinsonism, possibly acting in the striatum,[224] may largely reflect effects on the D1 direct pathway, while their actions on levodopa-induced response alterations may relate more to modulation of the D2 indirect striatal output pathway.

In MPTP lesioned primates, notwithstanding the apparently inconsistent effects of NBQX on parkinsonism,[201,225,226] a non-competitive antagonist at the AMPA allosteric modulation site (LY 300164; Talampanel) augments the antiparkinsonian action of levodopa, but attenuates its dyskinesiogenic effects; conversely, a positive modulator of AMPA receptors (CX516) by itself has no antiparkinsonian activity, but exacerbates levodopa-induced dyskinesias.[227]

Taken together with the reported efficacy of the glutamate release inhibitor riluzole,[204,228] it now appears that sensitization of striatal AMPA as well as NMDA receptors may contribute to the motor dysfunction associated with dopaminergic denervation and dopaminomimetic-induced response alterations.

Persistence of Striatal Neuronal Alterations

As already noted, in parkinsonian animals and patients with a sufficiently severe loss of DA neurons it takes only a few days to a few weeks of intermittent dopaminomimetic treatment to induce motor complications.[58,68,87,90,92,229] Similarly, in animal models as well as in patients with PD, only a few weeks to a few months are required for these response alterations to subside when intermittent treatment is replaced by relatively continuous and thus more physiological dopaminergic stimulation.[78–80] These latter observations suggest that the molecular and cellular changes responsible for the response modifications to intermittent levodopa therapy linger long after removal of the inciting stimulus. Recent studies in parkinsonian rats indicate that the expression and maintenance of levodopa-induced motor response alterations may be functionally associated with the regulation of cAMP response element-binding protein (CREB), a transcription factor commonly implicated in the formation and maintenance of long-term memory.[230–232] The transcriptional activation of CREB depends on its phosphorylation at Ser133 either directly or indirectly by such kinases as PKA.[233–235]

The unilateral destruction of the nigrostriatal DA system modestly increases Ser133 phosphorylation of CREB in ipsilateral medium spiny neurons in response to acute levodopa challenge.[236] Three weeks of twice-daily levodopa treatment of these hemiparkinsonian animals leads to a progressive shortening in the duration of the rotational response as well as to a large increase in both total pCREB expression and the number of pCREB-positive neurons in the ipsilateral striatum. Both changes persist for about 4 weeks after withdrawal of levodopa treatment. The time course of alterations in CREB phosphorylation thus correlates with the time course of alterations in motor behavior following cessation of dopaminomimetic therapy.[236] Agents that disrupt the activity of this transcription factor, such as CREB antisense or the PKA inhibitor Rp-cAMPS, attenuate both the change in motor response duration and the degree of CREB phosphorylation.

These findings, together with the observation that chronic intermittent stimulation of D1 receptors, but not of D2 receptors, increases the magnitude of striatal pCREB expression, indicate that the activation of D1/PKA-mediated phosphorylation of CREB family proteins may be involved in the persistence of levodopa-induced motor response alterations.

Differential Contribution of D1, D2, and D3 DA-bearing Spiny Neurons

Continuing controversy surrounds the degree of separation of D1 and D2 family DA receptors on striatal medium spiny neurons. Numerous histological, electrophysiological, and pharmacological studies support the concept that D1 receptors preferentially function on spiny neurons projecting directly to the pars reticulata of substantia nigra and internal globus pallidus, while DA D2 receptors mainly function on neurons that project indirectly to the internal globus via the external globus pallidus and subthalamic nucleus.[237–242] Recent observations on the differential phosphorylation changes on striatal NMDA NR2A and NR2B subunits as a consequence of selective D1 or D2 receptor stimulation add support to the functional significance of this dichotomization.[185] Nevertheless, other evidence, especially anatomic, suggests little if any separation actually exists, thus casting doubt on the rather simplistic models commonly used to depict indirect striatopallidal and direct striatonigral pathway contributions to symptom production in PD.[102,103,243]

Thus it is hardly surprising that preclinical studies have yet to clarify the differential contributions of these pathways to the pathogenesis of motor complications, not withstanding recent observations suggesting the participation of mechanisms mediated by the D3 subtype of D2 family DA receptors.[126,244,245] Determination of whether targeting one or another DA receptor subtype or interacting with all of them together, like the natural transmitter, maximizes therapeutic benefit while minimizing risk the risk of complications must await the development of drugs of sufficient DA receptor subtype specificity that are suitable for clinical use.[246–250]

Participation of Structures Downstream from the Striatum

The non-physiological stimulation of DA receptors initiates changes that affect spiny neuron firing rates and patterns in ways that degrade motor function.[139,140] Precisely how downstream structures are affected by these alterations in striatal output is not yet well understood. Moreover, whether such basal ganglionic structures as the external and internal segments of globus pallidus, subthalamic nucleus, and thalamus, that directly or indirectly receive striatal projections, make an independent contribution to the pathogenesis of the motor complication syndrome remains to be elucidated.

In PD patients, beyond inferences drawn from the examination of postmortem tissues or surgical interventions, cerebral imaging studies now offer the best potential for advancing our understanding of these questions. Positron emission tomography (PET) evaluations indicate that untreated PD is associated with specific regional changes that are reversed by levodopa therapy.[251–253] $H_2{}^{15}O$/PET studies have also begun to detail how different components of the motor cortico-striato-pallido-thalamo-cortical loop and related pathways contribute to the beneficial and adverse effects of levodopa.[254] Functional MRI evaluations that correlate blood oxygenation level-dependent (BOLD) signal changes with motor performance in hemiparkinsonian patients have shown that hypoactivation in contralateral primary motor cortex and bilateral supplementary motor area reflect a decreased input from the subcortical motor loop, which is normalized by levodopa.[255] Nevertheless, performance effect confounds, as well as the restricted ability to resolve basal ganglia structures of interest, limit the usefulness of these approaches to the clinical study of motor complications.

Other Spiny Neuron Receptor-mediated Mechanisms

Medium spiny neurons not only receive dopaminergic projections from substantia nigra and glutamatergic terminals from the cerebral cortex but also express receptors for numerous other striatal transmitter systems. These include serotonin 5-HT_{2A}, adrenergic α_2, adenosine A2a, cannabinoid CB-1, and metabotropic glutamatergic mGluR5. By signaling through common cascades, activity at certain of these receptors may have the potential for modulating the effects of DA receptor stimulation on glutamatergic receptor function. This possibility has important implications both for understanding the pathogenesis of and developing novel treatments for motor disability in PD.[149,256]

Serotonin 5-HT_{2A} Receptors

Serotonin receptors of the 5-HT_{2A} subtype are richly expressed along the dendrites of striatal medium spiny neurons.[257,258] 5-HT_{2A} receptor stimulation activates signaling pathways involving cAMP- and calcium-activated kinases such as PKA and PKC.[259–262] It is thus conceivable that drugs acting selectively at these receptors might influence striatal mechanisms and thus motor function. Indeed, quetiapine, an atypical antipsychotic with DA D2/D3 as well as 5-HT_{2A}/C antagonist activity, reportedly can ameliorate neuroleptic-induced tardive dyskinesia[263–265] and levodopa-induced dyskinesias.[266]

In parkinsonian rats, quetiapine has been found to normalize the shortening in response produced by levodopa.[267] Moreover, quetiapine cotreatment acts prophylactically to prevent onset of the levodopa-induced shortening in motor response duration. At a dose that was effective in reversing the shortened motor response to levodopa, the atypical neuroleptic diminished the enhanced Ser831 phosphorylation of spiny neuron GluR1 subunits produced by intermittent levodopa therapy,[267] an effect consistent with the reported ability of 5-HT_{2A} receptor stimulation to enhance S831 phosphorylation on AMPA receptor GluR1subunits via PKC activation.[259] Similarly, in parkinsonian monkeys quetiapine coadministration attenuates levodopa-induced dystonic as well as choreiform dyskinesias, at doses that do not interfere with the antiparkinsonian response to the dopamine precursor.[267] It is unlikely that DA receptor inhibition accounts for the ability of quetiapine to reduce levodopa-induced dyskinesias, since the same dose fails either to exacerbate parkinsonian signs when given alone or to attenuate the antiparkinsonian response to levodopa. Moreover, in parkinsonian rodents quetiapine prolongs rather than shortens the response to levodopa or DA agonists, as would be expected from a drug acting primarily via dopamine D2/D3 receptor blockade.

Based on these results, clinical evaluation of selective 5-HT_{2A} antagonists in combination with dopaminergic therapy of PD seems indicated.

α_2-Adrenergic Receptors

The relation of noradrenergic system dysfunction to the motor disabilities characterizing PD remains largely a matter of speculation due in large measure to a paucity of appropriate pharmacological tools.[268] Notwithstanding the sparse innervation of the striatum by adrenergic projections, α_2 adrenoceptors are highly expressed in this structure,[269,270] and α_2-adrenergic agents have potent effects on motor behavior.[271,272] Whether these effects are mediated by their interactions with postsynaptic α_2-adrenergic receptors on spiny neurons or by modulating striatal NE release through interactions with presynaptic α_2 adrenoceptors has yet to be established.[269,273] Nevertheless, in parkinsonian rats, the administration of idazoxan, a partial agonist at the α_2-adrenergic receptor, attenuates the shortening in motor response induced by chronic levodopa therapy.[274] This normalizing effect presumably occurs downstream from the nigrostriatal DA system, since it is also observed following D1 or D2 DA agonist challenge.

Studies of idazoxan in MPTP lesioned primates have found an enhanced antiparkinsonian action of levodopa and a reduction in levodopa-induced dyskinesias.[275–277] Unfortunately, pilot clinical evaluations of idazoxan revealed an unfavorable dose/response relation that halted further development.[51,278,279] Another NE antagonist, fipamezole (JP-1730) – which has high affinity at human $\alpha_{(2A)}$, $\alpha_{(2B)}$, and $\alpha_{(2C)}$ receptors – also has been found in parkinsonian marmosets to reduce dyskinesias induced by levodopa, while prolonging the duration but not diminishing the magnitude of its antiparkinsonian action.[280] Initial clinical studies of fipamezole suggest that effects in parkinsonian animal models may prove predictive of the activity of drugs of this type in parkinsonian patients.[274]

Adenosine A2a Receptors

Adenosine receptors of the A2a subtype are also abundantly expressed on medium spiny neurons, especially those with functioning D2 DA receptors.[281,282] A2a receptors signal in part through activation of PKA and PKC,[283,284] which in turn can alter the regulation of coexpressed inototropic glutamatergic receptors.[158,187] Drugs that block A2a receptors in parkinsonian rodents and primates possess both antiparkinsonian and antidyskinetic activity.[285–287] Specifically, studies in parkinsonian rats have shown that the selective A2a receptor antagonist KW-6002 normalizes levodopa-induced motor response alterations as well as the augmentation in Ser845 phosphorylation of striatal GluR1 subunits[89] that can be mediated by PKA.[186,288] KW-6002 also reverses parkinsonian disability in MPTP-lesioned marmosets, without inducing dyskinesias; even in parkinsonian primates previously primed by levodopa to manifest these abnormal movements, KW-6002 induces little if any dyskinesias.[286] Moreover, in MPTP-lesioned monkeys, coadministration of the selective A2a receptor antagonist KW-6002 with daily apomorphine injections acts prophylactically to prevent dyskinesia onset.[70]

Initial clinical studies with KW-6002 (istradefylline) have shown that at doses, which alone or in combination with a steady-state intravenous infusion of optimal-dose levodopa have no definite effect on parkinsonian severity, the A2a antagonist potentiates the antiparkinsonian response to low-dose levodopa with less dyskinesias than produced by optimal-dose levodopa monotherapy. KW-6002 also prolongs the duration of antiparkinsonian action of levodopa.[289] At a lower dose, KW-6002 reportedly reduces "off" time while increasing "on" time with dyskinesia.[290]

In addition to suggesting a novel approach to the treatment of PD, these findings lend additional support to the view that drugs that act at cell surface receptors on spiny neuron dendrites to modify signaling kinases affecting the regulation of ionotropic glutamatergic receptors can modify motor function in parkinsonian patients.

Cannabinoid Receptors

The basal ganglia are richly endowed with cannabinoid receptors and their activation is well known to influence motor behavior, although precise mechanisms remain obscure.[291] The effects of CB1 cannabinoid receptor modulation in relation to the treatment of levodopa-induced motor complications have received particular investigative attention.[292] Both CB1 cannabinoid receptor antagonists and agonists appear able to modulate the motor effects of levodopa in parkinsonian animals.[293,294] Coadministration of the cannabinoid receptor agonist nabilone with levodopa to MPTP-lesioned marmosets reduces levodopa-induced dyskinesia without altering the antiparkinsonian action of levodopa; the duration of antiparkinsonian action of levodopa is also prolonged.[295] Clinically, a pilot trial of the cannabinoid receptor agonist nabilone appeared to have some beneficial effects on levodopa-induced dyskinesias in parkinsonian patients.[296]

Metabotropic Receptors

Group I metabotropic receptors of the mGluR5 subtype are also situated on striatal spiny neurons where they function synergistically with coexpressed A2a receptors.[297–299] The recent development of selective ligands for these G protein-coupled glutamatergic receptors has revealed that they can enhance NMDA currents by triggering signaling cascades involving PKC and Src.[300–302] Chronic treatment with the selective metabotropic glutamate mGluR5 antagonist 2-methyl-6-(phenylethynyl)-pyridine (MPEP) reversed akinetic deficits in rats lesioned with 6-OHDA,[303] possibly by normalizing indirect striopallidal pathway dysfunction.[304]

CONCLUSIONS

Expanding insight into mechanisms contributing to symptom production in PD will undoubtedly accelerate the discovery of better approaches to therapy.

The clinical appearance of parkinsonism and later of motor response complications now appears to involve functional alterations in striatal medium spiny neurons. The non-physiological stimulation of their dopaminergic receptors, due to denervation as well as standard therapeutic interventions, activates signaling cascades linking them to nearby ionotropic glutamatergic receptors. As a result, the phosphorylation state of NMDA and AMPA subunits changes, their synaptic efficacy rises, and excitatory input from cortex to striatum intensifies. Under these circumstances, striatal spiny neuron output changes in ways that compromise motor function.

At present, there is no fully satisfactory treatment for late-stage PD. This situation largely reflects disability caused by motor response complications as well as other treatment-related adverse effects. To the extent that motor complications contribute to infirmity, future attempts to ameliorate this disorder should focus on approaches to correcting or preventing the deleterious consequences of dopaminergic deafferentation by restoring DA-mediated transmission in the most physiological manner possible. In parkinsonian animals as well as in patients with advanced disease, dopaminomimetic replacement strategies that provide continuous DA receptor stimulation appear to confer prophylactic as well as palliative benefit.[22,40] In view of the rapid progression of current research, practical means for the continuous normalization of striatal dopaminergic transmission can be expected in the not too distant future.

Novel DA replacement strategies now include the continuous administration of DA agonists either transcutaneously by means of skin patches[305,306] or subcutaneously by means of polymeric implants.[70] Alternatively, recent studies suggest that coadministration of 5-HT_{1A} agonists may also prove beneficial. Since in parkinsonian striatum, serotoninergic terminals serve as an important site for the decarboxylation of exogenous levodopa to DA, it is not surprising that drugs that selectively stimulate 5-HT_{1A} autoreceptors have been found to influence dopaminergic mechanisms.[35,307–309] In levodopa-treated parkinsonian rodents, for example, 5-HT_{1A} receptor stimulation tends to blunt the peak while prolonging the duration of DA release.[37,310,311] Administration of the selective 5-HT_{1A} agonist sarizotan to these animals reverses the shortened duration of motor response induced by intermittent levodopa treatment.[36] In MPTP-lesioned monkeys, sarizotan decreases levodopa-induced dyskinesias without diminishing the antiparkinsonian response to levodopa. Similarly, in PD patients sarizotan has no effect on parkinsonian severity when given alone or with levodopa, but appears to reduce dyskinesias and prolong the antiparkinsonian response to levodopa.[39] The promising results from these experimental approaches suggest that one or more could prove useful in the future treatment of PD.

But more fundamentally, the possibility that medium spiny neuron dysregulation contributes to the motor disabilities attending striatal dopaminergic denervation and intermittent stimulation has suggested a new therapeutic paradigm for PD.[149,256] Rather than continuing classical attempts to restore striatal dopaminergic transmission, it may prove safer and more effective to pursue alternative pharmacological approaches to the prevention or reversal of the reactive changes associated with current therapy. Potential strategies include the pharmaceutical targeting on medium spiny neurons of:

- protein kinases (including PKA, PKC, CaMKII and src isoforms) whose anomalous activation by the non-physiological stimulation of DA receptors alters the phosphorylation state of glutamatergic receptors;
- ionotropic glutamatergic receptors (NMDA and AMPA) whose dysregulation corrupts striatal output;
- other cell-surface receptors (such as A2a, 5-HT_{2A} and CB1) that are able to modulate signaling cascades that link dopaminergic and glutamatergic receptors;
- transcription factors (e.g. CREB) that promote retention of maladaptive responses to past stimuli.

The vigorous exercise of these and related therapeutic options may prove helpful not only for those suffering from PD but also for those disabled by other neurodysfunctional disorders.

REFERENCES

1. Papavasiliou PS, Cotzias GC, Duby SE et al. Levodopa in parkinsonism: potentiation of central effects with a peripheral inhibitor. N Engl J Med 1972;286:8–14.
2. Calne DB, Teychenne PF, Claveria LE et al. Bromocriptine in parkinsonism. Br Med J 1974;4:442–444.
3. Carlsson A. Basic concepts underlying recent developments in the field of Parkinson's disease. Contemp Neurol Ser 1971;8:1–31.
4. Hornykiewicz O. Neurochemical pathology and pharmacology of brain dopamine and acetylcholine: rational basis for the current drug treatment of parkinsonism. Contemp Neurol Ser 1971;8:33–65.
5. Zigmond MJ, Abercrombie ED, Berger TW, Grace AA, Stricker EM. Compensations after lesions of central dopaminergic neurons: some clinical and basic implications. Trends Neurosci 1990;13:290–296.
6. Calne DB, Zigmond MJ. Compensatory mechanisms in degenerative neurologic diseases: insights from parkinsonism. Arch Neurol 1991;48:361–363.
7. Stocchi F, Bonamartini A, Vacca L, Ruggieri S. Motor fluctuations in levodopa treatment: clinical pharmacology. Eur Neurol 1996;36(suppl. 1):38–42.
8. Quinn NP. Classification of fluctuations in patients with Parkinson's disease. Neurology 1998;51 (2 suppl. 2):s25–29.
9. Reardon KA, Shiff M, Kempster PA. Evolution of motor fluctuations in Parkinson's disease: a longitudinal study over 6 years. Mov Disord 1999;14:605–611.
10. Fabbrini G, Juncos J, Mouradian MM, Serrati C, Chase TN. Levodopa pharmacokinetic mechanisms and motor fluctuations in Parkinson's disease. Ann Neurol 1987;21:370–376.
11. Fabbrini G, Mouradian MM, Juncos JL et al. Motor fluctuations in Parkinson's disease: central pathophysiological mechanisms. Part I. Ann Neurol 1988;24:366–371.
12. Gancher ST, Nutt JG, Woodward W. Response to brief levodopa infusions in parkinsonian patients with and without motor fluctuations. Neurology 1988;38:712–716.
13. Marras C, Lang AE. Measuring motor complications in clinical trials for early Parkinson's disease. J Neurol Neurosurg Psychiatry 2003;74:143–146.
14. Shaw KM, Lees AJ, Stern GM. The impact of treatment with levodopa on Parkinson's disease. Q J Med 1980;49(195):283–293.
15. Shif M, Kempster PA. Response to L-dopa and evolution of motor fluctuations in the early phase of treatment of Parkinson's disease. Clin Exp Neurol 1994;31:38–42.
16. Miyawaki E, Lyons K, Pahwa R et al. Motor complications of chronic levodopa therapy in Parkinson's disease. Clin Neuropharmacol 1997;20:523–530.

17. Schrag A, Quinn N. Dyskinesias and motor fluctuations in Parkinson's disease: a community-based study. Brain 2000;123:2297–2305.
18. Ahlskog JE, Muenter MD. Frequency of levodopa-related dyskinesias and motor fluctuations as estimated from the cumulative literature. Mov Disord 2001;16:448–458.
19. Parkinson Study Group. Effect of deprenyl on the progression of disability in early Parkinson's disease. N Engl J Med 1989;321:1364–1371.
20. Peppe A, Dambrosia JM, Chase TN. Risk factors for motor response complications in L-dopa-treated parkinsonian patients. Adv Neurol 1993;60:698–702.
21. Parkinson Study Group. Impact of deprenyl and tocopherol treatment on Parkinson's disease in DATATOP patients requiring levodopa. Ann Neurol 1996;39:37–45.
22. Chase TN, Juncos J, Serrati C, Fabbrini G, Bruno G. Fluctuations in response to chronic levodopa therapy. Adv Neurol 1986;45:477–480.
23. Gancher ST, Nutt JG, Woodward WR. Peripheral pharmacokinetics of levodopa in untreated, stable, and fluctuating parkinsonian patients. Neurology 1987;37:940–944.
24. Nutt JG, Woodward WR, Gancher ST, Merrick D. 3-O-methyldopa and the response to levodopa in Parkinson's disease. Ann Neurol 1987;21:584–588.
25. Baas H, Harder S, Demisch L et al. Fluctuations in Parkinson's disease: pathogenetic significance of levodopa's cerebral pharmacokinetics and pharmacodynamics. J Neural Transm Suppl 1995;46:367–379.
26. van Laar T. Levodopa-induced response fluctuations in patients with Parkinson's disease: strategies for management. CNS Drugs 2003;17:475–489.
27. Juncos JL, Fabbrini G, Mouradian MM, Serrati C, Chase TN. Dietary influences on the antiparkinsonian response to levodopa. Arch Neurol 1987;44:1003–1005.
28. Nutt JG, Woodward WR, Carter JH, Trotman TL. Influence of fluctuations of plasma large neutral amino acids with normal diets on the clinical response to levodopa. J Neurol Neurosurg Psychiatry 1989;52:481–487.
29. Robertson DR, Higginson I, Macklin BS et al. The influence of protein containing meals on the pharmacokinetics of levodopa in healthy volunteers. Br J Clin Pharmacol 1991;31:413–417.
30. Alexander GM, Schwartzman RJ, Grothusen JR, Gordon SW. Effect of plasma levels of large neutral amino acids and degree of parkinsonism on the blood-to-brain transport of levodopa in naive and MPTP parkinsonian monkeys. Neurology 1994;44:1491–1499.
31. Mouradian MM, Juncos JL, Fabbrini G, Chase TN. Motor fluctuations in Parkinson's disease: pathogenetic and therapeutic studies. Ann Neurol 1987;22:475–479.
32. Horstink MW, Zijlmans JC, Pasman JW et al. Which risk factors predict the levodopa response in fluctuating Parkinson's disease? Ann Neurol 1990;27:537–543.
33. Zigmond MJ, Acheson AL, Stachowiak MK, Stricker EM. Neurochemical compensation after nigrostriatal bundle injury in an animal model of preclinical parkinsonism. Arch Neurol 1984;41:856–861.
34. Ng KY, Chase TN, Colburn RW, Kopin IJ. L-Dopa-induced release of cerebral monoamines. Science 1970;170:76–77.
35. Melamed E, Hefti F, Wurtman RJ. Nonaminergic striatal neurons convert exogenous L-dopa to dopamine in parkinsonism. Ann Neurol 1980;8:558–563.
36. Bibbiani F, Oh JD, Chase TN. Serotonin 5-HT_{1A} agonist improves motor complications in rodent and primate parkinsonian models. Neurology 2001;57:1829–1834.
37. Kannari K, Yamato H, Shen H et al. Activation of 5-HT(1A) but not 5-HT(1B) receptors attenuates an increase in extracellular dopamine derived from exogenously administered L-dopa in the striatum with nigrostriatal denervation. J Neurochem 2001;76:1346–1353.
38. Yamato H, Kannari K, Shen H, Suda T, Matsunaga M. Fluoxetine reduces L-dopa-derived extra cellular DA in the 6-OHDA-lesioned rat striatum. Neuroreport 2001;12:1123–1126.
39. Bara-Jimenez W, Sherzai A, Bibbiani F et al. $5HT_{1A}$ agonist effects in advanced Parkinson's disease. Neurology 2003;60(suppl. 1):A507.
40. Shoulson I, Glaubiger GA, Chase TN. On-off response: clinical and biochemical correlations during oral and intravenous levodopa administration in parkinsonian patients. Neurology 1975;25: 1144–1148.
41. Juncos J, Serrati C, Fabbrini G, Chase TN. Fluctuating levodopa concentrations and Parkinson's disease. Lancet 1985;2(8452):440.
42. Mouradian MM, Juncos JL, Fabbrini G et al. Motor fluctuations in Parkinson's disease: central pathophysiological mechanisms. Part II. Ann Neurol 1988;24:372–378.

43. Chase TN, Mouradian MM, Fabbrini G, Juncos JL. Pathogenetic studies of motor fluctuations in Parkinson's disease. J Neural Transm Suppl 1988;27:3–10.
44. de la Fuente-Fernandez R, Pal PK, Vingerhoets FJ et al. Evidence for impaired presynaptic dopamine function in parkinsonian patients with motor fluctuations. J Neural Transm 2000;107:49–57.
45. de la Fuente-Fernandez R, Lu JQ, Sossi V et al. Biochemical variations in the synaptic level of dopamine precede motor fluctuations in Parkinson's disease: PET evidence of increased dopamine turnover. Ann Neurol 2001;49:298–303.
46. Lees AJ. The on-off phenomenon. J Neurol Neurosurg Psychiatry 1989 (suppl.); June 29–37.
47. Rajput AH, Fenton ME, Birdi S et al. Clinical–pathological study of levodopa complications. Mov Disord 2002;17:289–296.
48. Obeso JA, Rodriguez-Oroz MC, Chana P et al. The evolution and origin of motor complications in Parkinson's disease. Neurology 2000;55(11 suppl. 4):s13–20.
49. Nutt JG. Motor fluctuations and dyskinesia in Parkinson's disease. Parkinsonism Relat Disord 2001;8:101–108.
50. Martignoni E, Riboldazzi G, Calandrella D, Riva N. Motor complications of Parkinson's disease. Neurol Sci 2003;24(suppl. 1):s27–29.
51. Rascol O, Fabre N. Dyskinesia: L-dopa-induced and tardive dyskinesia. Clin Neuropharmacol 2001;24:313–323.
52. Blanchet PJ. The fluctuating parkinsonian patient: clinical and pathophysiological aspects. Can J Neurol Sci 2003;(30 suppl. 1):s19–26.
53. Vidailhet M, Bonnet AM, Marconi R, Durif F, Agid Y. The phenomenology of L-dopa-induced dyskinesias in Parkinson's disease. Mov Disord 1999;14(suppl. 1):13–18.
54. Mouradian MM, Heuser IJ, Baronti F et al. Pathogenesis of dyskinesias in Parkinson's disease. Ann Neurol 1989;25:523–526.
55. Blanchet PJ, Allard P, Gregoire L, Tardif F, Bedard PJ. Risk factors for peak dose dyskinesia in 100 levodopa-treated parkinsonian patients. Can J Neurol Sci 1996;23(3):189–193.
56. Schrag A, Ben-Shlomo Y, Quinn N. How common are complications of Parkinson's disease? J Neurol 2002;249:419–423.
57. Kostic VS, Marinkovic J, Svetel M, Stefanova E, Przedborski S. The effect of stage of Parkinson's disease at the onset of levodopa therapy on development of motor complications. Eur J Neurol 2002;9(1):9–11.
58. Smith LA, Jackson MJ, Hansard MJ, Maratos E, Jenner P. Effect of pulsatile administration of levodopa on dyskinesia induction in drug-naive MPTP-treated common marmosets: effect of dose, frequency of administration, and brain exposure. Mov Disord 2003;18:487–495.
59. Rajput AH, Stern W, Laverty WH. Chronic low-dose levodopa therapy in Parkinson's disease: an argument for delaying levodopa therapy. Neurology 1984;34:991–996.
60. Grandas F, Galiano ML, Tabernero C. Risk factors for levodopa-induced dyskinesias in Parkinson's disease. J Neurol 1999;246:1127–1133.
61. Pearce RK, Heikkila M, Linden IB, Jenner P. L-dopa induces dyskinesia in normal monkeys: behavioural and pharmacokinetic observations. Psychopharmacology (Berl) 2001;156:402–409.
62. Juncos JL, Engber TM, Raisman R et al. Continuous and intermittent levodopa differentially affect basal ganglia function. Ann Neurol 1989;25:473–478.
63. Chase TN, Baronti F, Fabbrini G et al. Rationale for continuous dopaminomimetic therapy of Parkinson's disease. Neurology 1989;39(suppl. 2):7–10.
64. Engber TM, Susel Z, Juncos JL, Chase TN. Continuous and intermittent levodopa differentially affect rotation induced by D-1 and D-2 dopamine agonists. Eur J Pharmacol 1989;168:291–298.
65. Engber TM, Susel Z, Kuo S, Chase TN. Chronic levodopa treatment alters basal and dopamine agonist-stimulated cerebral glucose utilization. J Neurosci 1990;10:3889–3895.
66. Weick BG, Engber TM, Susel Z, Chase TN, Walters JR. Responses of substantia nigra pars reticulata neurons to GABA and SKF 38393 in 6-hydroxydopamine-lesioned rats are differentially affected by continuous and intermittent levodopa administration. Brain Res 1990;523:16–22.
67. Engber TM, Marin C, Susel Z, Chase TN. Differential effects of chronic dopamine D1 and D2 receptor agonists on rotational behavior and dopamine receptor binding. Eur J Pharmacol 1993;236: 385–393.
68. Papa SM, Engber TM, Kask AM, Chase TN. Motor fluctuations in levodopa treated parkinsonian rats: relation to lesion extent and treatment duration. Brain Res 1994;662:69–74.
69. Goulet M, Grondin R, Blanchet PJ, Bedard PJ, Di Paolo T. Dyskinesias and tolerance induced by chronic treatment with a D1 agonist administered in pulsatile or continuous mode do not correlate with changes of putaminal D1 receptors in drug-naive MPTP monkeys. Brain Res 1996;719:129–137.

70. Bibbiani F, Constantini L, Patel R, Chase TN. Continuous apomorphine administration with novel EVA implants reduces the risk of motor complications compared to pulsatile apomorphine in L-dopa naive MPTP lesioned primates. Neurology 2003;60(suppl. 1):A330.
71. Rinne UK. Early combination of bromocriptine and levodopa in the treatment of Parkinson's disease: a 5-year follow-up. Neurology 1987;37:826–828.
72. Rinne UK, Bracco F, Chouza C et al. Early treatment of Parkinson's disease with cabergoline delays the onset of motor complications: results of a double-blind levodopa controlled trial. The PKDS009 Study Group. Drugs 1998;55(suppl. 1):23–30.
73. Pearce RK, Banerji T, Jenner P, Marsden CD. De novo administration of ropinirole and bromocriptine induces less dyskinesia than L-dopa in the MPTP-treated marmoset. Mov Disord 1998;13:234–241.
74. Jenner P. Pathophysiology and biochemistry of dyskinesia: clues for the development of non-dopaminergic treatments. J Neurol 2000;247(suppl. 2):43–50.
75. Olanow W, Schapira AH, Rascol O. Continuous dopamine-receptor stimulation in early Parkinson's disease. Trends Neurosci 2000;23(suppl.):s117–126.
76. Nutt JG, Obeso JA, Stocchi F. Continuous dopamine-receptor stimulation in advanced Parkinson's disease. Trends Neurosci 2000;23(suppl.):s109–115.
77. Rascol O, Brooks DJ, Korczyn AD et al. A five-year study of the incidence of dyskinesia in patients with early Parkinson's disease who were treated with ropinirole or levodopa. 056 Study Group. N Engl J Med 2000;342:1484–1491.
78. Mouradian MM, Heuser IJ, Baronti F, Chase TN. Modification of central dopaminergic mechanisms by continuous levodopa therapy for advanced Parkinson's disease. Ann Neurol 1990;27:18–23.
79. Baronti F, Mouradian MM, Davis TL et al. Continuous lisuride effects on central dopaminergic mechanisms in Parkinson's disease. Ann Neurol 1992;32:776–781.
80. Hadj Tahar A, Gregoire L, Bangassoro E, Bedard PJ. Sustained cabergoline treatment reverses levodopa-induced dyskinesias in parkinsonian monkeys. Clin Neuropharmacol 2000;23:195–202.
81. Di Monte DA, McCormack A, Petzinger G et al. Relationship among nigrostriatal denervation, parkinsonism, and dyskinesias in the MPTP primate model. Mov Disord 2000;15:459–466.
82. Brooks DJ. PET studies and motor complications in Parkinson's disease. Trends Neurosci 2000;23(suppl.):s101–108.
83. Jenner P. The contribution of the MPTP-treated primate model to the development of new treatment strategies for Parkinson's disease. Parkinsonism Relat Disord 2003;9(3):131–137.
84. Diamond SG, Markham CH, Hoehn MM, McDowell FH, Meunter MD. Multicenter study of Parkinson's mortality with early versus late dopa treatment. Ann Neurol 1987;22:8–12.
85. Scigliano G, Musicco M, Soliveri P et al. Mortality associated with early and late levodopa therapy initiation in Parkinson's disease. Neurology 1990;40:265–269.
86. Schneider JS. Levodopa-induced dyskinesias in parkinsonian monkeys: relationship to extent of nigrostriatal damage. Pharmacol Biochem Behav 1989;34:193–196.
87. Blanchet PJ, Grondin R, Bedard PJ. Dyskinesia and wearing-off following dopamine D1 agonist treatment in drug-naivel-methy l-4-phenyl-1,2,3,6-tetrahydropyridine-lesioned primates. Mov Disord 1996;11:91–94.
88. Jenner P. The MPTP-treated primate as a model of motor complications in PD: primate model of motor complications. Neurology 2003;61(suppl 3):s4–11.
89. Bibbiani F, Oh JD, Petzer JP et al. A2A antagonist prevents dopamine agonist-induced motor complications in animal models of Parkinson's disease. Exp Neurol 2003;184:285–294.
90. Ballard PA, Tetrud JW, Langston JW. Permanent human parkinsonism due to 1-methyl-4-phenyl-1,2,3,6-tetrahydropyridine (MPTP): seven cases. Neurology 1985;35:949–956.
91. Markham CH. Major treatment problems in L-dopa therapy in Parkinson's disease. In: Barbeau A, McDowell FH (eds), L-Dopa and Parkinsonism. Philadelphia: FA Davis, 1970, pp. 10–12.
92. Onofrj M, Paci C, Thomas A. Sudden appearance of invalidating dyskinesia-dystonia and off fluctuations after the introduction of levodopa in two dopaminomimetic drug naive patients with stage IV Parkinson's disease. J Neurol Neurosurg Psychiatry 1998;65:605–606.
93. de Jong GJ, Meerwaldt JD, Schmitz PI. Factors that influence the occurrence of response variations in Parkinson's disease. Ann Neurol 1987;22:4–7.
94. Denny AP, Behari M. Motor fluctuations in Parkinson's disease. J Neurol Sci 1999;165(1):18–23.
95. Obeso JA, Rodriguez-Oroz M, Marin C et al. The origin of motor fluctuations in Parkinson's disease: importance of dopaminergic innervation and basal ganglia circuits. Neurology 2004;62 (1 suppl. 1):s17–30.
96. Bravi D, Mouradian MM, Roberts JW et al. Wearing-off fluctuations in Parkinson's disease: contribution of postsynaptic mechanisms. Ann Neurol 1994;36:27–31.

97. Verhagen Metman L, Locatelli ER, Bravi D, Mouradian MM, Chase TN. Apomorphine responses in Parkinson's disease and the pathogenesis of motor complications. Neurology 1997;48:369–372.
98. Bezard E, Brotchie JM, Gross CE. Pathophysiology of levodopa-induced dyskinesia: potential for new therapies. Nat Rev Neurosci 2001;2:577–588.
99. Kotter R. Postsynaptic integration of glutamatergic and dopaminergic signals in the striatum. Prog Neurobiol 1994;44:163–196.
100. McGeorge AJ, Faull RLM. The organization of the projection from the cerebral cortex to the striatum in the rat. Neuroscience 1989;29:503–537.
101. Kincaid A, Wilson CJ. Corticostriatal innervation of the patch and matrix in the rat striatum. J Comp Neurol 1996;374:578–592.
102. Albin RL, Young AB, Penney JB. The functional anatomy of disorders of the basal ganglia. Trends Neurosci 1995;18(2):63–64.
103. Obeso JA, Rodriguez-Oroz MC, Rodriguez M et al. Pathophysiology of the basal ganglia in Parkinson's disease. Trends Neurosci 2000;23(10 suppl.):s8–19.
104. Grace AA, Bunney BS. The control of firing pattern in nigral dopamine neurons: single spike firing. J Neurosci 1984;4:2866–2876.
105. Schultz W. Behavior-related activity of primate dopamine neurons. Rev Neurol (Paris) 1994;150:634–639.
106. Skirboll S, Wang J, Mefford I, Hsiao J, Bankiewicz KS. In vivo changes of catecholamines in hemi-parkinsonian monkeys measured by microdialysis. Exp Neurol 1990;110:187–193.
107. Sarre S, De Klippel N, Herregodts P, Ebinger G, Michotte Y. Biotransformation of locally applied L-dopa in the corpus striatum of the hemi-parkinsonian rat studied with microdialysis. Naunyn Schmiedebergs Arch Pharmacol 1994;350:15–21.
108. Zoli M, Torri C, Ferrari R et al. The emergence of the volume transmission concept. Brain Res Brain Res Rev 1998;26:136–147.
109. Bernheimer H, Birkmayer W, Hornykiewicz O, Jellinger K, Seitelberger F. Brain dopamine and the syndromes of Parkinson and Huntington: clinical, morphological and neurochemical correlations. J Neurol Sci 1973;20:415–455.
110. Chase TN. Cerebrospinal fluid monoamine metabolites and peripheral decarboxylase inhibitors in parkinsonism. Neurology 1970;20(12 suppl.):36–40.
111. Chase TN, Watanabe AM. Methyldopahydrazine as an adjunct to L-dopa therapy in parkinsonism. Neurology 1972;22:384–392.
112. Lloyd KG, Davidson L, Hornykiewicz O. The neurochemistry of Parkinson's disease: effect of L-dopa therapy. J Pharmacol Exp Ther 1975;195:453–464.
113. Rinne UK, Sonninen V, Marttila R. Brain dopamine turnover and the relief of parkinsonism. Adv Exp Med Biol 1977;90:267–275.
114. Davidson DL, Yates CM, Mawdsley C, Pullar IA, Wilson H. CSF studies on the relationship between dopamine and 5-hydroxytryptamine in Parkinsonism and other movement disorders. J Neurol Neurosurg Psychiatry 1977;40:1136–1141.
115. Centonze D, Picconi B, Gubellini P, Bernardi G, Calabresi P. Dopaminergic control of synaptic plasticity in the dorsal striatum. Eur J Neurosci 2001;13:1071–1077.
116. Chase TN, Oh JD. Striatal mechanisms and pathogenesis of parkinsonian signs and motor complications. Ann Neurol 2000;47(4 suppl. 1):s122–129.
117. Jenner P, Boyce S, Marsden CD. Receptor changes during chronic dopaminergic stimulation. J Neural Transm Suppl 1988;27:161–175.
118. Turjanski N, Lees AJ, Brooks DJ. In vivo studies on striatal dopamine D1 and D2 site binding in L-dopa-treated Parkinson's disease patients with and without dyskinesias. Neurology 1997;49:717–723.
119. Hurley MJ, Mash DC, Jenner P. Dopamine D(1) receptor expression in human basal ganglia and changes in Parkinson's disease. Brain Res Mol Brain Res 2001;87:271–279.
120. Kim YJ, Ichise M, Ballinger JR et al. Combination of dopamine transporter and D2 receptor SPECT in the diagnostic evaluation of PD, MSA, and PSP. Mov Disord 2002;17:303–312.
121. Nitsch C, Riesenberg R. Synaptic reorganisation in the rat striatum after dopaminergic deafferentation: an ultrastructural study using glutamate decarboxylase immunocytochemistry. Synapse 1995;19:247–263.
122. Arbuthnott GW, Ingham CA, Wickens JR. Dopamine and synaptic plasticity in the neostriatum. J Anat 2000;196:587–596.
123. Engber TM, Susel Z, Kuo S, Gerfen CR, Chase TN. Levodopa replacement therapy alters enzyme activities in striatum and neuropeptide content in striatal output regions of 6-hydroxydopamine lesioned rats. Brain Res 1991;552:113–118.

124. Taylor MD, De Ceballos ML, Rose S, Jenner P, Marsden CD. Effects of a unilateral 6-hydroxydopamine lesion and prolonged L-3,4-dihydroxyphenylalanine treatment on peptidergic systems in rat basal ganglia. Eur J Pharmacol 1992;219(2):183–192.
125. Schwarting RK, Huston JP. The unilateral 6-hydroxydopamine lesion model in behavioral brain research: analysis of functional deficits, recovery and treatments. Prog Neurobiol 1996;50:275–331.
126. Bordet R, Ridray S, Schwartz JC, Sokoloff P. Involvement of the direct striatonigral pathway in levodopa-induced sensitization in 6-hydroxydopamine-lesioned rats. Eur J Neurosci 2000;12:2117–2123.
127. Engber TM, Boldry RC, Kuo S, Chase TN. Dopaminergic modulation of striatal neuropeptides: differential effects of D1 and D2 receptor stimulation on somatostatin, neuropeptide Y, neurotensin, dynorphin and enkephalin. Brain Res 1992;581:261–268.
128. Herrero MT, Augood SJ, Hirsch EC et al. Effects of L-dopa on preproenkephalin and preprotachykinin gene expression in the MPTP-treated monkey striatum. Neuroscience 1995;68: 1189–1198.
129. Henry B, Crossman AR, Brotchie JM. Effect of repeated L-dopa, bromocriptine, or lisuride administration on preproenkephalin-A and preproenkephalin-B mRNA levels in the striatum of the 6-hydroxydopamine-lesioned rat. Exp Neurol 1999;155:204–220.
130. Winkler C, Kirik D, Bjorklund A, Cenci MA. L-dopa-induced dyskinesia in the intrastriatal 6-hydroxydopamine model of parkinson's disease: relation to motor and cellular parameters of nigrostriatal function. Neurobiol Dis 2002;10:165–186.
131. Morissette M, Goulet M, Soghomonian JJ et al. Preproenkephalin mRNA expression in the caudate-putamen of MPTP monkeys after chronic treatment with the D2 agonist U91356A in continuous or intermittent mode of administration: comparison with L-dopa therapy. Brain Res Mol Brain Res 1997;49(1/2):55–62.
132. Tel BC, Zeng BY, Cannizzaro C et al. Alterations in striatal neuropeptide mRNA produced by repeated administration of L-DOPA, ropinirole or bromocriptine correlate with dyskinesia induction in MPTP-treated common marmosets. Neuroscience 2002;115:1047–1058.
133. Quik M, Police S, Langston JW, Di Monte DA. Increases in striatal preproenkephalin gene expression are associated with nigrostriatal damage but not L-dopa-induced dyskinesias in the squirrel monkey. Neuroscience 2002;113:213–220.
134. Engber TM, Boldry RC, Chase TN. The kappa-opioid receptor agonist spiradoline differentially alters the rotational response to dopamine D1 and D2 agonists. Eur J Pharmacol 1991;200(1): 171–173.
135. Marin C, Chase TN. Effects of SCH 32615, an enkephalinase inhibitor, on D-1 and D-2 dopamine receptor-mediated behaviors. Neuropharmacology 1995;34:677–682.
136. Marin C, Engber TM, Chaudhuri P, Peppe A, Chase TN. Effects of kappa receptor agonists on D1 and D2 dopamine agonist and antagonist-induced behaviors. Psychopharmacology (Berl) 1996;123:215–221.
137. Vila M, Marin C, Ruberg M et al. Systemic administration of NMDA and AMPA receptor antagonists reverses the neurochemical changes induced by nigrostriatal denervation in basal ganglia. J Neurochem 1999;73(1):344–352.
138. Boules M, Warrington L, Fauq A, McCormick D, Richelson E. Antiparkinson-like effects of a novel neurotensin analog in unilaterally 6-hydroxydopamine lesioned rats. Eur J Pharmacol 2001;428(2):227–233.
139. Chen MT, Morales M, Woodward DJ, Hoffer BJ, Janak PH. In vivo extracellular recording of striatal neurons in the awake rat following unilateral 6-hydroxydopamine lesions. Exp Neurol 2001;171:72–83.
140. Boraud T, Bezard E, Bioulac B, Gross CE. From single extracellular unit recording in experimental and human Parkinsonism to the development of a functional concept of the role played by the basal ganglia in motor control. Prog Neurobiol 2002;66:265–283.
141. Paulsen O, Sejnowski TJ. Natural patterns of activity and long-term synaptic plasticity. Curr Opin Neurobiol 2000;10(2):172–179.
142. Braunewell KH, Manahan-Vaughan D. Long-term depression: a cellular basis for learning. Rev Neurosci 2001;12(2):121–140.
143. Silva AJ. Molecular and cellular cognitive studies of the role of synaptic plasticity in memory. J Neurobiol 2003;54:224–237.
144. Jay TM. Dopamine: a potential substrate for synaptic plasticity and memory mechanisms. Prog Neurobiol 2003;69:375–390.
145. Chapman PF, Ramsay MF, Krezel W, Knevett SG. Synaptic plasticity in the amygdala: comparisons with hippocampus. Ann NY Acad Sci 2003;985:114–124.

146. Cepeda C, Levine MS. Dopamine and *N*-methyl-D-aspartate receptor interactions in the neostriatum. Dev Neurosci 1998;20(1):1–18.
147. Reynolds JN, Wickens JR. Substantia nigra dopamine regulates synaptic plasticity and membrane potential fluctuations in the rat neostriatum, in vivo. Neuroscience 2000;99:199–203.
148. Chase TN, Engber TM, Mouradian MM. Contribution of dopaminergic and glutamatergic mechanisms to the pathogenesis of motor response complications in Parkinson's disease. Adv Neurol 1996;69:497–501.
149. Chase TN, Oh JD. Striatal dopamine- and glutamate-mediated dysregulation in experimental parkinsonism. Trends Neurosci 2000;23(10 suppl.):s86–91.
150. Lin JY, Dubey R, Funk GD, Lipski J. Receptor subtype-specific modulation by dopamine of glutamatergic responses in striatal medium spiny neurons. Brain Res 2003;959:251–262.
151. Barnes GN, Slevin JT. Ionotropic glutamate receptor biology: effect on synaptic connectivity and function in neurological disease. Curr Med Chem 2003;10:2059–2072.
152. Wollmuth LP, Kuner T, Seeburg PH, Sakmann B. Differential contribution of the NR1- and NR2A-subunits to the selectivity filter of recombinant NMDA receptor channels. J Physiol (Lond) 1996;491:779–797.
153. Koles L, Wirkner K, Illes P. Modulation of ionotropic glutamate receptor channels. Neurochem Res 2001;26:925–932.
154. Carroll RC, Zukin RS. NMDA-receptor trafficking and targeting: implications for synaptic transmission and plasticity. Trends Neurosci 2002;25:571–577.
155. Kwok KH, Tse YC, Wong RN, Yung KK. Cellular localization of GluR1, GluR2/3 and GluR4 glutamate receptor subunits in neurons of the rat neostriatum. Brain Res 1997;778:43–55.
156. Bernard V, Somogyi P, Bolam JP. Cellular, subcellular, and subsynaptic distribution of AMPA-type glutamate receptor subunits in the neostriatum of the rat. J Neurosci 1997;17:819–833.
157. Stefani A, Chen Q, Flores-Hernandez J et al. Physiological and molecular properties of AMPA/Kainate receptors expressed by striatal medium spiny neurons. Dev Neurosci 1998;20:242–252.
158. Swope SL, Moss SI, Raymond LA, Huganir RL. Regulation of ligand-gated ion channels by protein phosphorylation. Adv Second Messenger Phosphoprotein Res 1999;33:49–78.
159. Hatt H. Modification of glutamate receptor channels: molecular mechanisms and functional consequences. Naturwissenschaften 1999;86(4):177–186.
160. Kotecha SA, MacDonald JF. Signaling molecules and receptor transduction cascades that regulate NMDA receptor-mediated synaptic transmission. Int Rev Neurobiol 2003;54:51–106.
161. Dingledine R, Borges K, Bowie D, Traynelis SF. The glutamate receptor ion channels. Pharmacol Rev 1999;51(1):7–61.
162. Dunah AW, Yasuda RP, Luo J et al. Biochemical studies of the structure and function of the *N*-methyl-D-aspartate subtype of glutamate receptors. Mol Neurobiol 1999;19:151–179.
163. Cheung HH, Gurd JW. Tyrosine phosphorylation of the *N*-methyl-D-aspartate receptor by exogenous and postsynaptic density-associated Src-family kinases. J Neurochem 2001;78:524–534.
164. Kohr G, Seeburg PH. Subtype-specific regulation of recombinant NMDA receptor-channels by protein tyrosine kinases of the src family. J Physiol (Lond) 1996;492:445–452.
165. Rostas JA, Brent VA, Voss K et al. Enhanced tyrosine phosphorylation of the 2B subunit of the *N*-methyl-D-aspartate receptor in long-term potentiation. Proc Natl Acad Sci USA 1996;93: 10452–10456.
166. Yu XM, Askalan R, Keil GJ, Salter MW. NMDA channel regulation by channel-associated protein tyrosine kinase Src. Science 1997;275:674–678.
167. Lu WY, Xiong ZG, Lei S et al. G-protein-coupled receptors act via protein kinase C and Src to regulate NMDA receptors. Nat Neurosci 1999;2:331–338.
168. Ali DW, Salter MW. NMDA receptor regulation by Src kinase signalling in excitatory synaptic transmission and plasticity. Curr Opin Neurobiol 2001;11:336–342.
169. Nakazawa T, Komai S, Tezuka T et al. Characterization of Fyn-mediated tyrosine phosphorylation sites on GluR epsilon 2 (NR2B) subunit of the *N*-methyl-D-aspartate receptor. J Biol Chem 2001;276:693–699.
170. Zheng F, Gingrich MB, Traynelis SF, Conn PJ. Tyrosine kinase potentiates NMDA receptor currents by reducing tonic zinc inhibition. Nat Neurosci 1998;1(3):185–191.
171. Menegoz M, Lau LF, Herve D, Huganir RL, Girault JA. Tyrosine phosphorylation of NMDA receptor in rat striatum: effects of 6-OH-dopamine lesions. NeuroReport 1995;7:125–128.
172. Oh JD, Russell DS, Vaughan CL, Chase TN, Russell D. Enhanced tyrosine phosphorylation of striatal NMDA receptor subunits: effect of dopaminergic denervation and L-DOPA administration. Brain Res 1998;813:150–159.

173. Dunah AW, Wang Y, Yasuda RP et al. Alterations in subunit expression, composition, and phosphorylation of striatal *N*-methyl-D-aspartate glutamate receptors in a rat 6-hydroxydopamine model of Parkinson's disease. Mol Pharmacol 2000;57:342–352.
174. Lai SK, Tse YC, Yang MS, Wong CK, Chan YS, Yung KK. Gene expression of glutamate receptors GluR1 and NR1 is differentially modulated in striatal neurons in rats after 6-hydroxydopamine lesion. Neurochem Int 2003;43:639–653.
175. Seasack SR, Aoki C, Pickel VM. Ultrastructural localization of D2 receptor-like immunoreactivity in midbrain dopamine neurons and their striatal targets. J Neurosci 1994;14:88–106.
176. Suen PC, Wu K, Xu JL et al. NMDA receptor subunits in the postsynaptic density of rat brain: expression and phosphorylation by endogenous protein kinases. Brain Res Mol Brain Res 1998;59:215–228.
177. Nishi A, Bibb JA, Matsuyama S et al. Regulation of DARPP-32 dephosphorylation at PKA- and Cdk5-sites by NMDA and AMPA receptors: distinct roles of calcineurin and protein phosphatase-2A. J Neurochem 2002;81:832–841.
178. Song I, Huganir RL. Regulation of AMPA receptors during synaptic plasticity. Trends Neurosci 2002;25:578–588.
179. Fan XD, Li XM, Ashe PC, Juorio AV. Lesion of the substantia nigra pars compacta downregulates striatal glutamate receptor subunit mRNA expression. Brain Res 1999;850(1/2):79–86.
180. Leonard AS, Hell JW. Cyclic AMP-dependent protein kinase and protein kinase C phosphorylate *N*-methyl-D-aspartate receptors at different sites. J Biol Chem 1997;272:12107–12115.
181. Tingley WG, Ehlers MD, Kameyama K et al. Characterization of protein kinase A and protein kinase C phosphorylation of the *N*-methyl-D-aspartate receptor NR1 subunit using phosphorylation site-specific antibodies. J Biol Chem 1997;272:5157–5166.
182. Bayer KU, Schulman H. Regulation of signal transduction by protein targeting: the case for CaMKII. Biochem Biophys Res Commun 2001;289:917–923.
183. Liao GY, Wagner DA, Hsu MH, Leonard JP. Evidence for direct protein kinase-C mediated modulation of *N*-methyl-D-aspartate receptor current. Mol Pharmacol 2001;59:960–964.
184. Mayadevi M, Praseeda M, Kumar KS, Omkumar RV. Sequence determinants on the NR2A and NR2B subunits of NMDA receptor responsible for specificity of phosphorylation by CaMKII. Biochim Biophys Acta 2002;1598(1/2):40–45.
185. Oh JD, Vaughan CL, Chase TN. Effect of dopamine denervation and dopamine agonist administration on serine phosphorylation of striatal NMDA receptor subunits. Brain Res 1999;821:433–442.
186. Lee HK, Barbarosie M, Kameyama K, Bear MF, Huganir RL. Regulation of distinct AMPA receptor phosphorylation sites during bidirectional synaptic plasticity. Nature 2000;405:955–959.
187. Carvalho AL, Duarte CP, Carvalho AP. Regulation of AMPA receptors by phosphorylation. Neurochem Res 2000;25:1245–1255.
188. McDonald BJ, Chung HJ, Huganir RL. Identification of protein kinase C phosphorylation sites within the AMPA receptor GluR2 subunit. Neuropharmacology 2001;41:672–679.
189. Li AJ, Suzuki M, Suzuki S, Ikemoto M, Imamura T. Differential phosphorylation at serine sites in glutamate receptor-1 within neonatal rat hippocampus. Neurosci Lett 2003;341:41–44.
190. Esteban JA, Shi SH, Wilson C et al. PKA phosphorylation of AMPA receptor subunits controls synaptic trafficking underlying plasticity. Nat Neurosci 2003;6(2):136–143.
191. Chao SZ, Lu W, Lee HK, Huganir RL, Wolf ME. D(1) dopamine receptor stimulation increases GluR1 phosphorylation in postnatal nucleus accumbens cultures. J Neurochem 2002;81:984–992.
192. Oh JD, Geller AI, Zhang G, Chase TN. Gene transfer of constitutively active protein kinase C into striatal neurons accelerates onset of levodopa-induced motor response alterations in parkinsonian rats. Brain Res 2003;971:18–30.
193. Lee FJ, Xue S, Pei L et al. Dual regulation of NMDA receptor functions by direct protein–protein interactions with the dopamine D1 receptor. Cell 2002;111:219–230.
194. Oh JD, Del Dotto P, Chase TN. Protein kinase A inhibitor attenuates levodopa-induced motor response alterations in the hemi-parkinsonian rat. Neurosci Lett 1997;228(1):5–8.
195. Leonard AS, Hell JW. Cyclic AMP-dependent protein kinase and protein kinase C phosphorylate *N*-methyl-D-aspartate receptors at different sites. J Biol Chem 1997;272:12107–12115.
196. Grosshans DR, Browning MD. Protein kinase C activation induces tyrosine phosphorylation of the NR2A and NR2B subunits of the NMDAR. J Neurochem 2001;76:737–744.
197. MacDonald JF, Kotecha SA, Lu WY, Jackson MF. Convergence of PKC-dependent kinase signal cascades on NMDA receptors. Curr Drug Targets 2001;2:299–312.
198. Engber TM, Papa SM, Boldry RC, Chase TN. NMDA receptor blockade reverses motor response alterations induced by levodopa. Neuroreport 1994;5:2586–2588.

199. Papa SM, Boldry RC, Engber TM, Kask AM, Chase TN. Reversal of levodopa-induced motor fluctuations in experimental parkinsonism by NMDA receptor blockade. Brain Res 1995;701:13–18.
200. Marin C, Papa SM, Engber TM et al. MK801 prevents levodopa-induced motor response alterations in parkinsonian rats. Brain Res 1996;736:202–205.
201. Loschmann PA, Wullner U, Heneka MT et al. Differential interaction of competitive NMDA and AMPA antagonists with selective dopamine D-1 and D-2 agonists in a rat model of Parkinson's disease. Synapse 1997;26:381–391.
202. Boldry RC, Chase TN, Engber TM. Influence of previous exposure to levodopa on the interaction between dizocilpine and dopamine D1 and D2 agonists in rats with 6-hydroxydopamine-induced lesions. J Pharmacol Exp Ther 1993;267:1454–1459.
203. Fredriksson A, Palomo T, Chase T, Archer T. Tolerance to a suprathreshold dose of L-dopa in MPTP mice: effects of glutamate antagonists. J Neural Transm 1999;106(3/4):283–300.
204. Marin C, Jimenez A, Bonastre M, Chase TN, Tolosa E. Non-NMDA receptor mediated mechanisms are involved in levodopa-induced motor response alterations in parkinsonian rats. Synapse 2000;36:267–274.
205. Blanchet PJ, Konitsiotis S, Chase TN. Amantadine reduces levodopa-induced dyskinesias in parkinsonian monkeys. Mov Disord 1998;13:798–802.
206. Papa SM, Chase TN. Levodopa-induced dyskinesias improved by a glutamate antagonist in Parkinsonian monkeys. Ann Neurol 1996;39:574–578.
207. Blanchet PJ, Papa SM, Metman LV, Mouradian MM, Chase TN. Modulation of levodopa-induced motor response complications by NMDA antagonists in Parkinson's disease. Neurosci Biobehav Rev 1997;21:447–453.
208. Danysz W, Parsons CG, Kornhuber J, Schmidt WJ, Quack G. Aminoadamantanes as NMDA receptor antagonists and antiparkinsonian agents-preclinical studies. Neurosci Biobehav Rev 1997;21:455–468.
209. Verhagen Metman L, Del Dotto P, van den Munckhof P et al. Amantadine as treatment for dyskinesias and motor fluctuations in Parkinson's disease. Neurology 1998;50:1323–1326.
210. Verhagen Metman L, Del Dotto P, Natte R, van den Munckhof P, Chase TN. Dextromethorphan improves levodopa-induced dyskinesias in Parkinson's disease. Neurology 1998;51:203–206.
211. Metman LV, Del Dotto P, LePoole K et al. Amantadine for levodopa-induced dyskinesias: a 1-year follow-up study. Arch Neurol 1999;56:1383–1386.
212. Luginger E, Wenning GK, Bosch S, Poewe W. Beneficial effects of amantadine on L-dopa-induced dyskinesias in Parkinson's disease. Mov Disord 2000;15:873–878.
213. Ruzicka E, Streitova H, Jech R et al. Amantadine infusion in treatment of motor fluctuations and dyskinesias in Parkinson's disease. J Neural Transm 2000;107:1297–1306.
214. Snow BJ, Macdonald L, Mcauley D, Wallis W. The effect of amantadine on levodopa-induced dyskinesias in Parkinson's disease: a double-blind, placebo-controlled study. Clin Neuropharmacol 2000;23(2):82–85.
215. Del Dotto P, Pavese N, Gambaccini G et al. Intravenous amantadine improves levadopa-induced dyskinesias: an acute double-blind placebo-controlled study. Mov Disord 2001;16:515–520.
216. Wessell RH, Ahmed SM, Menniti FS et al. NR2B selective NMDA receptor antagonist CP-101,606 prevents levodopa-induced motor response alterations in hemi-parkinsonian rats. Neuropharmacology. 2004;47:181–194.
217. Nash JE, Fox SH, Henry B et al. Antiparkinsonian actions of ifenprodil in the MPTP-lesioned marmoset model of Parkinson's disease. Exp Neurol 2000;165(1):136–142.
218. Steece-Collier K, Chambers LK, Jaw-Tsai SS, Menniti FS, Greenmayre JT. Antiparkinsonian actions of CP-101,606, an antagonist of NR2B subunit-containing *N*-methyl-D-aspartate receptors. Exp Neurol 2000;163(1):239–243.
219. Blanchet PJ, Konitsiotis S, Whittemore ER et al. Differing effects of *N*-methyl-D-aspartate receptor subtype selective antagonists on dyskinesias in levodopa-treated 1-methyl-4-phenyl-tetrahydropyridine monkeys. J Pharmacol Exp Ther 1999;290:1034–1040.
220. Wachtel H, Kunow M, Loschmann PA. NBQX (6-nitro-sulfamoyl-benzo-quinoxaline-dione) and CPP (3-carboxy-piperazin-propyl phosphonic acid) potentiate dopamine agonist induced rotations in substantia nigra lesioned rats. Neurosci Lett 1992;142:179–182.
221. Stauch Slusher B, Rissolo KC, Anzilotti KF, Jackson PF. Centrally-administered AMPA antagonists increase locomotion in parkinsonian rats. J Neural Transm Park Dis Dement Sect 1995;9(2/3): 145–149.
222. Jimenez A, Bonastre M, Vila M et al. LY293558, an AMPA glutamate receptor antagonist, prevents and reverses levodopa-induced motor alterations in parkinsonian rats. Synapse 2001;42:40–47.

223. Marin C, Jimenez A, Bonastre M et al. LY293558, an AMPA glutamate receptor antagonist, prevents and reverses levodopa-induced motor alterations in Parkinsonian rats. Synapse 2001;42(1):40–47.
224. Boldry RC, Kelland MD, Engber TM, Chase TN. NBQX inhibits AMPA-induced locomotion after injection into the nucleus accumbens. Brain Res 1993;600:331–334.
225. Klockgether T, Turski L, Honore T et al. The AMPA receptor antagonist NBQX has antiparkinsonian effects in monoamine-depleted rats and MPTP-treated monkeys. Ann Neurol 1991;30: 717–723.
226. Luquin MR, Obeso JA, Laguna J, Guillen J, Martinez-Lage JM. The AMPA receptor antagonist NBQX does not alter the motor response induced by selective dopamine agonists in MPTP-treated monkeys. Eur J Pharmacol 1993;235:297–300.
227. Konitsiotis S, Blanchet PJ, Verhagen L, Lamers E, Chase TN. AMPA receptor blockade improves levodopa-induced dyskinesia in MPTP monkeys. Neurology 2000;54:1589–1595.
228. Merims D, Ziv I, Djaldetti R, Melamed E. Riluzole for levodopa-induced dyskinesias in advanced Parkinson's disease. Lancet 1999;353:1764–1765.
229. Boyce S, Clarke CE, Luquin R et al. Induction of chorea and dystonia in parkinsonian primates. Mov Disord 1990;5:3–7.
230. Riccio A, Ginty DD. What a privilege to reside at the synapse: NMDA receptor signaling to CREB. Nat Neurosci 2002;5:389–390.
231. Nestler EJ. Common molecular and cellular substrates of addiction and memory. Neurobiol Learn Mem 2002;78:637–647.
232. Balschun D, Wolfer DP, Gass P et al. Does cAMP response element-binding protein have a pivotal role in hippocampal synaptic plasticity and hippocampus-dependent memory? J Neurosci 2003;23: 6304–6314.
233. Mayr B, Montminy M. Transcriptional regulation by the phosphorylation-dependent factor CREB. Nat Rev Mol Cell Biol 2001;2:599–609.
234. Waltereit R, Weller M. Signaling from cAMP/PKA to MAPK and synaptic plasticity. Mol Neurobiol 2003;27:99–106.
235. Colombo PJ, Brightwell JJ, Countryman RA. Cognitive strategy-specific increases in phosphorylated cAMP response element-binding protein and c-Fos in the hippocampus and dorsal striatum. J Neurosci 2003;15:23:3547–3554.
236. Oh JD, Chartisathian K, Ahmed SM, Chase TN. Cyclic AMP responsive element binding protein phosphorylation and persistent expression of levodopa-induced response alterations in unilateral nigrostriatal 6-OHDA lesioned rats. J Neurosci Res 2003;72:768–780.
237. Gerfen CR, Engber TM, Mahan LC et al. D1 and D2 dopamine receptor-regulated gene expression of striatonigral and striatopallidal neurons. Science 1990;250:1429–1432.
238. Gerfen CR. The neostriatal mosaic: multiple levels of compartmental organization. Trends Neurosci 1992;15(4):133–139.
239. Robertson GS, Vincent SR, Fibiger HC. D1 and D2 dopamine receptors differentially regulate c-fos expression in striatonigral and striatopallidal neurons. Neuroscience 1992;49:285–296.
240. Anderson JJ, Chase TN, Engber TM. Differential effect of subthalamic nucleus ablation on dopamine D1 and D2 agonist-induced rotation in 6-hydroxydopamine-lesioned rats. Brain Res 1992;588:307–310.
241. Bergson C, Mrzljak L, Smiley JF et al. Regional, cellular, and subcellular variations in the distribution of D1 and D5 dopamine receptors in primate brain. J Neurosci 1995;15:7821–7836.
242. Wooten GF. Functional anatomical and behavioral consequences of dopamine receptor stimulation. Ann NY Acad Sci 1997;835:153–156.
243. Levesque M, Bedard A, Cossette M, Parent A. Novel aspects of the chemical anatomy of the striatum and its efferents projections. J Chem Neuroanat 2003;26:271–281.
244. Joyce JN. Dopamine D3 receptor as a therapeutic target for antipsychotic and antiparkinsonian drugs. Pharmacol Ther 2001;90:231–259.
245. Bezard E, Ferry S, Mach U et al. Attenuation of levodopa-induced dyskinesia by normalizing dopamine D3 receptor function. Nat Med 2003;9:762–767.
246. Braun A, Fabbrini G, Mouradian MM et al. Selective D-1 dopamine receptor agonist treatment of Parkinson's disease. J Neural Transm 1987;68:41–50.
247. Emre M, Rinne UK, Rascol A et al. Effects of a selective partial D1 agonist, CY 208-243, in de novo patients with Parkinson disease. Mov Disord 1992;7:239–243.
248. Chase TN, Verhagen Metman L, Bravi D et al. Dopamine receptor subtype receptor agonists in the treatment of Parkinson's disease. Clin Neuropharmacol 1995;18(suppl. 1):s207–221.

249. Blanchet PJ, Fang J, Gillespie M et al. Effects of the full dopamine D1 receptor agonist dihydrexidine in Parkinson's disease. Clin Neuropharmacol 1998;21:339–343.
250. Rascol O, Blin O, Thalamas C et al. ABT-431, a D1 receptor agonist prodrug, has efficacy in Parkinson's disease. Ann Neurol 1999;45:736–741.
251. Thobois S, Guillouet S, Broussolle E. Contributions of PET and SPECT to the understanding of the pathophysiology of Parkinson's disease. Neurophysiol Clin 2001;31:321–340.
252. Berding G, Odin P, Brooks DJ et al. Resting regional cerebral glucose metabolism in advanced Parkinson's disease studied in the off and on conditions with [(18)F]FDG-PET. Mov Disord 2001;16:1014–1022.
253. Ito K, Nagano-Saito A, Kato T et al. Striatal and extrastriatal dysfunction in Parkinson's disease with dementia: a 6-[18F]fluoro-L-dopa PET study. Brain 2002;125:1358–1365.
254. Feigin A, Ghilardi MF, Fukuda M et al. Effects of levodopa infusion on motor activation responses in Parkinson's disease. Neurology 2002;59:220–226.
255. Buhmann C, Glauche V, Sturenburg HJ et al. Pharmacologically modulated fMRI: cortical responsiveness to levodopa in drug-naive hemiparkinsonian patients. Brain 2003;126:451–461.
256. Chase TN, Oh JD, Blanchet PJ. Neostriatal mechanisms in Parkinson's disease. Neurology 1998;51(2 suppl. 2):s30–35.
257. Dwivedi Y, Pandey GN. Quantification of 5HT2A receptor mRNA in human postmortem brain using competitive RT-PCR. Neuroreport 1998;9:3761–3765.
258. Rodriguez JJ, Garcia DR, Pickel VM. Subcellular distribution of 5-hydroxytryptamine 2A and *N*-methyl-D-aspartate receptors within single neurons in rat motor and limbic striatum. J Comp Neurol 1999;413:219–231.
259. Rahimian R, Hrdina PD. Possible role of protein kinase C in regulation of 5-hydroxytryptamine 2A receptors in rat brain. Can J Physiol Pharmacol 1995;73:1686–1691.
260. Miller KJ, Mariano CL, Cruz WR. Serotonin 5HT2A receptor activation inhibits inducible nitric oxide synthase activity in C6 glioma cells. Life Sci 1997;61:1819–1827.
261. Inoue T, Itoh S, Kobayashi M et al. Serotonergic modulation of the hyperpolarizing spike afterpotential in rat jaw-closing motoneurons by PKA and PKC. J Neurophysiol 1999;82:626–637.
262. Hasuo H, Matsuoka T, Akasu T. Activation of presynaptic 5-hydroxytryptamine 2A receptors facilitates excitatory synaptic transmission via protein kinase C in the dorsolateral septal nucleus. J Neurosci 2002;22:7509–7517.
263. Gerber PE, Lynd LD. Selective serotonin-reuptake inhibitor-induced movement disorders. Ann Pharmacother 1998;32:692–698.
264. Parsa MA, Bastani B. Quetiapine (Seroquel) in the treatment of psychosis in patients with Parkinson's disease. J Neuropsychiatry Clin Neurosci 1998;10:216–219.
265. Farah A. Reduction of tardive dyskinesia with quetiapine. Schizophr Res 2001;47:309–310.
266. Henderson J, Yiannikas C, Graham JS. Effect of ritanserin, a highly selective 5-HT2 receptor antagonist, on Parkinson's disease. Clin Exp Neurol 1992;29:277–282.
267. Oh JD, Bibbiani F, Chase TN. Quetiapine attenuates levodopa-induced motor complications in rodent and primate parkinsonian models. Exp Neurol 2002;177:557–564.
268. Gesi M, Soldani P, Giorgi FS et al. The role of the locus coeruleus in the development of Parkinson's disease. Neurosci Biobehav Rev 2000;24:655–668.
269. Soldani P, Fornai F. The functional anatomy of noradrenergic neurons in Parkinson's disease. Funct Neurol 1999;14(2):97–109.
270. Holmberg M, Fagerholm V, Scheinin M. Regional distribution of alpha(2C)-adrenoceptors in brain and spinal cord of control mice and transgenic mice overexpressing the alpha(2C)-subtype: an autoradiographic study with [(3)H]RX821002 and [(3)H]rauwolscine. Neuroscience 2003;117:875–898.
271. Archer T, Fredriksson A. An antihypokinesic action of alpha2-adrenoceptors upon MPTP-induced behaviour deficits in mice. J Neural Transm 2003;110:183–200.
272. Invernizzi RW, Garavaglia C, Samanin R. The alpha 2-adrenoceptor antagonist idazoxan reverses catalepsy induced by haloperidol in rats independent of striatal dopamine release: role of serotonergic mechanisms. Neuropsychopharmacology 2003;28:872–879.
273. Zhang W, Ordway GA. The alpha2C-adrenoceptor modulates GABA release in mouse striatum. Brain Res Mol Brain Res 2003;112(1/2):24–32.
274. Bara-Jimenez W, Morris M, Dimitrova T et al. Alpha-2 adrenergic antagonist effects in advanced Parkinson's disease. Abstracts of International Congress of Parkinson's Disease and Movement Disorders, Rome, 2004.

275. Henry B, Fox SH, Peggs D, Crossman AR, Brotchie JM. The alpha2-adrenergic receptor antagonist idazoxan reduces dyskinesia and enhances anti-parkinsonian actions of L-dopa in the MPTP-lesioned primate model of Parkinson's disease. Mov Disord 1999;14:744–753.
276. Grondin R, Hadj Tahar A, Doan VD, Ladure P, Bedard PJ. Noradrenoceptor antagonism with idazoxan improves L-dopa-induced dyskinesias in MPTP monkeys. Naunyn Schmiedebergs Arch Pharmacol 2000;361(2):181–186.
277. Fox SH, Henry B, Hill MP et al. Neural mechanisms underlying peak-dose dyskinesia induced by levodopa and apomorphine are distinct: evidence from the effects of the alpha(2) adrenoceptor antagonist idazoxan. Mov Disord 2001;16:642–650.
278. Manson AJ, Iakovidou E, Lees AJ. Idazoxan is ineffective for levodopa-induced dyskinesias in Parkinson's disease. Mov Disord 2000;15:336–337.
279. Colosimo C, Craus A. Noradrenergic drugs for levodopa-induced dyskinesia. Clin Neuropharmacol 2003;26:299–305.
280. Savola JM, Hill M, Engstrom M et al. Fipamezole (JP-1730) is a potent alpha2 adrenergic receptor antagonist that reduces levodopa-induced dyskinesia in the MPTP-lesioned primate model of Parkinson's disease. Mov Disord 2003;18:872–883.
281. Hettinger BD, Lee A, Linden J, Rosin DL. Ultrastructural localization of adenosine A2A receptors suggests multiple cellular sites for modulation of GABAergic neurons in rat striatum. J Comp Neurol 2001;431:331–346.
282. Hillion J, Canals M, Torvinen M et al. Coaggregation, cointernalization, and codesensitization of adenosine A2A receptors and dopamine D2 receptors. J Biol Chem 2002;277:18091–18097.
283. Fredholm BB, Arslan G, Halldner L et al. Structure and function of adenosine receptors and their genes. Naunyn Schmiedebergs Arch Pharmacol 2000;362:364–374.
284. Shindou T, Nonaka H, Richardson PJ et al. Presynaptic adenosine A2A receptors enhance GABAergic synaptic transmission via a cyclic AMP dependent mechanism in the rat globus pallidus. Br J Pharmacol 2002;136:296–302.
285. Aoyama S, Kase H, Borrelli E. Rescue of locomotor impairment in dopamine D2 receptor-deficient mice by an adenosine A2A receptor antagonist. J Neurosci 2000;20:5848–5852.
286. Kanda T, Jackson MJ, Smith LA et al. Adenosine A2A antagonist: a novel antiparkinsonian agent that does not provoke dyskinesia in parkinsonian monkeys. Ann Neurol 1998;43:507–513.
287. Grondin R, Bedard PJ, Hadj Tahar A et al. Antiparkinsonian effect of a new selective adenosine A2A receptor antagonist in MPTP-treated monkeys. Neurology 1999;52:1673–1677.
288. Carvalho AL, Correia S, Faro CJ et al. Phosphorylation of GluR4 AMPA-type glutamate receptor subunit by protein kinase C in cultured retina amacrine neurons. Eur J Neurosci 2002;15:465–474.
289. Bara-Jimenez W, Sherzai A, Dimitrova T et al. Adenosine A(2A) receptor antagonist treatment of Parkinson's disease. Neurology 2003;61:293–296.
290. Hauser RA, Hubble JP, Truong DD. Randomized trial of the adenosine A(2A) receptor antagonist istradefylline in advanced PD. Neurology 2003;61:297–303.
291. Julian MD, Martin AB, Cuellar B et al. Neuroanatomical relationship between type 1 cannabinoid receptors and dopaminergic systems in the rat basal ganglia. Neuroscience 2003;119:309–318.
292. Brotchie JM. CB1 cannabinoid receptor signalling in Parkinson's disease. Curr Opin Pharmacol 2003;3(1):54–61.
293. Segovia G, Mora F, Crossman AR, Brotchie JM. Effects of CB1 cannabinoid receptor modulating compounds on the hyperkinesia induced by high-dose levodopa in the reserpine-treated rat model of Parkinson's disease. Mov Disord 2003;18:138–149.
294. Maccarrone M, Gubellini P, Bari M et al. Levodopa treatment reverses endocannabinoid system abnormalities in experimental parkinsonism. J Neurochem 2003;85:1018–1025.
295. Fox SH, Henry B, Hill M, Crossman A, Brotchie J. Stimulation of cannabinoid receptors reduces levodopa-induced dyskinesia in the MPTP-lesioned nonhuman primate model of Parkinson's disease. Mov Disord 2002;17:1180–1187.
296. Sieradzan KA, Fox SH, Hill M et al. Cannabinoids reduce levodopa-induced dyskinesia in Parkinson's disease: a pilot study. Neurology 2001;57:2108–2111.
297. Smith Y, Charara A, Hanson JE, Paquet M, Levey AI. GABA(B) and group I metabotropic glutamate receptors in the striatopallidal complex in primates. J Anat 2000;196(Pt 4):555–576.
298. Rouse ST, Marino MJ, Bradley SR et al. Distribution and roles of metabotropic glutamate receptors in the basal ganglia motor circuit: implications for treatment of Parkinson's disease and related disorders. Pharmacol Ther 2000;88:427–435.

299. Ferre S, Karcz-Kubicha M, Hope BT et al. Synergistic interaction between adenosine A2A and glutamate mGlu5 receptors: implications for striatal neuronal function. Proc Natl Acad Sci USA 2002;99:11940–11945.
300. Benquet P, Gee CE, Gerber U. Two distinct signaling pathways upregulate NMDA receptor responses via two distinct metabotropic glutamate receptor subtypes. J Neurosci 2002;22: 9679–9686.
301. Cosford ND, Roppe J, Tehrani L et al. [3H]-methoxymethyl-MTEP and [3H]-methoxy-PEPy: potent and selective radioligands for the metabotropic glutamate subtype 5 (mGlu5) receptor. Bioorg Med Chem Lett 2003;13:351–354.
302. Kotecha SA, Jackson MF, Al-Mahrouki A et al. Co-stimulation of mGluR5 and *N*-methyl-D-aspartate receptors is required for potentiation of excitatory synaptic transmission in hippocampal neurons. J Biol Chem 2003;278:27742–27749.
303. Breysse N, Baunez C, Spooren W, Gasparini F, Amalric M. Chronic but not acute treatment with a metabotropic glutamate 5 receptor antagonist reverses the akinetic deficits in a rat model of parkinsonism. J Neurosci 2002;22:5669–5678.
304. Ossowska K, Wardas J, Pietraszek M, Konieczny J, Wolfarth S. The striopallidal pathway is involved in antiparkinsonian-like effects of the blockade of group I metabotropic glutamate receptors in rats. Neurosci Lett 2003;342(1/2):21–24.
305. Metman LV, Gillespie M, Farmer C et al. Continuous transdermal dopaminergic stimulation in advanced Parkinson's disease. Clin Neuropharmacol 2001;24(3):163–169.
306. Hutton JT, Metman LV, Chase TN et al. Transdermal dopaminergic D(2) receptor agonist therapy in Parkinson's disease with N-0923 TDS: a double-blind, placebo-controlled study. Mov Disord 2001;16:459–463.
307. Nomikos GG, Arborelius L, Hook BB, Hacksell U, Svensson TH. The 5-HT1A receptor antagonist (S)-UH-301 decreases dopamine release in the rat nucleus accumbens and striatum. J Neural Transm Gen Sect 1996;103:541–554.
308. Santiago M, Matarredona ER, Machado A, Cano J. Influence of serotoninergic drugs on in vivo dopamine extracellular output in rat striatum. J Neurosci Res 1998;52:591–598.
309. Blier P, Pineyro G, El Mansari M, Bergeron R, De Montigny C. Role of somatodendritic 5-HT autoreceptors in modulating 5-HT neurotransmission. Ann NY Acad Sci 1998;861:204–216.
310. Gobert A, Lejeune F, Rivet JM et al. Modulation of the activity of central serotoninergic neurons by novel serotonin1A receptor agonists and antagonists: a comparison to adrenergic and dopaminergic neurons in rats. J Pharmacol Exp Ther 1995;273:1032–1046.
311. Maeda T, Kannari K, Shen H et al. Rapid induction of serotonergic hyperinnervation in the adult rat striatum with extensive dopaminergic denervation. Neurosci Lett 2003;343(1):17–20.

5

Clinical Features, Pathophysiology, and Management of Motor Complications in Parkinson's Disease

Jose A. Obeso, Maria C. Rodríguez-Oroz, and Ivana Zamarbide

INTRODUCTION

The treatment of Parkinson's disease (PD) has been evolving constantly and new therapeutic challenges emerge as older problems are resolved. Before the development of levodopa as standard treatment, the control of severe, generalized tremor was a major concern and a reason to undertake the risky surgical treatments available in the 1950s and 60s. The introduction of levodopa in 1967 provided great clinical benefit, but patients severely affected quickly developed sudden changes of the motor state ("on"/"off" fluctuations) and involuntary movements (dyskinesias) that had never been witnessed before. It took more than a decade to develop a coherent clinical and pathophysiological classification of motor complications (MC) in PD.[1,2,3] Motor fluctuations and dyskinesias still represent the most prevalent problem in the management of PD[4,5] and are the main reason for indicating surgical treatment.

However, as disease duration is prolonged in PD due to better treatments and quality of life, new complications have become more frequent and a major therapeutic challenge. Thus, a classification of complications associated with long-term treatment and evolution of PD has now been expanded to encompass not only the typical "levodopa-related" motor fluctuations and dyskinesias but also a variety of motor and non-motor features that were considered atypical for PD until recently. Among the former, one has to consider gait freezing, postural imbalance and falls, dysphagia and speech disturbances; and among the latter, dementia, dysautonomia, and sleep disorder. These are (apparently) becoming more prevalent, perhaps related to the increased lifespan and disease evolution of patients with PD.[6,7]

In this chapter we concentrate mainly on the more typical "levodopa-related" MCs as they are more amenable to therapeutic interventions.

CLINICAL FEATURES OF LEVODOPA-RELATED MOTOR COMPLICATIONS

The prevalence of motor fluctuations and dyskinesias increases with time after diagnosis and treatment with levodopa. Ten years after starting treatment, most patients (80–100%) with genuine PD have developed these problems.[8,9,10] Motor fluctuations and dyskinesias occur simultaneously in the majority of patients, although they have to be discussed separately for academic reasons.

Motor Fluctuations

Before the introduction of levodopa the mobility and severity of parkinsonian symptoms remained stable. Certainly, striking variations in the capacity to move ("paradoxical kinesia") or episodic freezing ("paradoxical akinesia") in the presence of intense stimuli (a fire, an accident, etc.) were well documented but they were not part of daily events in PD patients.[11] Motor fluctuations were readily recognized with the use of levodopa in the late 1960s and 70s but may actually be seen with any short-acting and potent antiparkinsonian agent, like apomorphine or quinpirole. There are two main types of motor responses to levodopa:

1. The "short-duration response" (SDR) is characterized by a short improvement in PD cardinal features, typically lasting some 3–4 hours. The SDR is the basis for the clinical phenomenon of "wearing-off."
2. The "long-duration response" (LDR) represents the time required to lose completely the antiparkinsonian effects of levodopa. The LDR has classically been measured in days (3–10 days), but a recent study (the ELLDOPA trial) in "de novo" patients suggests that it may actually last for several weeks after cessation of levodopa treatment.

Patients with PD typically enjoy several years (3–7 approximately) of treatment with dopaminergic (DA) drugs without experiencing major limitations. The standard therapeutic regimen during these early years consists of a dopamine agonist or levodopa (plus a peripheral decarboxylase inhibitor) three times a day. This is associated with a significant improvement in the major cardinal features of PD and in the quality of life. Patients do not notice a resurgence of parkinsonian symptoms when "off" medication for several hours and declare themselves "stable" (Figure 5.1). However, with increased disease duration and time under treatment, the benefit obtained after each dose becomes shorter and is clearly noticeable, giving rise to the "wearing-off" or "end-of-dose deterioration."[1,2] The beginning of this phenomenon may be subtle and take the form of mild sensory symptoms in a limb, a vague feeling of malaise or depressed mood. More typically it consists in a resurgence of motor features such as focal dystonic spasms (with or without associated pain), tremor, bradykinesia and rigidity. In most patients, the onset of the "wearing-off" phenomenon occurs by the most affected body part and is not associated with a marked deterioration of global motor capability. A frequent initial presentation of motor fluctuations is the "early morning akinesia," where patients suffer a resurgence of parkinsonian motor features before the initial morning dose.

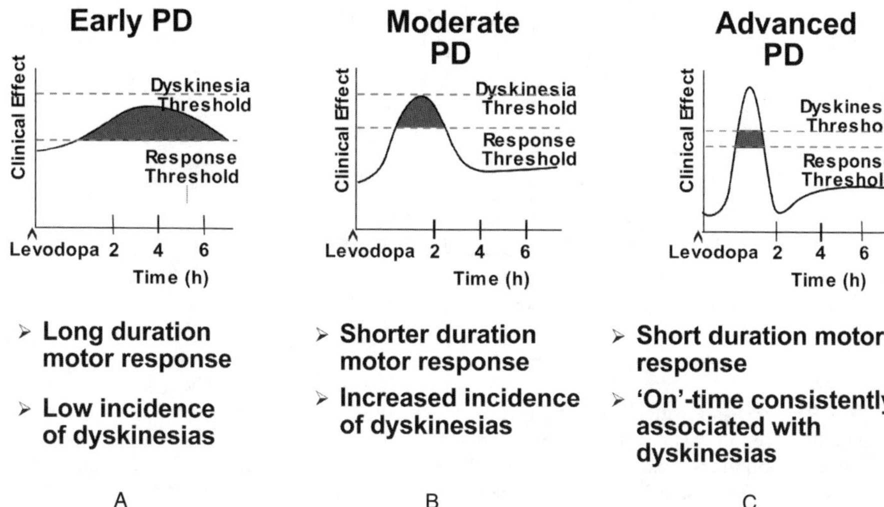

FIGURE 5.1 The short-duration response (SDR). In the early stages (A), disease severity is mild and the response to an acute challenge with levodopa is relatively long-lasting. The magnitude of the improvement is small. As disease progresses (B), the severity of the "off" medication state becomes worse (i.e. higher UPDRS motor scores). In parallel, the duration of the improvement is shorter and the magnitude larger. In very advanced PD (C), the SDR is very marked, giving rise to a very unstable pharmacological response that is the "on"/"off" phenomenon.

With increased disease progression, motor disability in the "off" medication state becomes less tolerable and more incapacitating giving rise, eventually, to incapacitating motor blocks or "off" periods. Initially at the onset of motor fluctuations, the response to levodopa lasts for some 4–6 hours and the changes in mobility are fairly predictable for patients taking medication regularly (i.e. 3–4 times a day) who therefore experience several "off/on/off" cycles per day. This situation may evolve into a more complex picture when the duration of each single dose is very short (less than 90–120 minutes) and the severity of the "off" period is very large – score >45 in the Unified Parkinson's Disease Rating Scale (UPDRS). This usually leads to increasing the number of daily doses and precipitating the occurrence of "levodopa dose failures." Such failures usually occur in the afternoon or early evening and are associated with food ingestion. Eventually, the relationship between levodopa intake and motor benefit may reach the point where many doses only induce a transient benefit or complete failure to produce motor improvement. Because, in some patients, changes in the motor state can occur suddenly and apparently unexpectedly, the terms "on"/"off" phenomenon or "yo-yo-ing" were originally applied to label this situation,[11] but in fact the changes in mobility are not usually that rapid or that unpredictable. Thus, the term "complex fluctuations" or "complicated end-of-dose deterioration" seems more appropriate. Indeed, it is now clear that "complex fluctuations" mainly represent a therapeutic artefact related to the use of small and too frequent doses of levodopa. As a result of a more careful

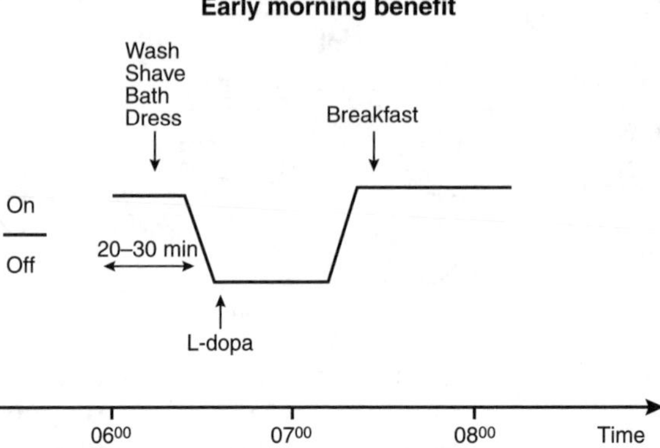

FIGURE 5.2 Early morning benefit. This is a practical example of a patient with moderately advanced PD. The self-made graph shows an initial early morning benefit followed by a deterioration in the motor state right after levodopa intake. Presumably, this effect occurred before levodopa plasma levels reached peak concentrations.

titration of levodopa and the widespread use of dopamine agonists, we have noticed a dramatic reduction in the last decade of the incidence of such seemingly random "on"/"off" fluctuations.

Interestingly, a proportion of patients with motor fluctuations exhibit a paradoxical "early morning benefit," where there is a short period (<2 hours) before taking the first morning dose when patients feel very well and capable of undertaking their daily life activities with what seems like normality (Figure 5.2). Following the first levodopa dose there is an "off" period, which subsides sometime later to give a full "on" response. The pharmacological basis of this phenomenon is not known. We believe it may represent the result of compensatory mechanisms capable of restoring the physiology of basal ganglia outflow temporarily.[12] Whether such compensations occur at the level of the nigrostriatal dopaminergic system, the internal circuits of the basal ganglia or elsewhere is not known.

Dyskinesias

Dyskinetic movements (with the exception of tremor, naturally) are not, as a rule, present in untreated PD. Dystonic spasms, usually taking the form of action dystonia of the foot, may be the presenting feature of PD particularly in young-onset PD.[13] Choreic dyskinesias may be induced in treated but stable patients under special conditions such as stress, arithmetics or during the performance of fine manipulative motor tasks. Dyskinesias in PD may be triggered in patients treated with a dopamine agonist in monotherapy but this is a relatively rare occurrence. More often, dyskinesias are observed in patients treated with levodopa who have developed motor fluctuations. Accordingly, levodopa-induced dyskinesias (LIDs) are conveniently classified according with their type and pattern of presentation (Figure 5.3) as follows.

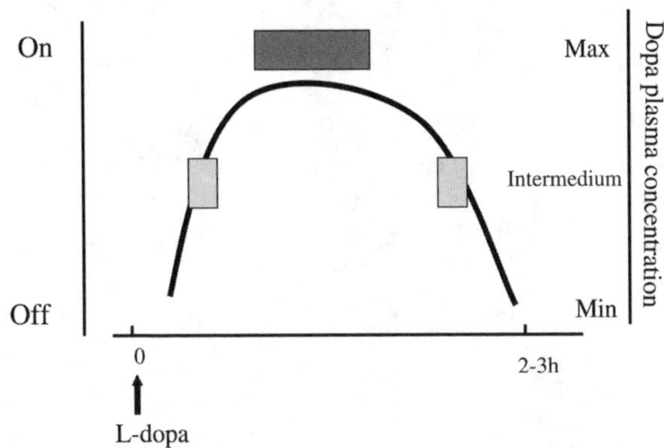

FIGURE 5.3 Presentation of levodopa-induced dyskinesias.

"On" dyskinesias

The onset of the involuntary movements coincides with the benefit of levodopa. They may appear at the time of maximum antiparkinsonian effect and highest levodopa plasma level ("peak dose")[14] or be present throughout the whole "on" period ("square wave").[1,2] The movements may be of the type of chorea, mobile dystonia (or athetosis) and myoclonus. The latter is very rare. Typically, choreic dyskinesias preferentially involve the face, neck, trunk and proximal upper-limb musculature, but the movements may affect any body part or become generalized. "On" dyskinesias become worse with increased levodopa doses and disappear with its withdrawal or with the administration of a dopamine blocking agent. The latter is at the cost of recurrence or exacerbation of parkinsonism.

Diphasic dyskinesias

Diphasic dyskinesias (DD) are characterized by a relatively abrupt onset of repetitive, rhythmic and slow (2–3 Hz) movements of the lower limbs heralding the onset and offset of the "on" period; thus they are typically associated with parkinsonian features in the upper half of the body (Figure 5.4). The stereotypic pattern of movements of DD may occasionally be replaced by rather large amplitude and less rhythmical movements, resembling ballism. Dystonic postures are the clinical manifestation of DD in a small proportion of patients.

Diphasic dyskinesias were originally described[14] and characterized by the so-called DID (dyskinesia–improvement–dyskinesia) pattern to indicate a dissociation between the involuntary movements and the beneficial effect of levodopa as well as the temporal pattern of presentation. It is now recognized that a diphasic pattern does not necessarily occur in every instance, so that dyskinesias may be present in only one phase of the cycle. More importantly, in

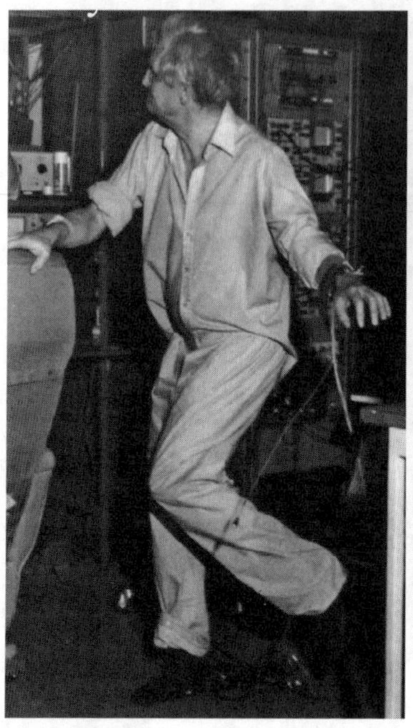
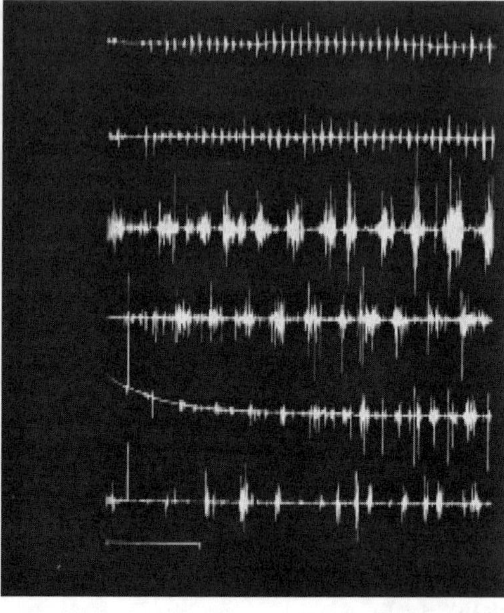

FIGURE 5.4 Electromyographic recording of movement during an episode of diphasic dyskinesias.

many patients the typical repetitive movements give way, when the patient turns "on," to a different type of dyskinetic movements (chorea or even ballism) in the affected leg. This is frequently a source of confusion in the assessment of patients with LIDs.

DD may be effectively abated by administering apomorphine (see Figure 5.3) or any other fast-acting dopaminergic drug.[15]

"Off"-period dystonia

This is due to co-contraction of antagonist muscles, twisting the body into fixed postures. It commonly consists of focal dystonic postures of a limb, such as extension of the foot and great toe or flexion of the toes, but may also be generalized. Dystonic postures in PD are pathognomonic of "off" periods, so they subside readily with the ensuing "on" response (see Figure 5.3).

Nocturnal myoclonus

Spontaneous myoclonic jerking of the leg at night occurs in patients treated with dopaminergic drugs and usually coincides with nightmares and other parasomnias. Nocturnal myoclonus is mainly related to the beginning of psychiatric complications, so it represents a very special category of LIDs from both pathophysiological and pharmacological viewpoints.

Special Presentations

In complicated patients the patterns of motor fluctuations and dyskinesias described above may not be recognizable. This frequently leads to serious clinical difficulties in the management of such situations.

Dyskinesias with parkinsonism

One body part is "on" and dyskinetic while the other half is "off." Typically the upper half of the body exhibits dyskinesias and coincidentally the patient is incapable of walking due to severe freezing of gait. This is the result of trying to overcome freezing and other gait problems with large levodopa doses.

Dyskinesias without benefit

This is a fairly uncommon situation described in the 1970s.[1,2] Patients suffer dyskinetic movements without having the antiparkinsonian benefit of levodopa. It would be similar to "off" dyskinesias. Our impression, from the few patients we have encountered, is that the dyskinesias correspond to DD but without the characteristic short-lasting and dual presentation. This is in fact relatively common with the use of continuous infusions of lisuride (see Figure 5.3) or apomorphine and long-acting dopamine agonists like cabergoline or controlled-release levodopa.

Graft-induced "off" dyskinesias

This is a new problem in the field of dyskinesias in PD. Focal or segmental dyskinesias similar to typical LIDs have now been reported in three transplantation studies and were not observed in any of the placebo-treated patients.[16–18] These dyskinesias thus appear to be specifically related to the transplantation procedure. Dyskinesias can persist for days or even weeks following withdrawal of dopaminergic medication – hence the use of the term "off-medication." However, careful evaluation indicates that in fact patients are not really "off" as compared to their baseline (pre-grafting) state but have improved by about 20–30%. In fact, the majority of patients with graft-induced dyskinesias in the study by Freed et al.[16] showed an excellent response to grafting.

The occurrence of graft-induced dyskinesias has enormous consequences for the field of cellular therapy in PD and requires further assessment.

PATHOPHYSIOLOGY OF LEVODOPA-RELATED MOTOR COMPLICATIONS

Motor Fluctuations: the Short-duration Response (SDR)

We shall discuss here the origin of the SDR, which is at the basis of the "wearing-off" phenomenon. The main features of the SDR (see Figure 5.1) are as follows:

1. There is a rapid onset (measured in minutes).
2. There follows a large magnitude of improvement. That is, the difference between the "off" and "on" motor scores is large and very noticeable.

3. A brief duration of improvement ensues, ranging from 15–30 minutes to a few (2–4) hours.
4. In severe patients, there is an aggravation of parkinsonian signs (below the "off" baseline state) at the end of the "on" period. This phenomenon has been labeled as "super off" when associated with very intense accentuation of motor features.

The origin of the SDR is mainly associated with the disease severity and the short half-life of standard levodopa. The former is determined by the degree of nigrostriatal dopamine deficit and the associated motor disability. The latter conveys a discontinuous and poorly regulated delivery of dopamine that plays a crucial pathophysiological role.

Presynaptic mechanisms

The extent of cell loss in the substantia nigra pars compacta (SNc) and the consequent depletion of striatal dopamine is the major determinant of motor severity in PD. Thus, there is an excellent correlation between dopaminergic innervation as measured by striatal 18-fluorodopa uptake by PET (positron emission tomography) and motor disability scored with the UPDRS.[19,20] The progressive loss of cells in the SNc is associated with further reduction in striatal dopamine availability and higher (i.e. more severe) motor scores in the UPDRS. In PD, replenishment of striatal dopamine concentrations depends on exogenous levodopa administration and levodopa plasma levels. Since the plasma half-life of levodopa is less than 90 minutes, striatal concentrations of dopamine are expected to oscillate in parallel with the variations in levodopa plasma concentrations. Thus, a SDR may be understood as "the normal" pharmacological response of a denervated system (i.e. the striatum) when challenged with a short-acting drug (levodopa). The SDR is less noticeable and not very relevant clinically in the early stages of PD (see Figure 5.1) and becomes more overt and disabling as disease progresses. Indeed, the SDR occurs immediately (with the first few doses) when dopamine deficit is very severe. This has been well documented in PD patients who are started on treatment after many years of evolution,[21] as well as in humans and monkeys intoxicated with the neurotoxin MPTP (1-methyl-4-phenyl-1,2,3,6-tetrahydropyridine).[22]

It is understood that, in such circumstances, the dopamine synthesized from levodopa becomes readily removed from the synaptic cleft and metabolized by COMT (catechol-O-methyltransferase) and MAO-B (monoamine oxidase B), thus readily explaining why the response duration to levodopa becomes shorter as disease progresses. In the striatum of rats with unilateral destruction of the nigrostriatal projection by 6-hydroxydopamine (6-OHDA) injection, dopamine striatal concentrations assessed by microdialysis reach lower peak values and decline more rapidly than in the normal (intact) striatum.[23,24] A recent study with PET measured raclopride binding (as an index of dopamine synaptic concentration) before and after levodopa administration in PD patients with and without motor fluctuations to assess the central kinetics of dopamine. De la Fuente et al.[25] reported that, in patients with motor fluctuations compared with stable patients, raclopride binding was decreased, reflecting higher synaptic dopamine levels due to a reduced number of terminals. However, the area under the curve was reduced due to shorter availability of dopamine. The net result is that the greater the cell loss in the SNc, the more altered is the central kinetics of dopamine in PD.

Postsynaptic mechanisms

In addition to presynaptic mechanisms, data indicate that the SDR and its clinical consequence, the "wearing-off" phenomenon, is mediated by striatal postsynaptic mechanisms and modifications in the output activity of the basal ganglia.[12,26]

The findings regarding response duration and disease severity that substantiated the "storage hypothesis" are replicated in patients given apomorphine,[27–29] which does not depend on presynaptic mechanisms to act. There is also experimental data indicating how the dopaminergic response is modified without intervening changes in the degree of dopamine depletion. For example, in the 6-OHDA lesioned rat the full lesion is established after 3 days but administration of levodopa twice a day is associated with a progressive shortening in the duration of the motor response over a treatment period of 3 weeks.[30] In this model, the accentuation of the "wearing off" cannot be explained by a progressive loss of dopamine storage and release capacity. Similarly, in the MPTP monkey model and in PD patients, repeated administration of a short-acting agonist such as apomorphine is associated with a shortening of the motor response duration that occurs within hours.[31]

It is not possible, therefore, to attribute the development of the SDR exclusively to presynaptic mechanisms. In fact, the major determinant of the SDR and the "wearing-off" phenomenon is the motor severity or degree of parkinsonism in the "off" medication state (see Figure 5.1) and the plastic changes induced by discontinuous or pulsatile dopaminergic delivery. Whereas the magnitude of the motor improvement becomes larger as disease severity increases, the duration of the motor response becomes shorter, but it is actually the magnitude of the response that determines the clinical recognition of the "wearing-off" phenomenon.[32,33]

The postsynaptic mechanisms include plastic changes at the striatal level as well as functional alterations in the output circuits of the basal ganglia. It must be understood that the more severe parkinsonism is associated with more pronounced hyperactivity in the STN/GPi, and vice versa.[34,35] Increased severity of the underlying parkinsonism and pulsatile dopaminergic stimulation associated with standard levodopa therapy are the most relevant variables associated with the induction of a short-duration response and the clinically recognizable "wearing-off" phenomenon. In our pathophysiological interpretation, presynaptic storage of dopamine plays no direct role. Instead, progressive reduction of dopaminergic terminals and the derangement of tonic dopaminergic activation is the essential component leading to: (a) increased motor severity, (b) disruption of basal ganglia autoregulatory mechanisms, and (c) the induction of pulsatile stimulation with the use of standard levodopa.

Dyskinesias

Levodopa-induced dyskinesias (LIDs) are an inducible phenomenon, secondary to abnormal dopaminergic activation. The sensitivity to develop LIDs is enhanced by dopaminergic denervation, but this is not an essential requirement. LIDs have been described in intact monkeys of two different species.[36,37] In this respect LIDs differ from motor fluctuations; the latter are the "expected" consequence of pharmacologically activating a denervated system, while the former need the abnormal activation of primary physiological mechanisms.

The anatomo-physiological basis of LIDs

Chorea/ballism and dystonia are primarily associated with dysfunction of the basal ganglia. The pathophysiological hallmark of LIDs is a reduction in neuronal activity in the subthalamic nucleus (STN), leading to disinhibition of the thalamocortical projection.[38–40] Pallidotomy, thalamotomy (when including the pallidal receiving area, VLo) and pyramidotomy abolish chorea/ballism or LIDs in the absence of hemiparesis.[41–43]

Dyskinesias identical to LIDs can be induced in patients with PD by lesion or high-frequency electrical stimulation (to block neuronal activity of the STN)[44–46] and by fetal cell grafting in the putamen.[16–18] Thus, the abnormal neuronal signals underlying LIDs are probably generated at the putamen and conveyed through the "indirect" circuit to the globus pallidus pars interna (GPi) – motor thalamus and cortical motor areas.[47–49] This is supported by molecular findings showing that pulsatile dopaminergic stimulation is associated with dyskinesias and augmented levels of striatal enkephalin-A and increased expression of the proenkephalin gene both in MPTP monkeys and patients with PD.[50,51] Enkephalin is known to co-express with D2 receptors in putaminal medium spiny neurons that project to the globus pallidus pars externa (GPe) in the "indirect" circuit. It is therefore believed that chronic levodopa treatment reduces the activity in the putamino-GPe projection, leading to disinhibition of the GPe. This renders the STN overinhibited and reduces the glutamatergic excitatory drive on to the GPi.[48,49] On the other hand, the role of the "direct" putamino-GPi projection in the pathophysiology of LIDs has also attracted attention.[52] The expression of pre-proenkephalin-B has also been found to increase in MPTP monkeys and PD patients who had developed LIDs.[53] The increment occurred specifically in the striosome, not in the matrix within the post-commissural putamen.

The relative roles of the "indirect" and "direct" circuits in the pathophysiology of LIDs remains uncertain. Efforts to ascribe the activation of D1 ("direct" circuit) or D2 ("indirect" circuit) have proved unsuccessful as selective receptor agonists of either family equally induce dyskinesias.[54] In any case, LIDs are mediated by hypoactivity in the GPi, which is the basic physiological feature of dyskinesias. Such abnormality cannot be the only mechanism mediating LIDs, since pallidotomy, which should bring GPi activity close to zero, abolishes chorea/ballism dyskinesias of any origin.[55]

We understand LIDs as the pathological counterpart of a basal ganglia mechanism involved in the suppression of unwanted actions and the running of automatic movements.[26] Accordingly, we suggest that LIDs may be mediated by neuronal activity in the SMA–area 6 loop within the motor circuit.[55] This includes the dorsal region of the post-commissural putamen, the anterior portion of the sensorimotor GPi, and the premotor areas. The expression of dyskinetic movements requires a reduction in GPi firing rate below normal levels but also the release of a pattern or code of neuronal activity. These signals or neuronal code activate the premotor cortical areas to involuntarily generate movement sequences (i.e. dyskinesias) probably encoded within the motor cortical areas.[56,57] This would explain why LIDs resemble so closely fragments of normal movements.

Pharmacological mechanisms

We have discussed the pathophysiology of LIDs from a unitary point of view as if the phenomenon were homogenous. However, the clinical features and temporal pattern of presentation indicate the putative involvement of different mechanisms. Let us summarize a number of important and well-established observations.

1. "Off" dystonia and DD most commonly affect, respectively, the foot and leg and are associated with periods of inadequate mobility. Both presentations are readily aborted by a potent and fast-acting dopaminergic drug like apomorphine.
2. "On" dyskinesias consist of choreic or dystonic movements that preferentially affect the face, neck, trunk and upper limbs. They are made worse by administering dopaminergic drugs and can only be effectively blocked with anti-dopaminergic agents (haloperidol, sulpiride, etc.).

This suggests that the spectrum of LIDs is associated with different degrees of dopaminergic striatal stimulation and different physiological states of the basal ganglia (Figure 5.5). Furthermore, it also suggests a half of the body's somatotopic sensitivity for the dopamine system. This would explain the heterogeneous pattern of response to different levels of dopaminergic stimulation and may also be relevant to understanding the pathophysiology of graft-induced dyskinesias.

In line with the above physiological conclusions, LIDs may be seen as a state where the probability of generating a motor or command signal from the putamen is abnormally enhanced. Normally, the dopaminergic system exerts a modulatory control of the corticostriatal glutamatergic (excitatory) input that probably serves to select and balance striatopallidal activity.

Under normal conditions, dopamine receptors are stimulated tonically, except for phasic bursts associated with behavioral events involving reward, motivation, or unexpected stimuli.[58,59] Phasic release of dopamine has a potent but brief effect that is spatially limited as dopamine is rapidly removed from the synapse.[58] Although the concentrations of dopamine associated with tonic release are much lower than after phasic release, they extend over a larger striatal volume[60] and exert a dual (inhibitory/facilitatory) modulatory effect on striatal activity.[61]

It is currently believed that the failure of standard levodopa therapy to mimic the tonic features of the dopaminergic nigrostriatal system induces plastic

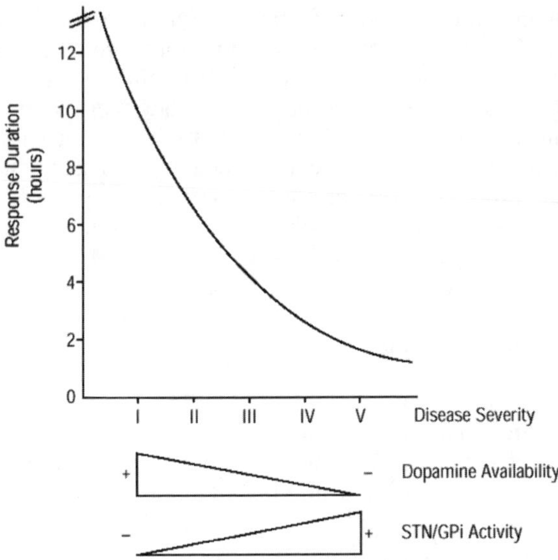

FIGURE 5.5 Schematic of the relationship between dopaminergic striatal depletion, firing activity in the output of the basal ganglia, and the types of LIDs.

changes in the striatum (e.g. abnormal long-term potentiation)[62] that modify and shift the striatal network towards a state that facilitates movement occurrence – that is, dyskinesias. The underlying physiological changes (still not well defined) may be mediated by a series of molecular abnormalities such as phosphorylation of NMDA and AMPA receptor subunits,[63] up-regulation of AMPA receptors,[64] as well as increased expression of neuropeptides in medium spiny striatal neurons that give rise to or aggravate the SDR and sensitize the striatum to induce dyskinesias.

TREATMENT OF MOTOR COMPLICATIONS

The treatment of motor complications embraces two main aspects:

- Prevention or retardation of their occurrence
- Practical management of patients who already suffer from these complications.

Prevention of Motor Complications

Undoubtedly, therapeutic developments in PD should be directed to control disease progression as well as to restore the consequences of dopaminergic depletion. This is not available yet. In practice, a reasonable therapeutic approach to prevent and treat motor complications consists in providing dopaminergic replacement therapy in a more continuous manner, thus avoiding the effects of pulsatility on an already deranged basal ganglia network.

Strategies to extend the half-life of levodopa and thereby avoid such pulsatile stimulation are therefore of considerable interest.

For example, the administration of levodopa/carbidopa with a COMT inhibitor extends its elimination half-life and leads to more stable and predictable plasma levels of levodopa. In the rat with 6-OHDA lesion and in MPTP monkeys, this strategy has proved strikingly effective in preventing the development of the "wearing-off" response and dyskinesias.[65,66] Similarly, a recent study showed that continuous subcutaneous administration of apomorphine provided similar antiparkinsonian efficacy but significantly less dyskinesias than a similar dose of apomorphine given intermittently.[67] Importantly, a similar study was conducted in patients with PD, using subcutaneous administration of the dopamine agonist lisuride.[68] The study also found a reduced incidence of motor complications in the group of patients treated with continuous dopaminergic stimulation.

The available data strongly suggest that it will be possible to adjust the delivery of dopaminergic drugs to provide a more physiological restoration of the dopaminergic deficit and, by doing so, the risk of developing motor complications will be reduced. Admittedly, a more definitive strategy would be to normalize the primary abnormality underlying the origin of PD. This, however, is a more complex challenge.

Practical Issues

Motor fluctuations and LIDs not only share by and large the same risk factors and etiopathogenic mechanisms, but also in fact usually coincide in most patients. Thus, the practical management of these two main motor complications has to be considered together. Here, we shall summarize the most common clinical presentations from more simple to complicated stages.

1. Early morning dystonia and akinesia – This occurs when the SDR becomes noticeable and occurs precisely after the maximal interval without medication intake. Thus, controlled-release levodopa or a higher dose of dopaminergic agonists late at night may effectively control this phenomenon.
2. Mild "wearing-off" in the morning with "occasional levodopa dose failures" in the afternoon – As the symptoms in the "off" state are frequently mild (muscle stiffness, pain, general discomfort, subtle motor worsening, etc.), the addition of entacapone or a dopamine agonist (if the patient is only on levodopa) can relieve the wearing-off. In patients already on these treatments, an increment of the dose of the dopamine agonist can ameliorate the "off" periods. The failure of an individual levodopa dose, usually the one(s) in the afternoon, may be managed by avoiding coincidental lunch with levodopa intake. This accounts for the typical reduction in levodopa absorption, and consequently the plasma levels, that is critical at this moment when the SDR does not allow maintenance of an appropriate motor situation after many hours without medication.
3. Established "wearing-off" with or without mild "peak dose dyskinesias." To minimize this situation, an adequate strategy is to use higher doses of a dopamine agonist and reduce the total daily dose of levodopa as well as the

number of doses (i.e. some 4–5 a day at most). The extended practice of using small and frequent doses of levodopa to manage the critically short duration response present in severe PD (see Figure 5.1) is not a desirable one. This in fact usually leads to a complex motor situation with unpredictable and/or inefficient doses giving rise to an "on"/"off" phenomenon. In a proportion of patients this strategy may also provoke a severe and continuous dyskinetic state without sufficient motor improvement that is related to an intermedium level of dopaminergic stimulation ("dyskinesia without benefit").

4. "Severe night and early morning 'off' and severe 'off' epidoses following each dose and frequent failures to respond to levodopa." This is an aggravated version of the above. "On" periods are associated with "peak-dose" dyskinesias. Diphasic dyskinesias and "off" period dystonia are also commonly present. This is a complex situation in which the theoretical pharmacological recommendations are similar to the ones discussed above. However, it is very difficult if not impossible in practice to control sufficiently this state even after careful titration of levodopa and dopamine agonists. Thus, surgical treatment, mainly deep-brain stimulation (DBS) of the subthalamic nucleus, is the therapy of choice. DBS is now well recognized to improve motor complication and the parkinsonian motor features in a sustained and stable manner. The possibility of installing a portable infusion pump to deliver apomorhine subcutaneously or levodopa intraintestinally is limited to very specialized teams.[69–71]
5. The above situation may get even more complicated by the coincidental occurrence of dyskinesia and parkinsonism as described above. The surgical treatment is the only way to try to resolve this situation.

REFERENCES

1. Marsden CD, Parkes JS, Quinn NP. Fluctuations of disability in Parkinson's disease clinical aspects. In: Marsden CD, Fahn S (eds), Neurology 2: Movement Disorders. London: Butterworth Scientific, 1981, pp. 96–122.
2. Fahn S. Fluctuations of disability in Parkinson's disease: pathophysiology. In: Marsden CD, Fahn S (eds), Neurology 2: Movement Disorders. London: Butterworth Scientific, 1981, pp. 123–145.
3. Obeso JA, Grandas F, Vaamonde J et al. Motor complications associated with chronic levodopa therapy in Parkinson's disease. Neurology 1989;39(Suppl.2):11–18.
4. Colosimo C, De Michele M. Motor fluctuations in Parkinson's disease: pathophysiology and treatment. Eur J Neurol 1999;6:1–21.
5. Obeso JA, Olanow CW, Nutt JG. Levodopa motor complications in Parkinson's disease. Trends Neurosci 2000;23(Suppl.):2–7.
6. Obeso JA, Rodriguez-Oroz MC, Chana P, Lera G, Rodriguez M, Olanow CW. The evolution and origin of motor complications in Parkinson's disease. Neurology 2000;55(Suppl. 4):13–23.
7. Aarsland D, Andersen K, Larsen J, Lolk A, Kragh-Sorensen P. Prevalence and characteristics of dementia in Parkinson's disease. Arch Neurol 2003;60:387–392.
8. Fahn S. The spectrum of levodopa-induced dyskinesias. Ann Neurol 2000;47:(Suppl. 1):2–11.
9. Grandas F, Galiano ML, Tabernero CJ. Risk factors for levodopa-induced dyskinesias in Parkinson's disease. J Neurol 1999;246:1127–1133.
10. Schrag A, Quinn N. Dyskinesias and motor fluctuations in Parkinson's disease: a community-based study. Brain 2000;123:2297–2305.
11. Marsden CD, Parkes JD. "On–off" effects in patients with Parkinson's disease on chronic levodopa therapy. Lancet 1976;i:292–296.

12. Obeso JA, Rodriguez-Oroz MC, Marin C, Alonso F, Zamarbide I, Lanciego JL, Rodriguez Diaz M: The origin of motor fluctuations in Parkinson's disease: importance of dopaminergic innervation and basal ganglia circuits. Neurology 2004; 62 (1 Suppl 1):S17–30.
13. Schrag A, Ben-Shlomo YB, Brown R, Marsden D. Young-onset Parkinson's disease revisited: clinical features, natural history, and mortality. Mov Disord 1998;13:885–894.
14. Muenter MD, Tyce GM. L-dopa therapy of Parkinson's disease: plasma L-dopa concentrations, therapeutic response, and side effects. Mayo Clinic Proc 1971;46:231–239.
15. Luquin MR, Scipioni O, Vaamonde J, Gershanik O, Obeso JA. Levodopa-induced dyskinesias in Parkinson's disease: clinical and pharmacological classification. Mov Disord 1992;7:117–124.
16. Freed CR, Greene PE, Breeze RE et al. Transplantation of embryonic dopamine neurons for severe Parkinson's disease. N Engl J Med 2001;344:710–719.
17. Hagell P, Piccini P, Bjorklund A et al. Dyskinesias following neural transplantation in Parkinson's disease. Nat Neurosci 2002;5:627–628.
18. Olanow CW, Goetz CG, Kordower JH et al. A double-blind placebo-controlled trial of bilateral fetal nigral transplantation in Parkinson's disease. Ann Neurol 2003;54:403–414.
19. Snow BJ, Toomaya I, McGeer EG et al. Human positron emission tomographic 18-F-fluorodopa studies correlate with dopamine cell counts and levels. Ann Neurol 1993;34:324–330.
20. Vingerhoets FGJ, Snow BL, Lees CS et al. Longitudinal fluorodopa positron emission tomographic studies of the evolution of idiopathic parkinsonism. Ann Neurol 1994;36:759–764.
21. Vaamonde J, Ibanez R, Gudin M, Hernandez A. Fluctuations and dyskinesias as early L-dopa-induced motor complications in severe parkinsonian patients. Neurologia 2003;18:162–165.
22. Ballard PA, Tetrud JW, Langston WJ. Permanent human parkinsonism due to one-methyl-4-phenyl-1,2,3,6-tetrahydropyridine (MPTP): seven cases. Neurology 1985;35:949–956.
23. Spencer SE, Wooten GF. Altered pharmacokinetics of L-dopa metabolism in rat striatum deprived of dopaminergic innervation. Neurology 1984;34:1105–1108.
24. Papa SM, Engber TM, Kask AM, Chase TN. Motor fluctuations in levodopa-treated parkinsonian rats: relation to lesion extent and treatment duration. Brain Res 1994;662:69–74.
25. De la Fuente-Fernandez R, Lu J-Q, Sossi V, Jivan S, Schulzer M et al. Biochemical variations in the synaptic level of dopamine precede motor fluctuations in Parkinson's disease: PET evidence of increased dopamine turnover. Ann Neurol 2001;49:298–303.
26. Obeso JA, Rodriguez-Oroz MC, Rodriguez M et al. Pathophysiology of the basal ganglia in Parkinson's disease. Trends Neurosci 2000;23(Suppl.):8–19.
27. Grandas F, Obeso JA. Motor response following repeated apomorphine administration is reduced in Parkinson's disease. Clin Neuropharm 1989;12:14–22.
28. Rodríguez M, Lera G, Vaamonde J, Luquin MR, Obeso JA. Motor response to apomorphine and levodopa in asymmetrical Parkinson's disease. J Neurol Neurosurg Psych 1994;57:562–566.
29. Bravi D, Mouradian MM, Roberts JW et al. Wearing-off fluctuations in Parkinson's disease: contribution of post-synaptic mechanisms. Ann Neurol 1994;36:27–31.
30. Engber TM, Papa SM, Boldry RC, Chase TN. NMDA receptor blockade reverses motor response alterations induced by levodopa. Neuroreport 1994:5: 2586–2588.
31. Luquin MR, Laguna J, Herrero MT, Obeso JA. Behavioral tolerance to repeated apomorphine administration in parkinsonian monkeys. J Neurolog Sci 1993;114:40–44.
32. Nutt JG. Effect of long-term therapy on the pharmacodynamics of L-dopa: Relation to on–off phenomenon. Arch Neurol 1992;49:1123–1130.
33. Zappia M, Colao R, Montesanti R. Long-duration response to levodopa influences the pharmacodynamics of short duration response in Parkinson's disease. Ann Neurol 1997;42:245–248.
34. Eidelberg D, Moeller K, Kazumata K et al. Metabolic correlates of pallidal neuronal activity in Parkinson's disease. Brain 1997;120:1315–1324.
35. Vila M, Levy R. Herrero MT, Ruberg M, Faucheux B, Obeso JA et al. Consequences of nigrostriatal denervation on the functioning of the basal ganglia in human and non-human primates: an in-situ hybridization study of cytochrome oxidase subunit I mRNA. J Neurosci 1997;17:765–773.
36. Pearce RK, Heikkila M, Linden OB, Jenner P. L-dopa induces dyskinesia in normal monkeys: behavioural and pharmacokinetic observations. Psychopharmacology 2001;156:402–409.
37. Quick M, Togasaki DM, Tan L, Protell P, Di Monte DA, Quik M, Langston JW. Levodopa induces dyskinesias in normal squirrel monkeys. Ann Neurol 2001;50:254–257.
38. Papa SM, Desimone R, Fiorani M, Oldfield EH. Internal globus pallidus discharge is nearly suppressed during levodopa-induced dyskinesias. Ann Neurol 1999;46:732–738
39. Merello M, Balej J, Delfino M, Cammarota A, Betti O, Leiguarda R. Apomorphine induces changes in GPi spontaneous outflow in patients with Parkinson's disease. Mov Disord 1999;14:45–49.

40. Lozano AM, Lang AE, Levy R, Hutchison W, Dostrovsky J. Neuronal recordings in patients with Parkinson's disease with dyskinesias induced by apomorphine. Ann Neurol 2000;47(Suppl. 1): S141–146.
41. Narabayashi H, Yokochi F, Nakajima Y. Levodopa-induced dyskinesia and thalamotomy. J Neurol Neurosurg Psychiat 1984;47:831–839.
42. Vitek JL, Giroux M. Physiology of hypokinetic and hyperkinetic movement disorders: model for dyskinesia. Ann Neurol 2000;(Suppl 1):131–140.
43. Page RD. The use of thalamotomy in the treatment of levodopa-induced dyskinesia. Acta Neurochir (Wien) 1992;114:77–117.
44. Benabid AL, Benazzouz A, Limousin P, Koudsie A, Krack P, Piallat B, Pollak P. Dyskinesias and the subthalamic nucleus. Ann Neurol 2000;47(Suppl. 1):S189–192.
45. Krack P, Pollak P, Limousin P, Benazzouz A, Deuschl G, Benabid AL. From off-period dystonia to peak-dose chorea: the clinical spectrum of varying subthalamic nucleus activity. Brain 1999;122:1133–1146.
46. Alvarez L, Macias R, Guridi J et al. Dorsal subthalamotomy for Parkinson's disease. Mov Disord 2001;16:72–78.
47. Crossman AR, Sambrook MA, Jackson A. Experimental hemichorea/hemiballismus in the monkey: studies on the intracerebral site of action in a drug-induced dyskinesia. Brain 1984;107:579–596.
48. Crossman AR. Primate models of dyskinesia: the experimental approach to the study of basal ganglia-related involuntary movement disorders. Neuroscience 1987;21:1–40.
49. Obeso JA, Rodriguez-Oroz MC, Rodriguez M, DeLong MR, Olanow W. Pathophysiology of levodopa-induced dyskinesias in Parkinson's disease: problems with the current model. Ann Neurol (Suppl. 1);2000:22–34.
50. Morissette M, Grondin R, Goulet M et al. Differential regulation of striatal pre-proenkephalin and pre-protachynin mRNA levels in MPTP monkeys chronically treated with dopamine D1 or D2 agonists. J Neurochem 1999;72:682–692.
51. Calon F, Birdi S, Rajput AH et al. Increase of pre-proenkephalin mRNA levels in the putamen of Parkinson's disease patients with levodopa-induced dyskinesias. J Neuropathol Exp Neurol 2002;61:186–196.
52. Bezard E, Brotchie JM, Gross CE. Pathophysiology of levodopa-induced dyskinesia in Parkinson's disease: opportunities for novel treatment. Nat Neurosci Rev 2001;2:577–588.
53. Henry B, Duty S, Fox SH, Crossman AR, Brotchie JM. Increased striatal pre-proenkephalin B expression is associated with dyskinesias in Parkinson's disease. Exp Neurol 2003;183:458–468.
54. Calon F, Tahar AH, Blanchet PJ et al. Dopamine-receptor stimulation: biobehavioral and biochemical consequences. Trends Neurosci 2000;23(Suppl.):92–100.
55. Guridi J, Lozano AM. A brief history of pallidotomy. Neurosurgery 1997;41:1169–1180.
56. Rizzolatti G, Luppino G. The cortical motor system. Neuron 2001;31:889–901.
57. Graziano M, Taylor Ch, Moore T, Cooke D. The cortical control of movement revisited. Neuron 2002;36:349–362.
58. Onn P, West AR, Grace AA. Dopamine-mediated regulation of striatal neuronal and network interactions. Trends Neurosci 2000;23(Suppl.):48–56.
59. Schultz W. Predictive reward signal of dopamine neurons. J Neurophysiol 1998;80:1–27.
60. Floresco SB, West AR, Ash B, Moore H, Grace AA. Afferent modulation of dopamine neurons firing differentially regulates tonic and phasic dopamine transmission. Nat Neurosci 2003;6:968–973.
61. Wilson CJ, Kawaguchi Y. The origins of two-state spontaneous membrane potential fluctuations of neostriatal spiny neurons. J Neurosci 1996;16:2397–2410.
62. Picconi B, Centonze D, Hakansson K, Bernardi G, Greengard P, Fisone G, Cenci MA, Calabresi P. Loss of bidirectional striatal synaptic plasticity in L-DOPA-induced dyskinesia. Nat Neurosci 2003;6:501–506.
63. Chase NT, Oh JD. Striatal dopamine- and glutamate-mediated dysregulation in experimental parkinsonism. Trends Neurosci 2000;23(Suppl.):86–91.
64. Bibbiani F, Oh JD, Petzer JP, Castagnoli N Jr, Chen JF, Schwarzschild MA, Chase TN. A2A antagonist prevents dopamine agonist-induced motor complications in animal models of Parkinson's disease. Exp Neurol 2003;184:285–294.
65. Jenner P, Obeso JA. Origin de las discinesias inducidas por levodopa: estudios en el modelo del mono tratado con MPTP. Neurologia 2003;18(Suppl. 1):19–23.
66. Marin C. Origen de las complicaciones motoras. Neurologia 2003;18(Suppl. 1):2–10.

67. Bibbiani F, Constantini L, Patel R, Chase T. Continuous apomorphine administration with novel EVA implants reduces the risk of motor complications compared to pulsatile apomorphine in L-dopa-naive, MPTP-lesioned primates. Neurology 2002;60(Suppl.):330.
68. Stocchi F. Prevention and treatment of motor fluctuations. Neurologia 2003;16(Suppl. 1):24–33.
69. Obeso JA, Luquin MR, Martínez Lage JM. Lisuride infusion pump: a device for the treatment of motor fluctuations in Parkinson's disease. Lancet 1986;i:467–470.
70. Stocchi F, Berardelli A, Vacca L, Barbato L, Monge A, Nordera G, Ruggieri S. Apomorphine infusion and the long-duration response to levodopa in advanced Parkinson's disease. Clin Neuropharmacol 2003;26:151–155.
71. Nyholm D, Askmark H, Gomes-Trolin C, Knutson T, Lennernas H, Nystrom C, Aquilonius SM. Optimizing levodopa pharmacokinetics: intestinal infusion versus oral sustained-release tablets. Clin Neuropharmacol 2003;26:156–163.

SECTION 2

OVERVIEW OF DRUG THERAPY FOR PARKINSON'S DISEASE

6

The Medical Management of Parkinson's Disease

Anthony H. V. Schapira
and C. Warren Olanow

INTRODUCTION

This chapter serves to integrate the various aspects of the medical management of Parkinson's disease (PD) that have been detailed in other parts of this book. In particular, it is intended to provide the reader with a practical approach to the treatment of PD, relevant to the various stages of the disease at which pharmacological intervention may be deemed appropriate. Reference is made to other chapters in this book for the reader to follow detailed analysis of drug profiles, efficacy, and trials.

TREATMENT AT DIAGNOSIS?

At present it is not possible to identify individuals with pre-symptomatic PD with any degree of certainty. Abnormal positron emission tomography (PET) scans have been observed in asymptomatic co-twins of PD patients who have subsequently developed PD themselves,[1] but this method cannot be regarded as a screening tool. Defective olfactory sense has been proposed as a potential screening method to define an "at risk" population,[2] but again the specificity of this technique is not sufficiently strong to enable it to be used as a method to identify pre-symptomatic patients. Therefore, at the time of writing, PD can be diagnosed only when the patient first manifests with appropriate clinical features.

The diagnostic accuracy of PD reaches 98.5% in the setting of a Movement Disorder Service based on clinical criteria alone.[3] The pathological features of PD are best supported by the presence of bradykinesia, rigidity, resting tremor, asymmetry, and a good and sustained response to levodopa. A clinical diagnosis can now, when necessary, be supported by single photon emission computerized tomographic (SPECT) scans using one of a variety of ligands that bind to the dopamine transporter. Accurate and early diagnosis of PD offers the patient and physician an opportunity to develop the foundations for a coherent long-term treatment strategy.

Traditionally, drugs for PD have been viewed as being only of symptomatic benefit and therefore their initiation has been restricted to the point at which the symptoms of PD interfere with social, domestic, or professional life. The patient best judges this time, although the physician must be alert to inappropriate reluctance to begin medication, and the unnecessary prolongation of disability and impaired quality of life. However, this traditional approach is now being re-evaluated, particularly in relation to the issues of whether treatment should be offered at diagnosis, and if so, which drug should be used for initial therapy. The potential advantages of early treatment include:

- Symptomatic relief
- Disease modification: neuroprotection.

Symptomatic Relief

Patients may themselves detect the early features of PD such as bradykinesia, pain, stiffness, or tremor and seek medical advice on their own account. Alternatively, family, friends, or colleagues are the first to detect changes and persuade the patient to attend. The severity of features at diagnosis depends, of course, on the duration and progression of disease, the elderly often falsely attributing PD symptoms to "growing old" and manifesting with more advanced symptoms. There is nothing to be gained from withholding treatment from those patients who have significant disability. Likewise, those patients with symptoms that may be mild but which impact significantly upon their social or professional lives will need treatment. The issue for these groups is which drug should be used for initiation. The current debate as to when to begin treatment centers on those patients with only mild dysfunction and no significant functional interference with life.

PD patients seek medical attention because of the significance of the symptoms of their disease and some argue that, on that basis alone, they should be offered treatment. It is important for the patient to be made aware of the potential improvements that they may derive from treatment. Bradykinesia, rigidity, pain, and sometimes even tremor respond dramatically to dopaminergic drugs. Drug treatment has often been delayed because of concern regarding a decline of medication efficacy over time, or alternatively the development of complications or side-effects. The introduction over the past few years of a range of effective and well-tolerated agents renders such concerns less critical. However, cost of medication, particularly in those health economies where the patient must bear some or all of the expense, can play a role in determining the timing of introduction. In this context it is legitimate for treatment to be delayed at the patient's request, but only to the point at which there is an effect upon social or professional life.

In conclusion, it is reasonable that the decision as to whether medication is initiated at diagnosis for symptomatic benefit should reside predominantly with the patient, but with appropriate guidance from the physician.

Disease Modification: Neuroprotection

The dominant early clinical features of PD are related to the motor deficits caused by the loss of dopaminergic neurons in the substantia nigra pars compacta. Recent reports suggest that PD pathology begins in the lower brainstem and ascends through the dorsal motor nucleus and locus ceruleus to the substantia nigra before progressing to affect other brainstem nuclei and the cortex.[4] Whatever the sequence of pathology, it is the loss of nigral neurons and the consequent motor abnormalities that is the most common reason for the patient to seek medical advice. In this context, drug treatment is highly successful. However, the widespread and progressive neurodegeneration in the PD brain leads to the gradual emergence of a variety of features that are collectively grouped under the title of "non-motor symptoms." These are predominantly, but not exclusively, the consequence of loss of non-dopaminergic pathways. The non-motor symptoms of PD range from cognitive problems such as apathy, depression, anxiety disorders, and hallucinations to sleep disorders, sexual dysfunction, and bowel problems, drenching sweats, sialorrhea, and pain. These symptoms are often the most troubling for patients and contribute significantly to morbidity and impaired quality of life and indeed come to dominate the later stages of PD. Treatment for these non-motor features is limited and often unsatisfactory.

It is the limitations of symptomatic dopaminergic treatment that has led to the search for agents to slow the progression of neurodegeneration in PD and thereby help prevent or slow clinical progression, or even reverse deficits by restoring normal function to defective neurons. It is accepted that such a strategy will be successful only if degeneration is ameliorated in multiple neurotransmitter systems, preventing the progression of both motor and non-motor features.

Advances in our understanding of the etiology and pathogenesis of PD have provided innumerable potential targets for developing neuroprotection. Numerous compounds have been investigated in the laboratory and several evaluated in clinical trials. Chapter 13 discusses the properties of each of these drugs in detail. Neuroprotection in PD is now reviewed in order that practicing clinicians can reach a judgment on whether the data available will influence their clinical practice, particularly in terms of when they would initiate treatment.

The drugs that have received most attention in relation to neuroprotection include the monoamine oxidase (MAO) type B inhibitors and dopamine agonists, although others including co-enzyme Q_{10}, growth factors, anti-apoptotic agents, and glutamate inhibitors have also been the subjects of clinical trials in PD.

MAO-B inhibitors

Two compounds of the pro-pargylamine group, selegiline (deprenyl) and rasagiline, both of which are MAO-B inhibitors, have demonstrated neuroprotective efficacy in the laboratory and have undergone clinical trials for a disease-modifying effect in early PD.

Selegiline can protect cultured dopaminergic neurons against the toxicity of 1-methyl-4 phenylpyridinium (MPP^+) and in animal models can reduce dopaminergic cell loss in response to 1-methyl-4-phenyl 1,2,3,6-tetrahydropyridine (MPTP).[5–9] Selegiline also protects against apoptotic cell death induced by serum and growth factor withdrawal,[10,11] possibly via an increased production of Bcl2. Selegiline, by virtue of its MAO-B activity, will reduce the turnover of dopamine and so reduce free radical generation. The production of reactive oxygen species and free-radical-mediated damage to lipids and proteins have been implicated in PD pathogenesis. Thus this property, together with the ability for selegiline to protect against MPTP toxicity, led to the evaluation of this drug in the first clinical trial for neuroprotection in PD.

The DATATOP study was a prospective, double-blind, placebo-controlled trial that investigated the effect of selegiline 5 mg twice daily and/or 2000 iu vitamin E as putative neuroprotective therapies.[12] The time until PD patients required levodopa was used as the primary endpoint. No beneficial effect of vitamin E was detected at the dose given. In contrast, selegiline significantly delayed the need for levodopa compared to placebo, an effect consistent with slowing of disease progression. However, selegiline was also found to exert a mild symptomatic effect that confounded interpretation of the study. To try to avoid this confound, selegiline was compared to placebo using as the primary endpoint the change in motor score between an untreated baseline visit and an untreated final visit performed after 12 months of treatment and 2 months of study drug withdrawal.[13] In this study, PD patients treated with selegiline had less deterioration from baseline than those receiving placebo, again suggesting that selegiline might be neuroprotective. However, in this study also, a long-lasting symptomatic effect of selegiline could not be excluded as contributing to the results. Nevertheless, in a long-term follow-up study of the DATATOP cohort, levodopa patients who had been taking selegiline for 7 years, compared to those who were changed to placebo after 5 years, had a significantly slower decline, less "wearing-off," "on"/"off," and freezing, but more dyskinesias in those on deprenyl.[14] Although one study did suggest that selegiline use might be associated with excess mortality, a recent large meta-analysis indicates that no such effect is evident and confirms the clinical efficacy of this drug in PD patients.[15]

Rasagiline is a more potent MAO-B inhibitor than selegiline. It too has demonstrated protective effects against a wide range of neurotoxins in both in-vitro and in-vivo studies. For instance, it protects against MPTP/MPP^+ and 6-hydroxydopamine toxicity and excitotoxic-mediated damage, and stabilizes the mitochondrial membrane potential to reduce apoptotic cell death.[16–19] Rasagiline has an advantage over selegiline in that both the parent compound and the aminoindan metabolite have neuroprotective actions, while selegiline-mediated neuroprotection appears to depend on its desmethyl metabolite. Furthermore, selegiline is metabolized to metamphetamine, a compound which itself has neurotoxic effects and which also blocks the protective action of rasagiline, aminoindan and selegiline. The isomer of rasagiline devoid of MAO-B inhibitory activity is also active in laboratory neuroprotective studies, indicating that this property is independent of MAO-B inhibition.[20]

Based on the pre-clinical data, rasagiline's potential for disease modification was assessed in a novel trial design of "wash-in" or "randomized start."

The TEMPO study randomized patients with early PD to placebo or rasagiline (1 or 2 mg) and evaluated progression with change from baseline in UPDRS scores over 6 months. After this time, patients in the placebo group were placed on 2 mg of rasagiline and all groups were followed for a further 6 months. At the end of the study, the change in UPDRS motor score between baseline and final visit was greater in patients who were randomized to the placebo group and received only 6 months of rasagiline in comparison to those who had received rasagiline for the entire 12-month period.[21] The interpretation of the TEMPO result is complex.[22] It cannot be explained by a symptomatic effect alone as patients in all groups were receiving the drug at the end of the study. At face value, they represent an early disease-modifying effect whereby 12 months of rasagiline had a greater effect than the same drug over 6 months. However, there are potential confounding effects, including differential dropout, although this was not apparent in the analysis. Further evaluation of rasagiline in a larger study, perhaps of similar design, is required to determine this drug's potential for neuroprotection in PD.

Dopamine agonists

Dopamine agonists were introduced for their ability to relieve the dopaminergic-related motor symptoms of PD. As a drug class, however, they have properties that have potential to provide disease modification. They have anti-oxidant activity as a result of their hydroxylated benzyl ring structure, and numerous laboratory studies have demonstrated neuronal protection against systems generating free radicals. These include attenuation of the effects of MPP^+, dopamine, 6-hydroxydopamine, and nitric oxide, and up-regulation of protective scavenging enzymes such as catalase and superoxide dismutase.[23–31] However, these benefits are predominantly seen at relatively high concentrations which may not be relevant in clinical practice.

Dopamine agonists have demonstrated anti-apoptotic activity in laboratory studies. For instance, pramipexole reduces cell death and prevents the release of cytochrome c and caspase activation in dopaminergic cells treated with MPP^+ or rotenone, and prevents a fall in mitochondrial membrane potential.[32–33] Importantly, this dopamine agonist has also shown protective effects in the MPTP primate model of PD.[34] Several studies suggest that dopamine agonists exert their protective effects not through stimulation of either D2 or D3 receptors, but rather via some alternative mechanism. For instance, pramipexole is still able to exert protective effects in cells exposed to MPP^+ or rotenone in cells devoid of dopamine receptors.[33] Blockade of dopamine receptors in dopaminergic cell cultures does not prevent the protective properties of pramipexole.[35,36] Further, the enantiomers of apomorphine and pramipexole, which do not bind to dopamine receptors, still protect dopaminergic neurons from MPP^+, H_2O_2, or 6-hydroxydopamine toxicity.[37,38] Other data, however, support a role for dopamine receptors in mediating at least some of the protective effects of agonists.[30,39–41] It appears increasingly likely that dopamine agonists may induce protection in different ways depending on the specific agonist, the model system, and the nature of the toxin. Nevertheless, the potential for dopamine agonists to protect non-dopaminergic cells, if translated to the clinic, would have profound implications for disease modification, and in particular for preventing the development of non-motor features in PD.

Two studies have sought to determine whether the neuroprotective benefits of dopamine agonists seen in the laboratory can be transferred to patients to modify the course of PD. The CALM-PD study used beta-CIT SPECT to follow the rate of loss of dopamine transporter as a marker of dopaminergic nigrostriatal cell density.[42] Patients with early PD were randomized to pramipexole or levodopa and followed for a total of four years, and levodopa supplementation was allowed in both arms. At 2, 3, and 4 years there was a significant reduction in the rate of transporter loss in the pramipexole group, averaging out at approximately 40%, consistent with the drug having a relatively protective effect in comparison to levodopa. A similar result was seen in the REAL-PET ropinirole study that used a similar trial design but utilized PET to follow loss of nigrostriatal cell density with fluorodopa.[43] This demonstrated a reduction of about 34% over two years in the ropinirole group compared to those on levodopa.

These studies have generated considerable interest and debate.[44,45] Both studies demonstrate that dopamine agonists are associated with a significant delay in the rate of decline of a surrogate imaging marker of nigrostriatal function. One interpretation of these findings is that these two dopamine agonists slow the rate of cell loss in the substantia nigra of PD patients, and this is consistent with the laboratory findings outlined above. However, neither showed a corresponding clinical benefit, but it can be argued that the time course of the trials was too short to permit such an effect to be detected in the context of viable compensatory mechanisms and powerful symptomatic effects, and this will only become apparent with longer follow-up. Another interpretation of these studies is that levodopa is toxic to nigral neurons. There is concern that levodopa might be toxic as it undergoes oxidative metabolism and has the potential to generate cytotoxic free radicals.[46] Levodopa has been shown to be toxic to cultured dopamine neurons, but there is no convincing evidence that levodopa is toxic in in-vivo models or in PD patients.[47] The ELLDOPA trial investigated the possibility that levodopa may be toxic in PD patients but produced conflicting results. In this study, untreated PD patients were randomized to a total daily dose of 150 mg, 300 mg, or 600 mg of levodopa or placebo. Beta-CIT SPECT was used as an endpoint for integrity of the nigrostriatal system. Levodopa was associated with a significant increase in the rate of decline of imaging marker over 9 months compared to placebo, consistent with a toxic effect.[48] Clinical evaluation, however, showed that those patients on levodopa had better UPDRS scores compared to placebo after 2 weeks of washout. This would, in contrast, be indicative of a protective effect of levodopa. However, intellectual parsimony would dictate that the simplest explanation for this clinical effect was that the washout period was too brief to eliminate the symptomatic benefits of levodopa. Finally, it has been proposed that the differences between the effects of levodopa and dopamine agonists seen in the CALM-PD and REAL-PET studies are not related to any direct effect of the drugs on dopamine neuron survival or degeneration, but rather to a pharmacological difference in the capacity of these drugs to regulate the dopamine transporter or fluorodopa metabolism.[45,49,50] However, a review of studies testing the effects of levodopa and dopamine agonists on transporter and fluorodopa metabolism reveals that the data are conflicting and that at present there is insufficient information for or against such an effect.[44]

In conclusion, dopamine agonists have an impressive portfolio of laboratory data demonstrating neuroprotective effects that might be capable of operating independently of the dopamine receptor. The results of the two clinical trials utilizing imaging endpoints support, but do not prove, a disease-modifying effect in patients.

Co-enzyme Q_{10}

Coenzyme Q10 has been evaluated in a pilot study of early PD patients to determine whether it might have disease-modifying capabilities.[51] The rationale for the use of co-enzyme Q_{10} in PD was based on the observation that mitochondrial complex I activity is decreased in the PD substantia nigra, PD patients have reduced levels of co-enzyme Q_{10}, and this compound protects against MPTP toxicity. Co-enzyme Q_{10} is both an anti-oxidant and an integral component of oxidative phosphorylation that has been shown to enhance electron transport. It is presumed not to have any symptomatic effect.

Patients were randomized to either a placebo arm or one of three doses of co-enzyme Q_{10} (300 mg, 600 mg, or 1200 mg) and followed for 16 months. There was a significant benefit for co-enzyme Q_{10} 1200 mg in terms of change from baseline in total UPDRS compared to placebo at 16 months, and a non-significant trend to benefit for lower doses. This interesting and important result is sufficient to support further study of co-enzyme Q_{10}, but insufficient at present to advocate that PD patients should use this compound.

Other agents

Other agents studied for potential neuroprotective action in PD include glial-derived nerve growth factor, riluzole, neuroimmunophyllin, CEP1437, and TCH346 (see Chapter 13). However, the results of these trials have been negative and will not be discussed further in this chapter.

Clinical Application of Neuroprotection Trials

None of the compounds discussed in detail above has been established to alter the course of PD, and none has been granted a license for neuroprotection from regulatory agencies. However, the clinician and patient need to consider the information available and integrate it into a management strategy that acknowledges the possibility of an effect, but does not depend on it. In this context, it is logical to assume that the earlier in the course of the disease any modifying drug is introduced, the more benefit it is likely to have.

Thus, in consideration of when to initiate treatment, the symptomatic benefit of a drug might be viewed in conjunction with its potential to provide neuroprotection and would favor its early rather than later introduction. For some patients this could be considered appropriate at diagnosis, for others later initiation might be preferable. Consideration should be given to balancing the benefits outlined above with the potential drawbacks, including side-effects of medication (discussed in detail below).

WHICH DRUG SHOULD BE USED FIRST?

Drugs available for the symptomatic relief of the motor features of PD include levodopa, dopamine agonists, MAOB inhibitors, and others such as anticholinergics and amantadine. The choice of which of these to use for initial therapy will be determined by a number of factors, most importantly the patient's characteristics. The benefits of a drug need to be offset against its short-term and long-term side-effects and complications, and these in turn may vary according to the patient population.

In order to help provide a practical approach for clinicians, the advantages and disadvantages of the major drugs used for symptomatic relief are briefly reviewed. The reader is also directed to the chapters that deal with these topics in greater detail. An updated algorithm for early treatment in PD is provided in Figure 6.1, which is incorporated into a subsequent version that deals with more advanced disease.

Levodopa

Levodopa is discussed in detail in Chapter 1. This was the first of the dopaminergic drugs and remains the "gold standard" against which the efficacy of others are judged. Levodopa and other dopaminergic agents improve the quality of life and life expectancy of PD patients.[52–54] It provides rapid and effective relief of bradykinesia, rigidity, and associated pain, and improves tremor in many patients. Symptoms such as postural instability, speech disturbance, sialorrhea etc. may not be improved and represent some of the non-dopaminergic components of PD. Clinical benefit as judged by improvement in total UPDRS score indicates that, in the setting of a clinical trial, levodopa improves early PD patients by 12–13 points after 3 months. Common early side-effects with levodopa are mainly gastrointestinal and comprise nausea, vomiting, and anorexia. These side-effects disappear with time, usually over 2–3 weeks, but may persist in some patients. They can be prevented or treated with domperidone 10–20 mg three times daily, taken usually for a period of 2–4 weeks. Constipation, orthostatic hypotension, akathisia, hallucinosis, and daytime sleepiness are less common and are seen more often in the elderly population. They can be managed by a variety of pharmacological and non-pharmacological measures (see Chapter 1 for details).

In early disease, levodopa has a long-duration response that enables adequate symptomatic control with dosage schedules of three times daily. Disease progression, however, erodes the utility of levodopa as 70% of patients develop motor complications within 6 years of initiation of the drug.[55,56] Wearing-off effects frequently require modification of dosage and/or dose frequency, or the introduction of additional or alternate therapies. Interestingly, so long as the plasma levodopa concentration is maintained, the clinical response will persist,[57–59] and "wearing-off" does not occur if the drug is given by continuous infusion.[60,61]

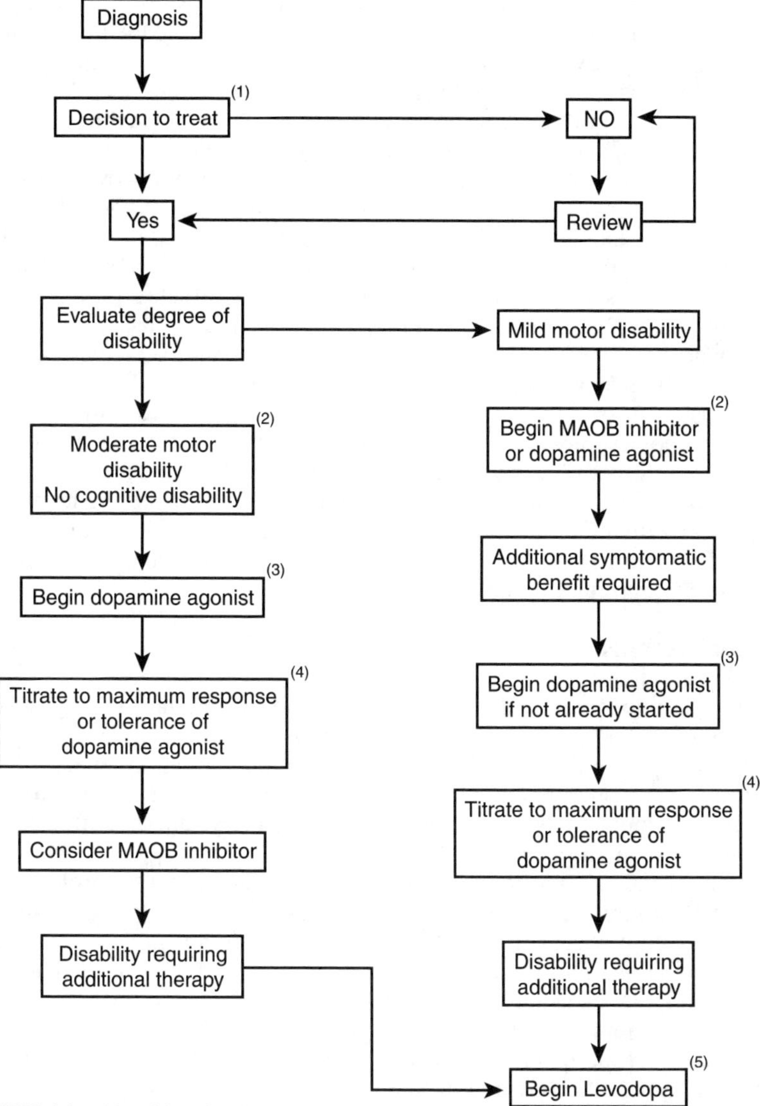

FIGURE 6.1 Algorithm for the management of early Parkinson's disease (see text for full explanations)

1. The decision as to when to treat is dealt with in detail in the text.
2. Dopamine agonists are relatively contraindicated in patients with cognitive disturbance.
3. Dose escalation as per manufacturer's recommendations is important for patient compliance and to limit side-effects.
4. Dose of dopamine agonist should be gradually increased over time to attempt to maintain motor control.
5. Levodopa introduction is inevitable for the majority of patients to maintain and optimize motor control. Consideration should be given as to whether to introduce dose frequency at four times per day with or without a COMT inhibitor in suitable patients.

Another significant long-term complication of levodopa use is the development of dyskinesias which, together with "wearing-off," constitute the motor complications caused by levodopa. Dyskinesias develop at a rate of approximately 10% per annum, although this rate is much greater in young-onset PD patients, 70% of whom will have dyskinesias within 3 years of levodopa initiation.[62] The mechanisms by which these motor complications develop are not completely understood, but pulsatile stimulation of dopamine receptors by short-acting agents including levodopa, and the degree of striatal denervation, have been implicated (see Chapters 4 and 5). Dyskinesias may occur at the time of maximal clinical benefit and peak concentration of levodopa (peak-dose dyskinesias) or appear at the onset and wearing-off of the levodopa effect (diphasic dyskinesias). Motor complications can be an important source of disability for some patients who cycle between "on" periods which are complicated by dyskinesias and "off" periods in which they suffer severe parkinsonism. The management of levodopa-related motor complications is discussed below and in Chapter 1.

Thus, levodopa offers a rapidly effective means to treat the motor symptoms of PD with a tolerable early side-effect profile, but more serious long-term complications. There is interest in the possibility that administering levodopa in combination with a COMT inhibitor in order to extend its elimination half-life might reduce the risk of motor complications, and clinical trials to test this hypothesis are currently under way.

Dopamine Agonists

Several dopamine agonists are available for use in PD and fall broadly into two groups: ergot and non-ergot. Ergot agonists include bromocriptine, cabergoline, lisuride, and pergolide; non-ergot agonists include apomorphine, piribedil, ropinirole, and pramipexole. These drugs have been subjected to extensive evaluation in clinical trials. Their characteristics, efficacy, and side-effect profiles are reviewed in detail in Chapter 2.

Bromocriptine, cabergoline, pergolide, pramipexole, and ropinirole have all been studied for monotherapy use in early PD,[63–71] as well as for adjunctive treatment in more advanced PD.[72–79] They have all demonstrated a significant beneficial effect on motor function and activities of daily living. Their side-effect profile is similar to levodopa in terms of inducing dopaminergic-related symptoms such as nausea, vomiting, and postural hypotension, but they are associated with a higher rate of peripheral edema, daytime somnolence, and hallucinosis particularly in the elderly. Somnolence with dopamine agonists is mainly seen during the early-dose escalation phase, so patients should be warned of this and the rare but important side-effect of sudden onset of sleep.[80] In patients with early PD, mean age 61 years, hallucinosis also occurred more frequently during dose escalation but, like sedation, settled to a rate no higher than levodopa during maintenance.[81]

The use of dopamine agonists is rarely associated with the development of pleural, pericardial, or peritoneal fibrosis.[82] A recent report has linked pergolide with fibrotic cardiac valvular disease[83] in a pattern similar to that seen with other agents that also stimulate the 5-HT_2 receptor, including methysergide and fenfluramine. There are insufficient data at present to know whether this complication is associated with ergot agonists alone, all dopamine agonists, or all dopaminergic drugs, and whether the effect is dose- and/or time-related. Until such time as additional information becomes available, vigilance is recommended; and when necessary, appropriate investigations (echocardiogram, chest x-ray, ESR) are warranted together with referral to a cardiologist.

Dopamine agonist monotherapy can effectively control dopaminergic symptoms for a period of time. Long-term follow-up indicates that approximately 85%, 68%, 55%, 43%, and 34% of PD patients initiated on pramipexole or ropinirole are still controlled on monotherapy at 1, 2, 3, 4, and 5 years, respectively.[81,84] However, this is dependent on the agonist being used at an appropriate dose. Nevertheless, patients will require levodopa supplementation at some point during their disease. If used correctly, they can produce symptom control comparable to levodopa. Although the two monotherapy studies quoted above showed superiority for levodopa in UPDRS scores by up to five points, patients in the agonist arms had comparable quality-of-life scores and could have taken supplemental levodopa if the physician or patient felt it was required. The explanation for this discrepancy might be because the UPDRS does not capture all the benefit that a patient might derive from a dopamine agonist, including possible non-motor effects such as an antidepressive action.

Several trials have now confirmed that bromocriptine, cabergoline, pergolide, pramipexole, and ropinirole are associated with a significantly reduced risk for the development of motor complications in comparison to levodopa.[66,70,84–86] In the pramipexole study, quality-of-life scores were also equivalent for the 4-year period.[81] This implies that the patients were equally well controlled on agonist (with levodopa supplementation when required) or levodopa alone. Of course, the levodopa group had more dyskinesias, but at 4 years these did not intrude significantly into patient quality of life, nor yet start to limit treatment options for motor control.

In conclusion, dopamine agonists provide effective control of PD-related motor symptoms, delay the onset of motor complications, delay the introduction of levodopa, enable a lower dose of levodopa to be used, and (in the case of pramipexole and ropinirole in particular) offer the possibility for some disease-modifying effect. They are well tolerated and, beyond the dose-escalation phase, their side-effect profile is similar to levodopa in patients under the age of 70 years.

MAO-B Inhibitors

Selegiline has been extensively studied for symptomatic benefit in early and advanced PD. Meta-analysis of 13 randomized trials showed that total UPDRS was improved by 2.7 points at 3 months.[15] As indicated above, this review confirmed that there is no excess mortality with selegiline. Selegiline delays the need for additional dopaminergic therapy by 9–12 months in early PD and, once introduced, levodopa dose is lower in those patients remaining on selegiline. There is no evidence at present that MAO-B inhibition itself delays the development of motor fluctuations other than through the delay in introduction of levodopa and an ability to use a lower dose.

Rasagiline improves total UPDRS by 3–4 points in early PD and this effect lasts about 6 months, at which point patients have returned to their baseline score.[87]

As discussed above, the TEMPO 12-month study results supported the possibility of a disease-modifying effect for rasagiline and would also presumably have the same benefits as selegiline for the delay in levodopa introduction.

Thus MAO-B inhibitors offer a viable option for initial therapy in early PD. The symptomatic benefit is significant but relatively modest. The ability to delay levodopa introduction is important in terms of retarding the development of motor complications. The disease-modifying effect, although unproven, offers an additional potential advantage.

Other Drugs

Non-dopaminergic drug therapy can be used in early PD, and these drugs are reviewed in detail in Chapter 3.

Anticholinergics were used to treat the symptoms of PD prior to the introduction of levodopa. Relatively little data are available on potency and tolerance. Clinical trials have shown a modest benefit for anticholinergics in improving bradykinesia and rigidity,[88–90] but this was at the expense of impaired cognitive function. Benztropine was equivalent to clozapine in producing a mild improvement in tremor.[91]

Amantadine produces mild and transitory improvement in PD symptoms, benefits usually lasting 6–9 months,[92] although some have suggested that in pure PD patients the effects are more long-lasting.[93] It is generally considered unsuitable for monotherapy in PD and is mostly used as an adjunct. Improvements in bradykinesia and rigidity are generally of the same order of magnitude as with anticholinergics, but their combination is additive.[94,95] Amantadine use is also limited by its potential to induce cognitive defects.

Practical Approach to the Initiation of Drug Treatment

The patient's age and the presence of any cognitive impairment or significant co-morbidity that is likely to influence life expectancy are important early considerations in deciding initial therapy for PD. Most PD patients come to diagnosis early in their seventh decade; patients recruited to the dopamine agonist monotherapy studies had a mean age of 61–62 years. For these, and also for the younger-onset patients, symptomatic control can be an important issue as many are still at work. They are also at risk of the development of motor complications with levodopa, and any possibility of disease modification will hold special attraction. Their disease is likely to run for 15–20 years or more and there is the opportunity early on to lay the foundations for an effective, safe and well-tolerated long-term treatment strategy.

Approaches to PD management in various stages are presented below. These represent the views of the authors.

Early PD with onset below age 70 years (see Figure 6.1)

1. In those patients whose PD symptoms are only mild but who desire some improvement in function, it is suggested that they should be offered a MAO-B inhibitor or a dopamine agonist as first-line therapy.

2. If PD symptoms are more significant and symptomatic improvement is required, patients with no evidence of cognitive impairment should be initiated on a dopamine agonist.

Early PD with onset over age 70 years

Generally, patients over age 70 years are increasingly less tolerant of dopamine agonists, although a significant proportion of patients this age and older can still benefit from agonist use with an acceptable side-effect profile.[96] Cognitive impairment can be considered a relative contraindication to dopamine agonist use as these drugs carry a high risk of exacerbating such problems. PD patients over age 70 have a relatively lower rate of onset of dyskinesias than younger patients, but these can still develop at about 5–10% a year.

1. Patients aged 70–75 years should be carefully evaluated and, if otherwise in good health, and without cognitive dysfunction, should be started on a dopamine agonist and followed-up to ensure they are able to tolerate the medication well.
2. It is proposed that patients with cognitive deficits who require symptomatic control of their PD should be initiated on levodopa.
3. Patients over the age of 75 years should be offered levodopa as first-line treatment for their PD symptoms.

The principle underlying these recommendations is to provide effective symptom control appropriate to the patient's needs and to minimize the short- and long-term side-effects of therapy.

SECOND-LINE THERAPY

Patients initiated on a MAO-B inhibitor will eventually require additional therapy to control their motor symptoms. The addition of a dopamine agonist is the most appropriate second-line treatment for these patients, provided they remain free of cognitive disturbance. However, studies addressing the degree of benefit provided by a dopamine agonist to patients receiving rasagiline have not yet been performed.

Patients initiated on a dopamine agonist should have their dose titrated to maximal effect in order to maintain their motor control. As indicated above, these patients will at some point require supplementary medication. A choice can then be made between introducing a MAO-B inhibitor or levodopa. Rasagiline has been shown to improve control in early patients[87] and those stable on levodopa, improving "on" time and reducing "off" time to a degree equivalent with entacapone.[97,98] Rasagiline is well tolerated in both early and more advanced patients. Introduction of rasagiline at this stage will probably enable a further delay in the introduction of levodopa. Inevitably, however, levodopa will be required as disease progression results in accumulating motor deficit.

Levodopa is often begun as a thrice-daily regimen, usually with 100 mg of levodopa and 25 mg of a dopa-decarboxylase inhibitor. The development of dyskinesias is probably related to dose of levodopa,[99,100] as well as its duration.[101,102] Continuation of the dopamine agonist will allow the levodopa dose to be kept low. Another factor considered significant in the generation of dyskinesias is the pulsatile stimulation of receptors with drugs having a short half-life, such as levodopa. In this context, it is noteworthy that continuous levodopa administration eliminates dyskinesias and fluctuations. Thus there is a case for using a more frequent dosage schedule or, alternatively, preparations of levodopa that have a longer half-life. Evaluation of delayed-release Sinemet (Sinemet CR™) did not demonstrate any benefit over standard-release Sinemet in prevention of motor fluctuations.[103] However, this study used the CR preparation only three times a day and, given its erratic absorption and marginally improved half-life, this protocol probably did not test the hypothesis of "continuous dopaminergic stimulation" with sufficient rigor.

The simultaneous administration of a catechol-O-methyl transferase (COMT) inhibitor with levodopa, either separately as entacapone or tolcapone, or in combination as Stalevo (levodopa and a dopadecarboxylase inhibitor with entacapone), offers an alternate approach to prolongation of the action of levodopa. A study in the MPTP primate model of PD showed that administration of levodopa with entacapone four times daily significantly protected against the development of dyskinesias compared to the same total daily dose as the standard preparation given twice daily with or without entacapone, or standard levodopa four times daily.[104] The hypothesis that introduction of levodopa with entacapone will reduce the risk for, or delay the onset of, motor complications is now being tested in a large clinical trial.

MANAGEMENT OF "WEARING-OFF"

Wearing-off equates to the loss of effectiveness of a given dose of dopaminergic therapy and the emergence of the primary motor features of PD (i.e. bradykinesia and rigidity) that still remain responsive to dopaminergic treatment. Patients recognize this as a return of symptoms prior to their next dose ("end-of-dose failure"), although some mistakenly associate it with the administration of the next dose, given the medication's latency of effect. As noted above, wearing-off is eliminated by continuous administration of either levodopa or a dopamine agonist.[60,61,105,106] While these methods are effective, they are not practical for the majority of patients. The simplest strategy is to increase the frequency of administration of levodopa, although this too may become difficult as dosage regimens increase to six or more times per day. Controlled-release formulations have proved disappointing with often little improvement in duration of response and problems with unpredictability of absorption and motor response. One open-label study demonstrated that the addition of cabergoline, a long-acting ergot, to patients taking pramipexole or ropinirole, both non-ergots, resulted in improved motor control.[107]

The introduction of a dopamine agonist should be considered in those patients on levodopa experiencing wearing-off who remain candidates for this treatment; that is, those with no significant cognitive disturbance. All dopamine agonists have demonstrated improvement in motor control as an adjunct to levodopa (see Chapter 2), and may allow a reduction in levodopa dose.

COMT inhibitors

Two selective COMT inhibitors are available for clinical use for the treatment of PD. These drugs exert profound influences on levodopa kinetics by increasing its bioavailability and elimination half-life. This allows more stable levodopa plasma levels to be obtained via the oral route and, conceivably, more sustained brain dopaminergic stimulation to be attained.

Entacapone is a selective, reversible inhibitor of COMT. It does not cross the blood–brain barrier and acts primarily in the gut. Entacapone essentially increases both the peripheral and central availability of levodopa. The plasma elimination of a 200-mg oral dose of entacapone is 1–2 hours. The pharmacokinetics of entacapone, particularly its elimination characteristics, are similar to those of levodopa, allowing co-administration of these agents. The recommended dose of entacapone is a 200-mg tablet administered with each dose of levodopa/carbidopa, up to a maximum of 10 times daily (in Europe) and 8 times daily in the United States. It should be noted that only the dose of levodopa should be titrated; the dose of entacapone administered with each dose of levodopa should remain the same (200 mg). Entacapone is effective in patients with wearing-off-type motor fluctuations and can produce an increase in "on" time and a reduction in "off" time by an average of 90 minutes a day.[108] The most common adverse event seen with entacapone is dyskinesia, which reflects increased central dopaminergic activity. Reducing the daily levodopa dosage by about 25% may be necessary to minimize possible dopaminergic adverse effects. This reduction may be made at the time of entacapone introduction in those patients on more than 800 mg of levodopa daily or in those with dyskinesias, but generally it is better to delay changing the levodopa dose until the patient's response can be evaluated. Physicians should be aware that dopaminergic adverse events generally occur within 24 hours of initiating entacapone and may require an immediate adjustment of the levodopa dosage. Entacapone may be combined with both standard and controlled-release formulations of levodopa/carbidopa and may be administered with or without food.

The introduction of Stalevo in 2003 offered an opportunity to simplify the dosage regimen for patients on entacapone. Patients stable on levodopa and entacapone given separately can be converted straight over to the equivalent dose of Stalevo. Stalevo tablets should not be cut or crushed; only one should be taken at each dose time and must not be combined with additional entacapone.

Tolcapone can cross the blood–brain barrier[109] and produces some central COMT inhibition. In practice this is likely to have minimal effect. A study in newly diagnosed, levodopa-naive patients with PD failed to show any clinical efficacy with the introduction of tolcapone either alone or with selegiline.[110] Tolcapone has a similar half-life to entacapone; however, due to a greater bioavailability and smaller volume of distribution, tolcapone produces a greater inhibition of COMT and is required only on a thrice-daily regimen.[111] Although tolcapone is available now in both Europe and North America, its use is restricted by its potential to cause severe hepatic toxicity.[112] It should not be given to patients with impaired liver function, and those PD patients taking tolcapone require regular monitoring of hepatic enzymes. This effect on liver function is not seen with entacapone, which probably reflects their differing potency in inducing mitochondrial permeabilization.[113]

Both entacapone and tolcapone can induce diarrhea, which is more common and may be severe and explosive with the latter.[114]

In conclusion, the introduction of second-line therapy in PD may be necessary in order to maintain control of motor features and improved quality of life. The choice of drug used at this stage depends on the characteristics of the patient and the medication used to date, as well as the nature of the motor decline and the presence or absence of motor fluctuations. The following is recommended by the authors as a practical guide for clinicians.

1. Patients initiated on a MAO-B inhibitor should be supplemented with a dopamine agonist when additional therapy becomes necessary, unless they are cognitively impaired or over 75 years of age, in which case they should be given levodopa as the second drug.
2. Patients initiated on a dopamine agonist who reach the stage of requiring additional therapy may derive some additional benefit from MAO-B inhibitor.
3. Levodopa will be necessary for those on a dopamine agonist with or without a MAO-B inhibitor who require additional symptom control. If possible we suggest that this be introduced as a regimen four times a day. There are theoretical reasons and some experimental data to support the introduction of levodopa in combination with entacapone, although this position cannot formally be advocated pending the results of clinical trials under way.
4. The greatest choice is for those patients already on levodopa who require additional control or who are experiencing wearing-off. If started on levodopa because of cognitive impairment or age over 75 years, the simplest approach is to increase the daily dose of levodopa with a frequency of administration four to six times daily. However, this may be impractical for some patients in this group and for them the use of Stalevo offers the benefit of extended and enhanced symptom control with the potential for a simplified dose regimen. Other patients who would still qualify for dopamine agonist treatment would benefit from their introduction at this point, thereby improving control, maintaining a lower dose of levodopa and delaying dyskinesias. Finally, if not already undertaken, the use of a MAO-B inhibitor is another option and will provide additional benefit to those on levodopa. The course of action selected will depend much on the characteristics of the patient and the severity and stage of the PD.

MANAGEMENT OF DYSKINESIAS

Dyskinesias are typically choreiform, occasionally dystonic, involuntary movements induced predominantly by exposure to levodopa. Their cause and management are discussed in detail in Chapters 4 and 5.

At first, patients may be unaware of them, but they may be noticed by relatives or friends who are frequently more troubled by them than the patient. However, they progress with time and not only cause difficulty and embarrassment, but also begin to restrict options for improving motor control. The impact of dyskinesias on quality of life is limited in the beginning; the four-year CALM-PD study results showed that quality of life was equivalent for those initiated on pramipexole or levodopa at this time point.[81] The implication is that both the agonist and levodopa groups had similar motor control and that the dyskinesias in the levodopa group did not intrude significantly into quality of life at 4 years. However, this would be likely to change as dyskinesias became more severe and options for motor control limited. A more arcane interpretation of the CALM-PD results would be that the motor benefits of levodopa were offset by the effect of the dyskinesias.

The practical management of dyskinesias depends on the severity of the involuntary movements and their relationship to medication dosage schedule. They may be peak-dose, biphasic or random. Peak-dose dyskinesias are related to high plasma concentrations of levodopa and can be managed by fractionating levodopa doses to avoid such peaks. This may or may not require an increase in the total daily dose. Alternative strategies include the introduction of a dopamine agonist if the patient is not already taking such an agent and if he or she remains a suitable candidate. Long-acting agonists are particularly useful in the management of dyskinesias, presumably due to their ability to provide more continuous dopaminergic stimulation while avoiding rapid fluctuations in receptor stimulation.[115] Biphasic dyskinesias occur when plasma levodopa concentration is rising or falling, and are associated with generally lower plasma levodopa concentrations. They tend to be more stereotypic and repetitive and to involve the lower extremeties. They are more troublesome to manage but may respond to higher levodopa doses designed to keep the plasma concentrations above a critical level.[116]

Amantadine has demonstrated efficacy in improving peak-dose dyskinesias.[117–120] The effective dose is 200–400 mg per day in two divided doses. The severity of dyskinesias may be reduced by 24–56% and the effect sustained at one year.

The potential for the continuous parenteral administration of dopamine agonists or levodopa to improve or abolish motor fluctuations including dyskinesias has been discussed above. This is dealt with in detail in Chapter 2.

Surgery with deep-brain stimulation or pallidotomy offers an important alternative to patients with dyskinesias that fail medical therapy. This is covered in detail in Chapters 7, 8 and 10 and in the overview by Olanow and Schapira in this book. The fact that surgery is considered for this group of patients emphasizes the importance of dyskinesias in terms of limiting options for motor control, and in affecting quality of life. The clear implication is that dyskinesias are best avoided or delayed if at all possible.

NON-MOTOR SYMPTOMS IN PD

Chapters 11 and 12 deal with the issues of depression, psychoses, cognitive dysfunction, gastrointestinal, urological, and sleep problems in detail. The difficulties that these create in the management of PD will be only summarized here.

It is the widespread and progressive neurodegeneration in the PD brain that leads to the emergence of non-motor symptoms. These are predominantly, but not exclusively, the consequence of loss of non-dopaminergic pathways. The non-motor symptoms of PD range from cognitive problems such as apathy, depression, anxiety disorders, and hallucinations, to sleep disorders, sexual dysfunction, bowel problems, drenching sweats, sialorrhea, and pain. As PD progresses these symptoms come to dominate and contribute significantly to morbidity and impaired quality of life.[121]

Depression, and to some extent apathy (anhedonia), may respond to tricyclics such as amitriptyline, or to selective serotonin re-uptake inhibitors (SSRIs). Pramipexole may be useful as an antidepressant, separate from its action to improve the motor features of PD.[122,123] Anxiety and panic attacks can be prominent in PD and these may sometimes relate to "wearing-off" and so respond to strategies outlined above for this complication. However, additional anxiolytic therapy may be needed in some patients.

Hallucinations can arise as a consequence of both the neurodegeneration of PD and the dopaminergic drugs used in treatment. Studies have shown that dopamine agonists, more than levodopa, are associated with the development of hallucinations particularly in the elderly. If troublesome, modification of existing therapy is the easiest strategy to reduce or stop hallucinations. However, in some patients this is difficult due to re-emergence of motor features and they may respond to clozapine or quetiapine.[124–126] Hallucinations are, of course, an important symptom of diffuse Lewy body disease, and their emergence early in the course of PD is a risk factor for dementia. PD patients who demonstrated dementia after 2 years diagnosis showed a modest but significant improvement in cognitive function with rivastigmine, to a degree similar to that seen with this drug in Alzheimer's disease.[127]

Abnormalities of sleep are common in PD and are the result of the natural consequences of aging, the underlying disease pathology,[128] motor and non-motor complications,[129,130] and drugs.[131] Disordered sleep often results in excessive daytime drowsiness and this in turn may be compounded by the sedative effect of dopaminergic drugs.[132] Several strategies are available to improve both night-time sleep and daytime alertness in PD and include improving sleep hygiene, treating nocturnal motor problems, better management of nocturia, modifying medication,[80] and the use of modafinil in refractory patients with daytime drowsiness.[133]

Sexual and bladder dysfunction are common and occur in both sexes. The dopaminergic treatment of PD may lead to increased sex drive but the effects of the disease often result in impaired sexual performance.[134] This combination not surprisingly may cause frustration, and sildenafil or apomorphine can usefully manage this in selected cases.[135–137] Bladder abnormalities particularly cause problems at night but can be successfully managed by a range of options that include non-pharmacological as well as pharmacological strategies.[138] The latter include the use of oxybutinin or detrusitol, or amitriptyline in patients with concommitent depression. Sialorrhea and drooling is often the result of reduced frequency of swallowing and may be helped by simple things such chewing gum or sucking sweets. Anticholinergic drugs may sometimes help, but often cause unwanted side-effects. Botulinum toxin can be used for refractory cases.[139]

Pain is a frequent symptom in PD and some patients manifest especially with shoulder pain. Pain, anxiety, akathisia, respiratory distress, depressive mood swings, and slowed and impaired thought are symptoms that may be experienced during "off" periods and will respond, at least in part, to dopaminergic therapy.[140–142] The recognition that a number of "non-motor" features may improve with dopaminergic drugs is important in improving the quality of life of PD patients.[143]

CONCLUSIONS

This chapter has sought to provide a practical guide to management options for the various stages of PD. It has already been emphasized by us and the other contributors to this book that treatment needs to conform to the individual needs of the patient. In addition, the patient must be involved as much as is both possible and reasonable in the decision-making process, particularly in the timing of the initiation of drug treatment and the nature of first-line therapy. The physician and patient have several options available, each with their own advantages and disadvantages.

REFERENCES

1. Piccini P, Burn DJ, Ceravolo R, Maraganore D, Brooks DJ. The role of inheritance in sporadic Parkinson's disease: evidence from a longitudinal study of dopaminergic function in twins. Ann Neurol 1999;45:577–582.
2. Ponsen MM, Stoffers D, Booij J, Eck-Smit BL, Wolters EC, Berendse HW. Idiopathic hyposmia as a preclinical sign of Parkinson's disease. Ann Neurol 2004;56:173–181.
3. Hughes AJ, Daniel SE, Ben Shlomo Y, Lees AJ. The accuracy of diagnosis of parkinsonian syndromes in a specialist movement disorder service. Brain 2002;125(Pt 4):861–870.
4. Braak H, Del Tredici K, Rub U, de Vos RA, Jansen Steur EN, Braak E. Staging of brain pathology related to sporadic Parkinson's disease. Neurobiol Aging 2003;24(2):197–211.
5. Mytilineou C, Cohen G. Deprenyl protects dopamine neurons from the neurotoxic effect of 1-methyl-4-phenylpyridinium ion. J Neurochem 1985;45:1951–1953.
6. Tatton WG, Greenwood CE. Rescue of dying neurons: a new action for deprenyl in MPTP parkinsonism. J Neurosci Res 1991;30:666–672.
7. Chiueh CC, Huang SJ, Murphy DL. Enhanced hydroxyl radical generation by 2′-methyl analog of MPTP: suppression by clorgyline and deprenyl. Synapse 1992;11:346–348.
8. Wu RM, Chiueh CC, Pert A, Murphy DL. Apparent antioxidant effect of L-deprenyl on hydroxyl radical formation and nigral injury elicited by MPP^+ *in vivo*. Eur J Pharmacol 1993;243(3):241–247.
9. Wu RM, Chen RC, Chiueh CC. Effect of MAO-B inhibitors on MPP^+ toxicity *in vivo*. Ann NY Acad Sci 2000;899:255–261.
10. Tatton WG, Ju WY, Holland DP, Tai C, Kwan M. (–)-Deprenyl reduces PC12 cell apoptosis by inducing new protein synthesis. J Neurochem 1994;63:1572–1575.
11. Wadia JS, Chalmers-Redman RM, Ju WJ, Carlile GW, Phillips JL, Fraser AD et al. Mitochondrial membrane potential and nuclear changes in apoptosis caused by serum and nerve growth factor withdrawal: time course and modification by (–)-deprenyl. J Neurosci 1998;18:932–947.
12. Effects of tocopherol and deprenyl on the progression of disability in early Parkinson's disease. The Parkinson Study Group. N Engl J Med 1993;328:176–183.
13. Olanow CW, Hauser RA, Gauger L, Malapira T, Koller W, Hubble J et al. The effect of deprenyl and levodopa on the progression of Parkinson's disease. Ann Neurol 1995;38:771–777.
14. Shoulson I, Oakes D, Fahn S, Lang A, Langston JW, LeWitt P et al. Impact of sustained deprenyl (selegiline) in levodopa-treated Parkinson's disease: a randomized placebo-controlled extension of the deprenyl and tocopherol antioxidative therapy of parkinsonism trial. Ann Neurol 2002;51:604–612.
15. Ives NJ, Stowe RL, Marro J, Counsell C, Macleod A, Clarke CE et al. Monoamine oxidase type B inhibitors in early Parkinson's disease: meta-analysis of 17 randomised trials involving 3525 patients. Br Med J 2004;329:593.

16. Akao Y, Maruyama W, Yi H, Shamoto-Nagai M, Youdim MB, Naoi M. An anti-Parkinson's disease drug, N-propargyl-1(R)-aminoindan (rasagiline), enhances expression of anti-apoptotic bcl-2 in human dopaminergic SH-SY5Y cells. Neurosci Lett 2002;326(2):105–108.
17. Maruyama W, Takahashi T, Youdim M, Naoi M. The anti-Parkinson drug, rasagiline, prevents apoptotic DNA damage induced by peroxynitrite in human dopaminergic neuroblastoma SH-SY5Y cells. J Neural Transm 2002;109:467–481.
18. Jenner P. Preclinical evidence for neuroprotection with monoamine oxidase-B inhibitors in Parkinson's disease. Neurology 2004;63(7 Suppl. 2):S13–22.
19. Am OB, Amit T, Youdim MB. Contrasting neuroprotective and neurotoxic actions of respective metabolites of anti-Parkinson drugs rasagiline and selegiline. Neurosci Lett 2004;355(3):169–172.
20. Youdim MB, Wadia A, Tatton W, Weinstock M. The anti-Parkinson drug rasagiline and its cholinesterase inhibitor derivatives exert neuroprotection unrelated to MAO inhibition in cell culture and *in vivo*. Ann NY Acad Sci 2001;939:450–458.
21. Parkinson's Study Group. A controlled, randomized, delayed-start study of rasagiline in early Parkinson disease. Arch Neurol 2004;61:561–566.
22. Rascol O. Monoamine oxidase inhibitors: is it time to up the TEMPO? Lancet Neurol 2003; 2(3):142–143.
23. Ogawa N, Tanaka K, Asanuma M, Kawai M, Masumizu T, Kohno M et al. Bromocriptine protects mice against 6-hydroxydopamine and scavenges hydroxyl free radicals *in vitro*. Brain Res 1994;657(1/2):207–213.
24. Muralikrishnan D, Mohanakumar KP. Neuroprotection by bromocriptine against 1-methyl-4-phenyl-1,2,3,6-tetrahydropyridine-induced neurotoxicity in mice. FASEB J 1998;12:905–912.
25. Kondo T, Ito T, Sugita Y. Bromocriptine scavenges methamphetamine-induced hydroxyl radicals and attenuates dopamine depletion in mouse striatum. Ann NY Acad Sci 1994;738:222–229.
26. Finotti N, Castagna L, Moretti A, Marzatico F. Reduction of lipid peroxidation in different rat brain areas after cabergoline treatment. Pharmacol Res 2000;42(4):287–291.
27. Yoshioka M, Tanaka K, Miyazaki I, Fujita N, Higashi Y, Asanuma M et al. The dopamine agonist cabergoline provides neuroprotection by activation of the glutathione system and scavenging free radicals. Neurosci Res 2002;43(3):259–267.
28. Nishibayashi S, Asanuma M, Kohno M, Gomez-Vargas M, Ogawa N. Scavenging effects of dopamine agonists on nitric oxide radicals. J Neurochem 1996;67:2208–2211.
29. Gomez-Vargas M, Nishibayashi-Asanuma S, Asanuma M, Kondo Y, Iwata E, Ogawa N. Pergolide scavenges both hydroxyl and nitric oxide free radicals *in vitro* and inhibits lipid peroxidation in different regions of the rat brain. Brain Res 1998;790(1/2):202–208.
30. Iida M, Miyazaki I, Tanaka K, Kabuto H, Iwata-Ichikawa E, Ogawa N. Dopamine D2 receptor-mediated antioxidant and neuroprotective effects of ropinirole, a dopamine agonist. Brain Res 1999;838(1/2):51–59.
31. Clow A, Freestone C, Lewis E, Dexter D, Sandler M, Glover V. The effect of pergolide and MDL 72974 on rat brain CuZn superoxide dismutase. Neurosci Lett 1993;164(1/2):41–43.
32. Kakimura J, Kitamura Y, Takata K, Kohno Y, Nomura Y, Taniguchi T. Release and aggregation of cytochrome c and alpha-synuclein are inhibited by the antiparkinsonian drugs, talipexole and pramipexole. Eur J Pharmacol 2001;417(1/2):59–67.
33. Gu M, Irvani M, Cooper JM, King D, Jenner P, Schapira AH. Pramipexole protects against apoptotic cell death by non-dopaminergic mechanisms. J Neurochem 2004;91:1075–1081.
34. Jenner P, Iravani MM, Haddon CO et al. Pramipexole protects against MPTP-induced nigral dopaminergic cell loss in primates. Neurology 2002;58:494.
35. Zou L, Jankovic J, Rowe DB, Xie W, Appel SH, Le W. Neuroprotection by pramipexole against dopamine- and levodopa-induced cytotoxicity. Life Sci 1999;64:1275–1285.
36. Kitamura Y, Kosaka T, Kakimura JI, Matsuoka Y, Kohno Y, Nomura Y et al. Protective effects of the antiparkinsonian drugs talipexole and pramipexole against 1-methyl-4-phenylpyridinium-induced apoptotic death in human neuroblastoma SH-SY5Y cells. Mol Pharmacol 1998;54:1046–1054.
37. Gassen M, Gross A, Youdim MB. Apomorphine enantiomers protect cultured pheochromocytoma (PC12) cells from oxidative stress induced by H_2O_2 and 6-hydroxydopamine. Mov Disord 1998; 13:242–248.
38. Vu TQ, Ling ZD, Ma SY et al. Pramipexole attenuates the dopaminergic cell loss induced by intraventricular 6-hydroxydopamine. J Neural Transm 2000;107(2):159–176
39. Takashima H, Tsujihata M, Kishikawa M, Freed WJ. Bromocriptine protects dopaminergic neurons from levodopa-induced toxicity by stimulating D(2)receptors. Exp Neurol 1999;159:98–104.

40. Nair VD, Olanow CW, Sealfon SC. Activation of phosphoinositide 3-kinase by D2 receptor prevents apoptosis in dopaminergic cell lines. Biochem J 2003;373(Pt 1):25–32.
41. Sawada H, Ibi M, Kihara T et al. Dopamine D2-type agonists protect mesencephalic neurons from glutamate neurotoxicity: mechanisms of neuroprotective treatment against oxidative stress. Ann Neurol 1998;44:110–119.
42. Parkinson's Study Group. Dopamine transporter brain imaging to assess the effects of pramipexole vs levodopa on Parkinson disease progression. JAMA 2002;287:1653–1661.
43. Whone AL, Watts RL, Stoessl AJ, Davis M, Reske S, Nahmias C et al. Slower progression of Parkinson's disease with ropinirole versus levodopa: The REAL-PET study. Ann Neurol 2003; 54:93–101.
44. Schapira AH, Olanow CW. Neuroprotection in Parkinson disease: JAMA 2004;291:358–364
45. Ahlskog JE. Slowing Parkinson's disease progression: recent dopamine agonist trials. Neurology 2003;60:381–389.
46. Olanow CW. A radical hypothesis for neurodegeneration. Trends Neurosci 1993;16:439–444.
47. Agid Y, Olanow CW, Mizuno Y. Levodopa: why the controversy? Lancet 2002;360:575.
48. Fahn S, Oakes D, Shoulson I, Kieburtz K, Rudolph A, Lang A et al. Levodopa and the progression of Parkinson's disease. N Engl J Med 2004;351:2498–2508.
49. Albin RL, Frey KA. Initial agonist treatment of Parkinson disease: a critique. Neurology 2003; 60:390–394.
50. Wooten GF. Agonists vs levodopa in PD: the thrilla of whitha. Neurology 2003;60:360–362.
51. Shults CW, Oakes D, Kieburtz K, Beal MF, Haas R, Plumb S et al. Effects of coenzyme Q_{10} in early Parkinson disease: evidence of slowing of the functional decline. Arch Neurol 2002;59:1541–1550.
52. Rajput AH. Levodopa prolongs life expectancy and is non-toxic to substantia nigra. Parkinsonism Relat Disord 2001;8:95–100.
53. Karlsen KH, Tandberg E, Arsland D, Larsen JP. Health-related quality of life in Parkinson's disease: a prospective longitudinal study. J Neurol Neurosurg Psychiatry 2000;69:584–589.
54. Clarke CE, Zobkiw RM, Gullaksen E. Quality of life and care in Parkinson's disease. Br J Clin Pract 1995;49:288–293.
55. Fahn S. Adverse effects of levodopa. In: Olanow CW (ed), The Scientific Basis for the Treatment of Parkinson's Disease. Carnforth: Parthenon Publishing Group, 1992, pp. 89–112.
56. Contin M, Riva R, Martinelli P. A levodopa kinetic-dynamic study of the rate of progression in Parkinson's disease. Neurology 1998;51:1075–1080.
57. Shoulson I, Glaubiger GA, Chase TN. On–off response: clinical and biochemical correlations during oral and intravenous levodopa administration in parkinsonian patients. Neurology 1975;25: 1144–1148.
58. Hardie RJ, Lees AJ, Stern GM. On–off fluctuations in Parkinson's disease: a clinical and neuropharmacological study. Brain 1984;107(Pt 2):487–506.
59. Mouradian MM, Heuser IJ, Baronti F, Chase TN. Modification of central dopaminergic mechanisms by continuous levodopa therapy for advanced Parkinson's disease. Ann Neurol 1990;27:18–23.
60. Nutt JG. On–off phenomenon: relation to levodopa pharmacokinetics and pharmacodynamics. Ann Neurol 1987;22:535–540.
61. Kurth MC, Tetrud JW, Tanner CM, Irwin I, Stebbins GT, Goetz CG et al. Double-blind, placebo-controlled, crossover study of duodenal infusion of levodopa/carbidopa in Parkinson's disease patients with "on–off" fluctuations. Neurology 1993;43:1698–1703.
62. Kostic V, Przedborski S, Flaster E, Sternic N. Early development of levodopa-induced dyskinesias and response fluctuations in young-onset Parkinson's disease. Neurology 1991;41(2 Pt 1):202–205.
63. Olanow CW. Single blind double observer-controlled study of carbidopa/levodopa vs bromocriptine in untreated Parkinson patients. Arch Neurol 1988;45:205.
64. Staal-Schreinemachers AL, Wesseling H, Kamphuis DJ, vd BW, Lakke JP. Low-dose bromocriptine therapy in Parkinson's disease: double-blind, placebo-controlled study. Neurology 1986;36: 291–293.
65. Rinne UK, Bracco F, Chouza C, Dupont E, Gershanik O, Marti Masso JF et al. Cabergoline in the treatment of early Parkinson's disease: results of the first year of treatment in a double-blind comparison of cabergoline and levodopa. The PKDS009 Collaborative Study Group. Neurology 1997;48:363–368.
66. Rinne UK, Bracco F, Chouza C, Dupont E, Gershanik O, Marti Masso JF et al. Early treatment of Parkinson's disease with cabergoline delays the onset of motor complications: results of a double-blind levodopa controlled trial. The PKDS009 Study Group. Drugs 1998;55(Suppl. 1):23–30.

67. Barone P, Bravi D, Bermejo-Pareja F, Marconi R, Kulisevsky J, Malagu S et al. Pergolide monotherapy in the treatment of early PD: a randomized, controlled study. Pergolide Monotherapy Study Group. Neurology 1999;53:573–579.
68. Parkinson's Disease Study Group. Safety and efficacy of pramipexole in early Parkinson disease: a randomized dose-ranging study. JAMA 1997;278:125–130.
69. Shannon KM, Bennett JP, Friedman JH. Efficacy of pramipexole, a novel dopamine agonist, as monotherapy in mild to moderate Parkinson's disease. The Pramipexole Study Group. Neurology 1997;49:724–728.
70. Korczyn AD, Brunt ER, Larsen JP, Nagy Z, Poewe WH, Ruggieri S. A 3-year randomized trial of ropinirole and bromocriptine in early Parkinson's disease. The 053 Study Group. Neurology 1999; 53:364–370.
71. Adler CH, Sethi KD, Hauser RA, Davis TL, Hammerstad JP, Bertoni J et al. Ropinirole for the treatment of early Parkinson's disease. The Ropinirole Study Group. Neurology 1997;49: 393–399.
72. Hoehn MM, Elton RL. Low dosages of bromocriptine added to levodopa in Parkinson's disease. Neurology 1985;35:199–206.
73. Toyokura Y, Mizuno Y, Kase M, Sobue I, Kuroiwa Y, Narabayashi H et al. Effects of bromocriptine on parkinsonism: a nationwide collaborative double-blind study. Acta Neurol Scand 1985;72(2): 157–170.
74. Inzelberg R, Nisipeaunu P, Rabey JM. Double-blind comparison of cabergoline and bromocriptine in Parkinson's disease patients with motor fluctuations. Neurology 1996;47:785–788.
75. Olanow CW, Fahn S, Muenter M, Klawans H, Hurtig H, Stern M et al. A multicenter double-blind placebo-controlled trial of pergolide as an adjunct to Sinemet in Parkinson's disease. Mov Disord 1994;9:40–47.
76. Diamond SG, Markham CH, Treciokas LJ. Double-blind trial of pergolide for Parkinson's disease. Neurology 1985;35:291–295.
77. Guttman M. Double-blind comparison of pramipexole and bromocriptine treatment with placebo in advanced Parkinson's disease. International Pramipexole/Bromocriptine Study Group. Neurology 1997;49:1060–1065.
78. Lieberman A, Ranhosky A, Korts D. Clinical evaluation of pramipexole in advanced Parkinson's disease: results of a double-blind, placebo-controlled, parallel-group study. Neurology 1997;49: 162–168.
79. Lieberman A, Olanow CW, Sethi K, Swanson P, Waters CH, Fahn S et al. A multicenter trial of ropinirole as adjunct treatment for Parkinson's disease. Ropinirole Study Group. Neurology 1998; 51:1057–1062.
80. Schapira AH. Excessive daytime sleepiness in Parkinson's disease. Neurology 2004;63:S24–27.
81. Holloway RG, Shoulson I, Fahn S, Kieburtz K, Lang A, Marek K et al. Pramipexole vs levodopa as initial treatment for Parkinson disease: a 4-year randomized controlled trial. Arch Neurol 2004; 61:1044–1053.
82. Muller T, Fritze J. Fibrosis associated with dopamine agonist therapy in Parkinson's disease. Clin Neuropharmacol 2003;26:109–111.
83. Van Camp G, Flamez A, Cosyns B, Weytjens C, Muyldermans L, Van Zandijcke M et al. Treatment of Parkinson's disease with pergolide and relation to restrictive valvular heart disease. Lancet 2004; 363:1179–1183.
84. Rascol O, Brooks DJ, Korczyn AD, De Deyn PP, Clarke CE, Lang AE. A five-year study of the incidence of dyskinesia in patients with early Parkinson's disease who were treated with ropinirole or levodopa. 056 Study Group. N Engl J Med 2000;342:1484–1491.
85. Oertel WH. Pergolide versus levodopa (PELMOPET). Mov. Disord 2000:15(Suppl. 3):4.
86. Parkinson's Disease Study Group. Pramipexole vs levodopa as initial treatment for Parkinson disease: a randomized controlled trial. JAMA 2000;284:1931–1938.
87. Parkinson's Disease Study Group. A controlled trial of rasagiline in early Parkinson disease: the TEMPO Study. Arch Neurol 2002;59:1937–1943.
88. Cantello R, Riccio A, Gilli M, Delsedime M, Scarzella L, Aguggia M et al. Bornaprine vs placebo in Parkinson disease: double-blind controlled cross-over trial in 30 patients. Ital J Neurol Sci 1986;7(1):139–143.
89. Martin WE, Loewenson RB, Resch JA, Baker AB. A controlled study comparing trihexyphenidyl hydrochloride plus levodopa with placebo plus levodopa in patients with Parkinson's disease. Neurology 1974;24:912–919.

90. Cooper JA, Sagar HJ, Doherty SM, Jordan N, Tidswell P, Sullivan EV. Different effects of dopaminergic and anticholinergic therapies on cognitive and motor function in Parkinson's disease: a follow-up study of untreated patients. Brain 1992;115(Pt 6):1701–1725.
91. Friedman JH, Koller WC, Lannon MC, Busenbark K, Swanson-Hyland E, Smith D. Benztropine versus clozapine for the treatment of tremor in Parkinson's disease. Neurology 1997;48:1077–1081.
92. Schwab RS, England AC, Poskanzer DC, Young RR. Amantadine in the treatment of Parkinson's disease. JAMA 1969;208:1168–1170.
93. Factor SA, Molho ES. Transient benefit of amantadine in Parkinson's disease: the facts about the myth. Mov Disord 1999;14:515–517.
94. Parkes JD, Baxter RC, Marsden CD, Rees JE. Comparative trial of benzhexol, amantadine, and levodopa in the treatment of Parkinson's disease. J Neurol Neurosurg Psychiatry 1974;37:422–426.
95. Walker JE, Albers JW, Tourtellotte WW, Henderson WG, Potvin AR, Smith A. A qualitative and quantitative evaluation of amantadine in the treatment of Parkinson's disease. J Chronic Dis 1972; 25:149–182.
96. Shulman LM, Minagar A, Rabinstein A, Weiner WJ. The use of dopamine agonists in very elderly patients with Parkinson's disease. Mov Disord 2000;15:664–668.
97. Rabey JM, Sagi I, Huberman M, Melamed E, Korczyn A, Giladi N et al. Rasagiline mesylate, a new MAO-B inhibitor for the treatment of Parkinson's disease: a double-blind study as adjunctive therapy to levodopa. Clin Neuropharmacol 2000;23:324–330.
98. Parkinson's Disease Study Group. A randomized placebo-controlled trial of rasagiline in levodopa-treated patients with Parkinson disease and motor fluctuations. Arch Neurol 2005;62:241–248.
99. Poewe WH, Lees AJ, Stern GM. Low-dose L-dopa therapy in Parkinson's disease: a 6-year follow-up study. Neurology 1986;36:1528–1530.
100. Fabbrini G, Mouradian MM, Juncos JL, Schlegel J, Mohr E, Chase TN. Motor fluctuations in Parkinson's disease: central pathophysiological mechanisms: I. Ann Neurol 1988;24:366–371.
101. Horstink MW, Zijlmans JC, Pasman JW et al. Which risk factors predict the levodopa response in fluctuating Parkinson's disease? Ann Neurol 1990;27:537–543.
102. Roos RA, Vredevoogd CB, van der Velde EA. Response fluctuations in Parkinson's disease. Neurology 1990;40:1344–1346.
103. Koller WC, Hutton JT, Tolosa E, Capilldeo R. Immediate-release and controlled-release carbidopa/levodopa in PD: a 5-year randomized multicenter study. Carbidopa/Levodopa Study Group. Neurology 1999;53:1012–1019.
104. Jenner P, Al-Barghouthy G, Smith L, Koupamaki M, Jackson M. Entacapone combined with L-dopa enhances antiparkinsonian activity and avoids dyskinesia in the MPTP-treated primate model of Parkinson's disease. Mov Disord 2002;17(Suppl. 5):S57–58.
105. Sage JI, Trooskin S, Sonsalla PK et al. Experience with continuous enteral levodopa infusions in the treatment of 9 patients with advanced Parkinson's disease. Neurology 1989;39(11 Suppl. 2): 60–63; discussion 72–73.
106. Stocchi F, Ruggieri S, Vacca L, Olanow CW. Prospective randomized trial of lisuride infusion versus oral levodopa in patients with Parkinson's disease. Brain 2002;125:2058–2066.
107. Stocchi F, Vacca L, Berardelli A, Onofrj M, Manfredi M, Ruggieri S. Dual dopamine agonist treatment in Parkinson's disease. J Neurol 2003;250:822–826.
108. Rinne UK, Larsen JP, Siden A, Worm-Petersen J. Entacapone enhances the response to levodopa in parkinsonian patients with motor fluctuations. Nomecomt Study Group. Neurology 1998;51: 1309–1314.
109. Russ H, Muller T, Woitalla D, Rahbar A, Hahn J, Kuhn W. Detection of tolcapone in the cerebrospinal fluid of parkinsonian subjects. Naunyn Schmiedebergs Arch Pharmacol 1999;360: 719–720.
110. Hauser RA, Molho E, Shale H, Pedder S, Dorflinger EE. A pilot evaluation of the tolerability, safety, and efficacy of tolcapone alone and in combination with oral selegiline in untreated Parkinson's disease patients. Tolcapone De Novo Study Group. Mov Disord 1998;13:643–647.
111. Jorga KM. COMT inhibitors: pharmacokinetic and pharmacodynamic comparisons. Clin Neuropharmacol 1998;21(Suppl.):S9–16.
112. Assal F, Spahr L, Hadengue A, Rubbia-Brandt L, Burkhard PR. Tolcapone and fulminant hepatitis. Lancet 1998;352:958.
113. Korlipara LV, Cooper JM, Schapira AH. Differences in toxicity of the catechol-O-methyl transferase inhibitors, tolcapone and entacapone, to cultured human neuroblastoma cells. Neuropharmacology 2004;46:562–569.

114. Tasmar [package insert]. Nutley, NJ: Roche Laboratories Inc., 1998.
115. Marco AD, Appiah-Kubi LS, Chaudhuri KR. Use of the dopamine agonist cabergoline in the treatment of movement disorders. Expert Opin Pharmacother 2002;3:1481–1487.
116. Lhermitte F, Agid Y, Signoret JL. Onset and end-of-dose levodopa-induced dyskinesias. Possible treatment by increasing the daily doses of levodopa. Arch Neurol 1978;35:261–263.
117. Verhagen ML, Del Dotto P, van den MP, Fang J, Mouradian MM, Chase TN. Amantadine as treatment for dyskinesias and motor fluctuations in Parkinson's disease. Neurology 1998;50: 1323–1326.
118. Metman LV, Del Dotto P, van den Munckhof P et al. Amantadine as treatment for dyskinesias and motor fluctuations in Parkinson's disease. Neurology 1998;50:1323–1326.
119. Metman LV, Del Dotto P, LePoole K, Konitsiotis S, Fang J, Chase TN. Amantadine for levodopa-induced dyskinesias: a 1-year follow-up study. Arch Neurol 1999;56:1383–1386.
120. Snow BJ, Macdonald L, Mcauley D, Wallis W. The effect of amantadine on levodopa-induced dyskinesias in Parkinson's disease: a double-blind, placebo-controlled study. Clin Neuropharmacol 2000;23:82–85.
121. Hely MA, Morris JG, Reid WG, Trafficante R. Sydney multicenter study of Parkinson's disease: non-L-dopa-responsive problems dominate at 15 years. Mov Disord 2005;20(2):190–199.
122. Corrigan MH, Denahan AQ, Wright CE, Ragual RJ, Evans DL. Comparison of pramipexole, fluoxetine, and placebo in patients with major depression. Depress Anxiety 2000;11(2):58–65.
123. Rektorova I, Rektor I, Bares M, Dostal V, Ehler E, Fanfrdlova Z et al. Pramipexole and pergolide in the treatment of depression in Parkinson's disease: a national multicentre prospective randomized study. Eur J Neurol 2003;10(4):399–406.
124. Pollak P, Tison F, Rascol O, Destee A, Pere JJ, Senard JM et al. Clozapine in drug induced psychosis in Parkinson's disease: a randomised, placebo controlled study with open follow up. J Neurol Neurosurg Psychiatry 2004;75:689–695.
125. Fernandez HH, Trieschmann ME, Burke MA, Jacques C, Friedman JH. Long-term outcome of quetiapine use for psychosis among Parkinsonian patients. Mov Disord 2003;18:510–514.
126. Mancini F, Tassorelli C, Martignoni E, Moglia A, Nappi G, Cristina S et al. Long-term evaluation of the effect of quetiapine on hallucinations, delusions and motor function in advanced Parkinson disease. Clin Neuropharmacol 2004;27:33–37.
127. Emre M, Aarsland D, Albanese A et al. Rivastigmine for dementia associated with Parkinson's disease. N Engl J Med 2004;351:2509–2518.
128. Jellinger KA. Pathology of Parkinson's disease: changes other than the nigrostriatal pathway. Mol Chem Neuropathol 1991;14:153–197.
129. Lees AJ, Blackburn NA, Campbell VL. The nighttime problems of Parkinson's disease. Clin Neuropharmacol 1988;11:512–519.
130. van Hilten B, Hoff JI, Middelkoop HA, van der Velde EA, Kerkhof GA, Wauquier A et al. Sleep disruption in Parkinson's disease: assessment by continuous activity monitoring. Arch Neurol 1994;51:922–928.
131. Paus S, Brecht HM, Koster J, Seeger G, Klockgether T, Wullner U. Sleep attacks, daytime sleepiness, and dopamine agonists in Parkinson's disease. Mov Disord 2003;18:659–667.
132. Hobson DE, Lang AE, Martin WR, Razmy A, Rivest J, Fleming J. Excessive daytime sleepiness and sudden-onset sleep in Parkinson disease: a survey by the Canadian Movement Disorders Group. JAMA 2002;287:455–463.
133. Happe S, Pirker W, Sauter C, Klosch G, Zeitlhofer J. Successful treatment of excessive daytime sleepiness in Parkinson's disease with modafinil. J Neurol 2001;248:632–634.
134. Basson R. Sex and idiopathic Parkinson's disease. Adv Neurol 2001;86:295–300.
135. Hussain IF, Brady CM, Swinn MJ, Mathias CJ, Fowler CJ. Treatment of erectile dysfunction with sildenafil citrate (Viagra) in parkinsonism due to Parkinson's disease or multiple system atrophy with observations on orthostatic hypotension. J Neurol Neurosurg Psychiatry 2001;71:371–374.
136. Raffaele R, Vecchio I, Giammusso B, Morgia G, Brunetto MB, Rampello L. Efficacy and safety of fixed-dose oral sildenafil in the treatment of sexual dysfunction in depressed patients with idiopathic Parkinson's disease. Eur Urol 2002;41(4):382–386.
137. O'sullivan JD. Apomorphine as an alternative to sildenafil in Parkinson's disease. J Neurol Neurosurg Psychiatry 2002;72:681.
138. Stocchi F, Carbone A, Inghilleri M, Monge A, Ruggieri S, Berardelli A et al. Urodynamic and neurophysiological evaluation in Parkinson's disease and multiple system atrophy. J Neurol Neurosurg Psychiatry 1997;62:507–511.

139. Mancini F, Zangaglia R, Cristina S, Sommaruga MG, Martignoni E, Nappi G et al. Double-blind, placebo-controlled study to evaluate the efficacy and safety of botulinum toxin type A in the treatment of drooling in parkinsonism. Mov Disord 2003;18:685–688.
140. Marsden CD. Problems with long-term levodopa therapy for Parkinson's disease. Clin Neuropharmacol 1994;17(Suppl. 2):S32–44.
141. Rabinstein AA, Shulman LM. Management of behavioral and psychiatric problems in Parkinson's disease. Parkinsonism Relat Disord 2001;7:41–50.
142. Goetz CG, Tanner CM, Levy M, Wilson RS, Garron DC. Pain in Parkinson's disease. Mov Disord 1986;1:45–49.
143. Hillen ME, Sage JI. Nonmotor fluctuations in patients with Parkinson's disease. Neurology 1996;47:1180–1183.

SECTION 3

SURGERY FOR PARKINSON'S DISEASE

7

Ablative Surgery for Parkinson's Disease

Ryan J. Uitti, John D. Putzke, and
Robert E. Wharen, Jr

INTRODUCTION

Ablative surgery for Parkinson's disease (PD) has been the most commonly performed form of surgical treatment for any neurodegenerative disorder. Advances in stereotactic neurosurgical technology, in conjunction with imperfect outcomes despite an expanding battery of pharmacological therapy, led to reemergence in performance of ablative surgery in the 1990s. While other surgical forms of therapy evolved in the late 1990s, ablative treatments continue to have unique characteristics that may make them appropriate therapeutic considerations for selected patients.

HISTORICAL REVIEW

Initial attempts to treat PD and other movement disorders surgically included a wide assortment of anatomic targets. However, ablative procedures such as motor cortex ablation, pedunculotomy, pyramidal tract sectioning of the spinal cord, and extirpation of cerebellar cortex carried with them significant morbidity (hemiparesis) and mortality, as they were carried out through an open surgical approach. Interest in surgical treatment was cultivated by Meyers' report in 1942 that interruption of pallidofugal fibers could modify the rigidity and tremor of PD, and by Cooper's report of improvement in parkinsonian signs and symptoms following ligation of the anterior choroidal artery causing a pallidal infarct (pallidotomy). These and other observations led to further delineation of neuroanatomic targets in the surgical treatment of movement disorders. The first stereotactic surgical treatment of movement disorders were performed in the 1950s and further development in techniques reduced perioperative risks.[1,2] Because of significant successes, thousands of patients were treated surgically for tremor and parkinsonism with ablation of the thalamus or pallidum throughout the 1960s.

Historically, ablative surgery was accomplished through a variety of means. Initially, alcohol injections were employed, followed later by cryocoagulation and finally by radiofrequency-induced thermal lesioning. Additionally, within the past decade some centers have used γ radiation to produce lesions.

Prior to 1967 and the widespread use of levodopa therapy, thalamotomy was the most commonly performed surgery for PD. While the intended target was the thalamus, it is clear that neurosurgeons, without the benefit of modern image-guided stereotaxis, may have inadvertently made lesions in other adjacent structures in the course of usual surgical practice. Some neurosurgeons recognized that PD patients undergoing "thalamotomy" in the early 1960s, who developed several days' worth of contralateral hemi-chorea immediately postoperatively, appeared to have the best surgical outcomes (personal communication, Ross Miller, M.D., Mayo Clinic neurosurgeon). In retrospect, it seems likely that such individuals may have had subthalamotomy lesions placed, as short-lived hemiballismus/chorea is frequently seen in lesioning or stimulation of this nucleus.

Following the advent of levodopa therapy, surgical procedures were infrequently performed in the late 1960s and 1970s. Computed tomography (CT)-guided stereotactic technology developed in the 1980s allowed for more precise lesioning procedures and more patients with tremor-predominant parkinsonism were once again treated with thalamotomy. Tremor was and continues to be the one parkinsonian sign that is typically more amenable to surgical rather than pharmacological management. Laitinen's report published in 1995, describing positive results from pallidotomy, is generally credited with revitalizing interest in performing pallidotomy for PD. He documented benefits following pallidotomy including not only tremor reduction but improvement in other signs of parkinsonism, namely rigidity and bradykinesia.[2] Pallidotomy has been the most common ablative procedure performed for PD since 1990. Thalamotomy has become less frequently performed with the advent of deep brain stimulation therapy aimed at this neuroanatomic target. Recently, some institutions have begun performing subthalamotomy, a topic discussed later in this chapter.

SCIENTIFIC BASIS

Somatotopically arranged thalamo-cortico-basal ganglia circuits have been well described over the past 20 years.[3] Basal ganglia output is centralized through the internal segment of the globus pallidum (GPi), substantia nigra reticulata (SNR), and thalamus before feeding back to the motor and supplementary motor cortices and the dorsal cingulate region. The major output from the basal ganglia (GPi and SNR) is thought to be modulated via "indirect" and "direct" pathways.[4,5] The "direct" pathway involves stimulation from the striata (caudate and putamen) directly to GPi/SNR. Activation of the "direct" pathway typically inhibits GPi neurons, while that of the indirect pathway, via the external segment of the globus pallidus (GPe) and the subthalamic nucleus (STN), stimulates GPi neurons, which in turn influence thalamic output nuclei. The direct pathway purportedly provides positive feedback to precentral motor fields while the indirect pathway provides negative feedback. Primate animal models of PD, using N-methyl-4-phenyl-1,2,3,6-tetrahydropyridine (MPTP)-treated monkeys, demonstrate that dopaminergic cell loss results in increased output from GPi as a result of excessive excitatory input from the subthalamic nucleus.[6] Increased GPi output leads to excessive inhibition of the ventrolateral nucleus of the thalamus, an electrophysiological finding that is associated clinically with bradykinesia.[6] Electrophysiological studies have also detected tremor cells (i.e. neurons firing at a frequency of 4–6 Hz) within GPi[7] and STN[8] in animal models of, and patients with, PD, providing electrophysiological evidence of these structures' role in producing signs of parkinsonism.

Current circuitry diagram models of parkinsonism have struggled to explain some of the paradoxes in clinical outcome from pallidotomy. Specifically, why patients may experience elimination of levodopa-induced dyskinesia and improvement in akinesia and bradykinesia are not easily explained by most physiological models.[9] Thus, electrophysiological models continue to be modified with ongoing observations.

Recent observations from deep brain stimulation studies[10,11] in PD patients have suggested the presence of at least two functionally distinct zones within GPi. Stimulation of the ventral margin (or marginally inferior to GPi) leads to improvement in rigidity and cessation of levodopa-induced dyskinesia. However, there is also blunting of antiparkinsonian effects of levodopa with such stimulation. In contrast, stimulation of the dorsal margin of GPi or within GPe leads to improvement in bradykinesia and may induce chorea. Our own studies in patients undergoing pallidotomy also confirm this observation.[12] Improvement in bradykinesia, documented with clinical ratings and quantitative reaction time measures,[13,14] following pallidotomy may stem from removal of excessive inhibitory output from the pallidum, allowing improved cortical influence on voluntary movement.[4] In conclusion, there appears to be segregation of pallidofugal fibers from the outer portion of GPi forming the ventral ansa lenticularis and from the inner portion of GPi, forming the dorsal lenticular fasciculus.

Functional imaging studies, with fluorodeoxyglucose–positron emission tomography (FDG–PET), delineate increased cerebral blood flow to the prefrontal and supplementary cortices following pallidotomy, supporting the concept that the pallidothalamic circuitry is important for the modulation of cortically generated movements.[15,16] Additionally, FDG–PET studies in patients with pallidal deep brain stimulation may show increased glucose metabolism in the premotor cortex ipsilateral to stimulation and in the cerebellum bilaterally, suggesting that clinical improvement stems from impact on elements of the cortico-striato-pallido-thalamocortical and cerebello-cortical motor loops.[17,18]

Lesions placed in the subthalamic nucleus, or deep brain stimulation of this nucleus, appears to allow release of inhibition of GPi. In a study employing apomorphine, a quick-acting dopamine agonist with a short half-life that improves parkinsonism and may cause dyskinesia (chorea), neural activity was recorded from both GPi and GPe and from the STN in patients undergoing surgery in this location. The results suggested that dopaminergic agents actby decreasing GPi and STN activity, and increasing GPe activity, and that drug-induced dyskinesias result from a large reduction in GPi firing.[19] Lesions in the subthalamic nuclei of MPTP-treated monkeys result in a reduction of all contralateral parkinsonian symptoms, supporting the concept that has been subsequently documented in PD patients.[5,20,21]

Moreover, studies employing deep brain stimulation in PD have shown the stimulation above and below STN produce functionally similar results in terms of antiparkinsonian effects to STN lesions.[22] These findings suggest that a volume of tissue encompassing the zona incerta, Forel's fields, and the lowermost portion of the anterior thalamus all produce the same functional result.

While the ventrolateral nucleus of the thalamus has been the best-studied target, thalamotomy is now reserved for only tremor-predominant PD patients. The ventrolateral nucleus of the thalamus is divided into the ventralis oralis posterior and ventralis intermedius nuclei. The ventralis intermedius nucleus of the thalamus receives input from somatosensory pathways and deep cerebellar nuclei, and projects to the motor cortex. Electrophysiological oscillations in neuronal activity may be routed through the ventralis intermedius nucleus, resulting in pathological tremor.[23] It is also possible that the ventralis intermedius nucleus itself is the generator of oscillations that drive tremor.[24] Others propose that tremor originates in the globus pallidus, based on the factthat tremor lessens when probes are introduced into the pallidum during pallidotomy.[2]

In summary, current electrophysiological models require further refinement to render a full understanding of why certain procedures, such as thalamotomy and pallidotomy, improve the symptoms of PD, do not cause involuntary movements, and typically reduce drug-induced chorea or dyskinesia.[25]

ABLATION METHODS

Prior to any ablative surgery for PD (thalamotomy, pallidotomy, subthalamotomy) most clinicians will obtain thorough preoperative motor, speech, and neuropsychological assessments in order to document a baseline functioning to facilitate future postoperative comparisons. CT or magnetic resonance (MR) imaging of the brain is obtained prior to (with stereotactic headframe in place) and following the procedure, with postoperative brain imaging being useful to assess for hematoma and edema and to verify lesion placement. Because pallidotomy may result in visual field deficits, pre- and postoperative assessment of visual fields may be useful.[26]

Radiologically guided planning methodology for neurosurgical stereotactic procedures represents the single most important advancement in ablative surgery methodology that has occurred over the past two decades. Stereotaxic surgery was developed to better determine the relationship of the surgical target to nearby structures, which can be visualized radiographically, and then to direct an electrode or other probe, to the target with minimal damage to surrounding structures.[27] The optimal means for targeting continues to be the subject of debate,[28] but it always includes neural imaging guided by integration of CT or MR imaging, with frames for stereotactic surgery, via specially designed computer software (Figure 7.1).[2,29] While MR imaging tends to be preferred, CT imaging can also be used and the only randomized study evaluating this issue found no difference between MR and CT for preoperative localization (in pallidotomy).[30] CT and MR also afford the opportunity to confirm appropriate placement of an ablative lesion postoperatively. Prior to sophisticated CT and MR stereotactic planning programs being available, surgeons depended upon relationships among anatomical landmarks defined by ventriculography, brain atlases based on a small number of brains, and clinical and electrophysiological guidance.

Small statistical differences in MR- versus CT-derived targets have been identified and although direct comparison with clinical outcomes have not been made, most institutions have concluded that MR-based target localization is superior to CT.[31] Comparisons of MRI-guided and ventriculography-based stereotactic surgery for PD have concluded that each results in similar clinical outcomes.[32]

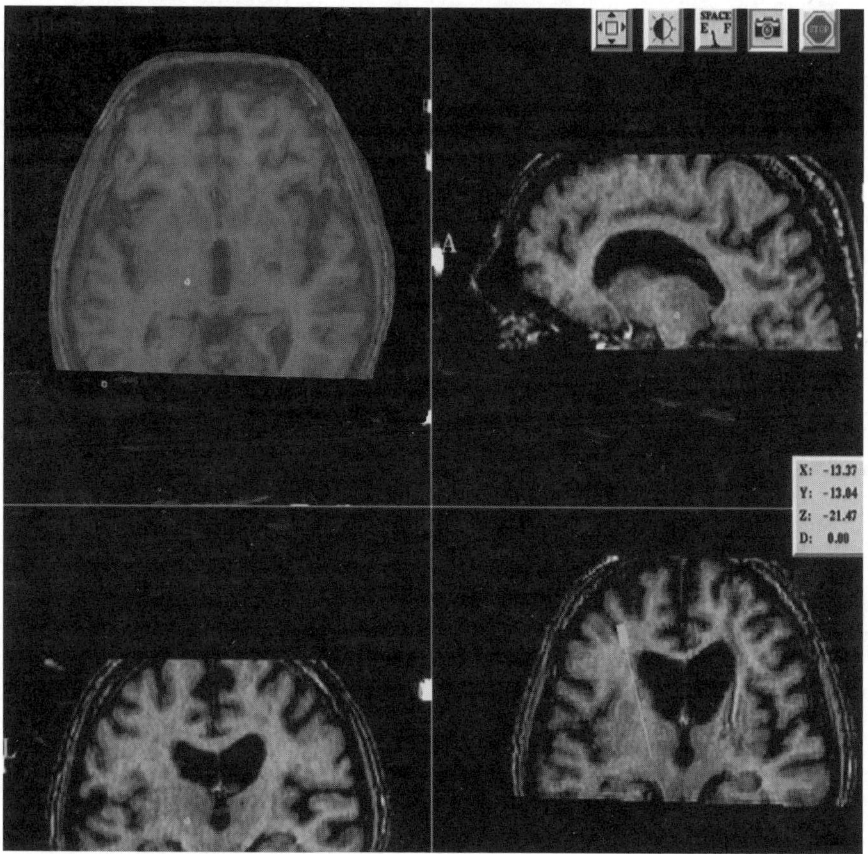

FIGURE 7.1 Stereotactic planning for thalamotomy.

Certain anatomic regions will demonstrate characteristic electrical discharge patterns that help to clarify the precise location of a microelectrode within the brain. There is debate regarding the utility of microelectrode recordings. Most institutions conclude that their own particular method has its advantages. When CT-guided stereotaxis was the only imaging modality employed, many institutions who continue to favor microelectrode recordings found that these studies were very useful in helping to determine the appropriate ablative target. These institutions were reduced to superimposing their electrophysiological findings upon anatomy templates derived from brain atlases rather than imaging from their own patient. Electrophysiological recordings obtained from microelectrodes placed at the radiological target may confirm the presence of characteristic neuronal activity for a particular target. For example, patients with disabling tremor may have "tremor cells" within the ventrointermediate (VIM) nucleus, that discharge coincident with clinical tremor.

Pallidotomy and thalamotomy lesions are made using stereotactic radiofrequency ablation, often following electrophysiologic recordings, and stimulation procedures.[33] It has been determined that electrophysiologic recording typically leads to final placement of lesions posterior and lateral to targets chosen by MRI (2–3 mm in mediolateral and anterior–posterior coordinates), with the actual lesion overlapping the MR theoretical target in 40–50% of patients.[34] Experienced centers using MR and microelectrode recordings typically require only one or two trajectories for performance of pallidotomy.[35] Occasionally, deep brain stimulation electrodes are employed in the process of directly making lesions.[36]

With improved MR-guided stereotaxis, the ability to identify a particular anatomic target has improved dramatically, lessening the necessity for microelectrode recordings in some targets, particularly the VIM thalamus. Improved anatomical targeting has resulted in reduced number of microelectrode recording tracks required and this may correlate with fewer adverse effects and reduced operating time.

In performing a thalamotomy, a monopolar microelectrode (or array of electrodes) is advanced through a burrhole to identify somatotopy in the thalamic somatosensory nucleus, ventralis posterior (Figure 7.2). Moving anteriorly to sensory recordings made following tactile stimulation of the contralateral hand or face leads to stimulation of the ventralis intermedius nucleus, which has a characteristic spontaneous discharge coincident with tremor activity.[27] A separate, monopolar, stimulating electrode may subsequently be used, noting tremor suppression once the correct area is reached.[27] The operation is monitored clinically in terms of speech, manual and foot dexterity, sensation, tone, and tremor, and electrically, in response to proprioceptive, kinesthetic, and electrical stimulation of the involved limb.[24,29,37] Once appropriate coordinates are determined, a lesion is made with a semi-microelectrode.[27,37] This electrode is hollow to allow the insertion of a thermocouple device, which uses radiofrequency current to create the lesion with 70–80°C heating for 1 minute at a single or multiple sites along the length of the electrode track.[27]

In performing a pallidotomy, a microelectrode recording probe is introduced through a frontal burrhole and advanced to confirm somatotopic localization within GPi, which has been previously targeted with stereotactic information

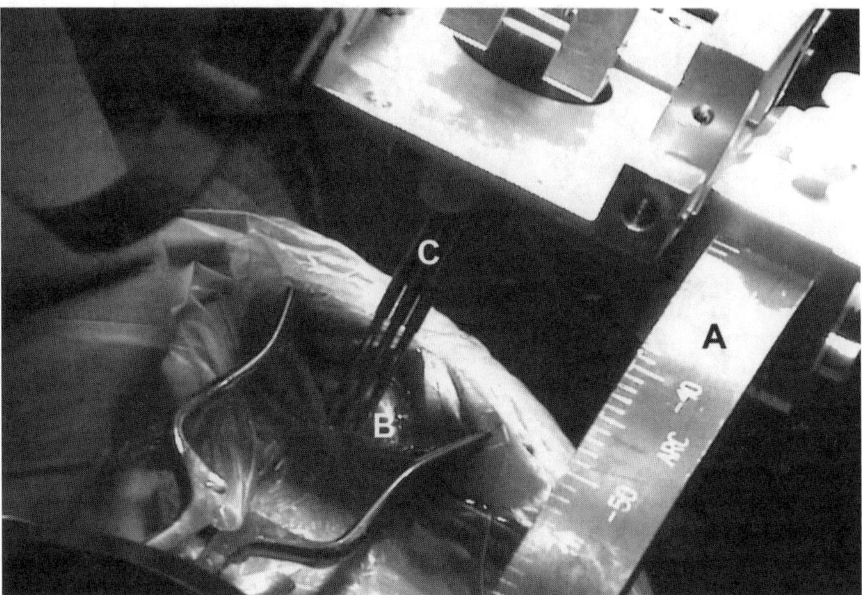

FIGURE 7.2 Surgical field showing: (A) stereotactic headframe, (B) burrhole, (C) three-cannulae for microelectrode recording/lesioning electrode placement.

from CT or MR imaging.[2,26] Single-cell electrical recording is performed using tungsten-tip, disposable microelectrodes, and analyzed for responses during passive and active movement.[33] Electrical stimulation prior to lesioning is performed, to prevent injury to the internal capsule and optic tracts adjacent to the globus pallidus interna.[33] Specific clinical signs have also been described that may occur and influence targeting decisions during surgery. For example, authors have reported a patient who had marked, sustained, contraversive eye deviation by stimulation during pallidal surgery. The authors suggest that this occurred as a result of excitation of internal capsular fiber by volume conducted current spread. Such conjugate eye deviation therefore may not necessarily indicate incorrect electrode placement.[38] If electrical stimulation does not result in weakness or visual field loss, a lesion is made.[2] The probe is then withdrawn several millimeters, with repeated lesioning, creating a three-dimensional lesion (Figure 7.3).[2,26] This is performed based on clinical response measured in the contralateral hemibody (i.e. reduction in parkinsonian signs). Some believe that bilateral pallidotomy can be safely done during the same procedure, and that the localization information from the first lesion is helpful in determining that of the second.[39] However, most centers favor performing only unilateral pallidotomy. Visual evoked potentials to photic stimulation of the eyes intraoperatively during pallidotomy are believed by some to facilitate the accuracy of the determination of the globus pallidus interna.[40,41] A consensus statement regarding pallidotomy has been reported suggesting, among other conclusions, that

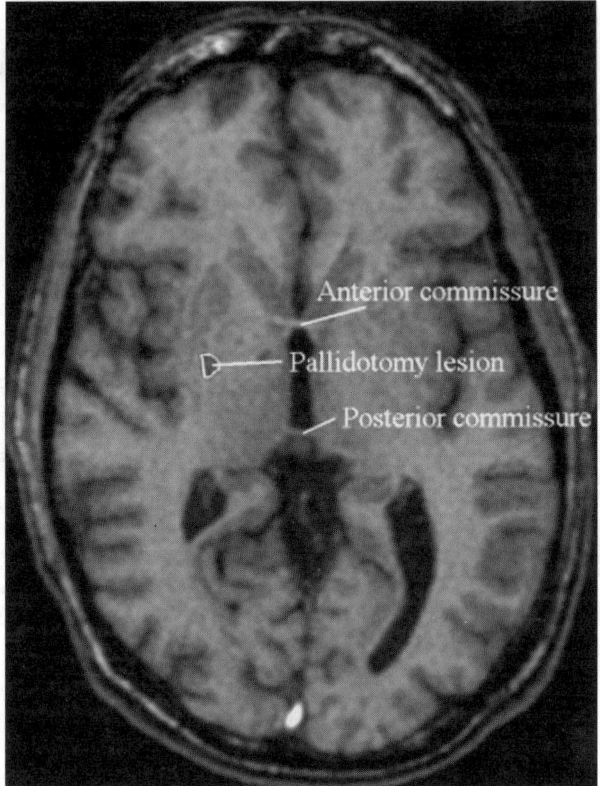

FIGURE 7.3 MRI showing pallidotomy lesion (outlined).

pallidotomy should be performed only at centers where a dedicated team of physicians has compiled substantial experience in the field.[42]

Microelectrode recordings in the subthalamic nucleus suggest a somatotopic arrangement that may aid in electrode placement.[43] Lesions of the subthalamic nucleus could be created in a similar fashion to those in pallidotomy and thalamotomy, but these lesions are considered technically more difficult because neuroimaging techniques are less able to localize this target. While lesioning of the subthalamic nucleus may cause hemiballismus and chorea, this is uncommon. Stimulation of STN is routinely performed in European and North American centers and offers significant advantage in allowing the possibility of performing a bilateral procedure due to the relative lack of risk of irreversible dysphonia. The actual risk for bilateral subthalamotomy producing dysphonia is unknown as most reported series include small numbers of patients.

Issues still debated regarding ablative surgery methodology include the need for microelectrode recording,[33,44–46] the number of lesions and lesion size, and the wisdom of making bilateral lesions. In a survey of 28 centers performing pallidotomy in North America, most centers were using MRI alone (50%) or with CT ($n = 6$) to localize the target. The median values of pallidal coordinates were stated as: 2 mm anterior to the midcommissural point, 21 mm lateral to the midsagittal plane, and 5 mm below the intercommissural line, with a total of three permanent lesions placed 2 mm apart. According to the survey, lesions are typically made employing a median temperature of 75°C for 1 minute. Microelectrode recording was performed by 50% of the centers surveyed, with the main target defining criteria being (1) the firing pattern of spontaneous neuronal discharge, and (2) the response to passive manipulation of a limb. Proponents for microelectrode recordings indicate that such recordings altered the final target in almost every instance, one of nine targets being more than 4 mm from the image-guided site.[35] Motor and visual evaluations were also performed intraoperatively.[47] Other studies have concluded that thalamotomy and pallidotomy have comparable accuracy, judging by postoperative multiplanar MRI data collected.[48]

Microvascular Doppler evaluation, performed in order to identify intracerebral vessels in proximity to targets for thermocoagulation (in thalamotomy or pallidotomy), has been described as a means to minimize risk of vascular injury. A prominent vascular sound was identified in 3 of 13 cases in one series.[49] It is unclear whether use of this technique significantly impacts on safety in these lesioning operations.

The effects of intravenous anesthesia with propofol on intraoperative electrophysiologic monitoring were studied in patients during pallidotomy and thalamotomy. Infusion of this agent may need to be reduced to detect neural noise levels required for targeting in some patients, but generally serves as a useful anesthetic agent for electrophysiological monitoring during functional neurosurgery.[50]

Gamma knife thalamotomy has been reported using stereotactic guidance.[51–53] Ohye and colleagues used 140–150 Gy and 4-mm collimators.[51] Pan and colleagues have used slightly higher doses of radiation (160–180 Gy maximum dose), also with 4-mm collimators.[52] Because of the delay in response and relative unpredictability of radiation lesions, most specialists suggest other modes of surgical treatment be used in most instances.[54]

INDICATIONS FOR ABLATIVE SURGERY

The goal of surgical treatment of movement disorders is amelioration or relief of this disorder with improvement in functional capacity. Consequently, patients considering ablative surgery must have significant limitations in functional capacities to justify the risks associated with an irreversible ablative surgical procedure. The specific definition of significant limitation will vary between patients. Most patients desire surgery when they find that more than half of their waking hours are dysfunctional, despite the optimization of pharmacological therapy. Patients who are incapacitated for a majority of their day usually believe that the risks associated with ablative surgery, generally reported to be around 2% for significant adverse effects, are worth taking in the context of potential surgical benefit. The main adverse effects with ablative surgery consist of death and hemiparesis from hemorrhage deep within basal ganglia structures. Other potential adverse effects include visual field deficits, sensory deficits, diplopia, and dysarthria.

Ablation surgery has generally targeted the sensorimotor portions of the thalamus, VIM nucleus, pallidum – internal (GPi) and external (GPe) – and the STN. A single optimal surgical target remains a subject of debate and is probably best determined on a case-by-case basis. Studies published in the past several years have focused on the optimal location and size of permanent lesions as they relate to minimizing movement disorder symptoms and signs and potential ill effects.

Is one surgical approach clearly superior to another? This question has no simple answer. Theoretically, a surgical procedure such as grafting or neural growth therapy that might lead to restitution of basal ganglia neurons and their neural connections would probably be ideal. Deep brain stimulation procedures have the advantage of apparent reversibility. The true long-term repercussions of deep brain stimulation and ablative lesioning surgery are not precisely known. If ablative surgery produced a solely predictable and beneficial long-term response one might be able to justify this surgery as being superior to deep brain stimulation that necessarily will require upkeep, at the very least, with sequential pulse generator placements over time, and ongoing minimal risks associated with a permanently implanted device.

Having discussed the limitations of interpretation of outcome for ablative surgery relative to medical or other forms of surgical treatment, it is clear that developing rigid guidelines for selection of patients for ablative surgery is unwise. There are patients who clearly may benefit from ablative surgery and perhaps many more who might benefit. The discussion that follows will initially focus upon scenarios where ablative surgery is clearly indicated. Thereafter, we will suggest other instances where ablative surgery could be considered, particularly in light of the lack of valid comparative data.

Persuasive arguments can be made that ablative surgery can be performed with minimal risk when such surgery is restricted to unilateral use. With improved MR and electrophysiological guidance, the number of patients experiencing unexpected side-effects with ablative surgery is acceptably low. However, bilateral ablative surgery focused upon any target, as it is routinely performed today, carries with it unavoidable potential adverse effects. We believe that there may be methods for further safeguarding ablative surgery in order to limit otherwise unanticipated irreversible side-effects. We have actually performed staged bilateral thalamotomies in an HIV-positive individual who had disabling essential tremor and in whom AIDS had not yet developed. The thalamotomy lesioning process was guided by initial placement of a deep brain stimulation electrode, employed as a macroelectrode. Having found the precise site where the smallest amount of stimulation led to complete resolution of contralateral tremor, we subsequently placed a lesioning electrode into the same location and produced a thalamotomy. Using the same method, this time paying close attention to the possibility of speech difficulties being produced while stimulating through the deep brain stimulation electrode, we were able to determine a small region where stimulation produced complete resolution of contralateral tremor without any disruption of speech or production of other side-effects. Subsequent lesioning at this location with a radiofrequency lesioning electrode produced an excellent result with complete resolution in tremor bilaterally with no adverse effects. Such practices have not been carried out in a large number of patients and therefore we can only speculate on how useful this may be. It is conceivable that patients might be best treated with initial ablative surgeries with deep brain stimulation or other modalities being applied in the context of symptomatic disease progression that outstrips the ablative surgery's therapeutic scope.

Today, ablative surgery represents the surgical option for which the least amount of ongoing adjustments in treatment is anticipated. For example, following ablative surgery most patients can begin taking a stable amount of antiparkinsonian medication with relatively predictable effects (improvement in the cardinal signs of parkinsonism and reduction in levodopa-induced dyskinesia). This is in clear contrast to patients who are treated with deep brain stimulation and transplantation in whom one would expect to necessarily reduce amounts of antiparkinsonian medication. Hence, patients who are incapable of assisting in modification of their treatment regimens or who are, for other logistical reasons, unable to return for neurological follow-up on a regular basis should be considered for ablative surgery. This group would include patients who are intellectually challenged and unable to communicate potential side-effects from deep brain stimulation for example. Additionally, patients in whom an implanted electrical device is contraindicated would potentially be ablative surgery candidates. This would include patients with deep brain stimulators that have become infected with ongoing skin breakdown that precludes further implantations due to potential risk of further infections. We have had several such patients in our clinic with this type of problem. Other patients with immune disorders that escalate the risk for infection would also be included in this group. For example, we have chosen to use ablative surgery over deep brain stimulation in patients with HIV (with or without AIDS) in whom the eventual risk for infection of an implanted brain device is increased. Other patients in whom ablative surgery is indicated would include patients with a long-standing stable amount of parkinsonism – for example, the 50-year old patient who has a 10-year history of tremor-predominant parkinsonism with unilateral hand tremor that proves disabling. Such a patient may enjoy excellent benefits from a unilateral ablative operation (thalamotomy, pallidotomy, or subthalamotomy) without the prospects of requiring multiple pulse generators and/or brain electrodes requiring replacement (Table 7.1).

Other Circumstances for Considering Ablative Surgery

At the present time, deep brain stimulation is necessarily limited to influencing a volume of tissue that is linearly related to the long axis of the deep brain stimulation electrode. Consequently, the "reversible lesion" or scope of influence of deep brain stimulation is limited to the tissue immediately adjacent to each electrode employed at the angle of introduction. At present, very few patients have more than a single electrode in one side of the brain. In contrast, ablative surgery can be performed along multiple tracks and consequently can produce lesions with greater volume and irregularity of shape. This may be important as some patients may have neuronal distributions that are more loosely organized within nuclear target regions. Additionally, some targets, such as the internal segment of the pallidum, have been shown to be large enough to have regions

TABLE 7.1 Patients in whom ablative surgery is indicated

Indication	*Comments*
Relatively isolated, disabling tremor Stable and incompletely responsive to medical therapy	For example, long-standing, disabling unilateral tremor – sole parkinsonian sign that is more amenable to surgical therapy than pharmacological
Deep brain stimulation contraindicated	Cannot return for follow-up; previous DBS infection: high risk for skin, brain, device infection
Cognitive difficulties	Patients in whom it may be impossible to determine all side-effects from deep brain stimulation
Parkinsonism is incompletely influenced by deep brain stimulation	Larger tissue volume/multiple tracks are required to produce significant improvement
Disabling dyskinesia following transplantation surgery	"Runaway" dyskinesia may infrequently occur, usually years following transplantation

that are functionally distinct. For example, deep brain stimulation studies[10,11] have led to the conclusion that there are at least two functional zones within the internal segment of the globus pallidus that may explain some of the paradoxes of outcome from pallidotomy (e.g. elimination of levodopa-induced dyskinesia with improvement of akinesia) as discussed early under "Scientific Basis." Clearly, while pallidotomy with multiple lesioning tracks can influence all regions within the GPi, a single deep brain stimulation electrode may not have this ability.

Speculatively, ablation surgery may be successfully combined with other forms of surgical therapy. While no prospective studies have evaluated such a design, it may be a reasonable consideration. For example, patients with predominantly unilateral parkinsonian signs could be treated initially with contralateral pallidotomy or subthalamotomy. At a later date, if contralateral parkinsonism develops and progresses, a second-sided surgery with deep brain stimulation could be undertaken. The deep brain stimulation surgery could be performed with less risk for producing irreversible side-effects, including dysarthria, than would be expected with bilateral ablative surgery. This type of surgical plan would most likely be considered employing the same target on each side of the brain. Using mixed targets, such as GPi and STN, might produce problems regarding concurrent antiparkinsonian medication use. Whereas influencing the GPi typically requires similar postoperative antiparkinsonian medication use, the same amount of medications in a patient with STN surgery would often produce disabling levodopa-induced dyskinesia. Hence, mixing surgical targets with ablative and DBS surgery might prove problematic. However, there may be scenarios where this is actually advisable depending upon the clinical aspects of a given patient. There are also instances where patients with transplantation therapy may require subsequent ablative surgery. This has taken place in the context of patients developing progressively more severe dyskinesia years after striatal transplantation of fetal tissues. Pallidal ablative surgery has led to resolution of disabling dyskinesia in this context.

CLINICAL CONSIDERATIONS REGARDING SPECIFIC ANATOMIC TARGETS OF ABLATIVE SURGERY

Pallidotomy is typically considered in patients with Parkinson's disease who have failed traditional pharmacotherapy and are suffering from severe motor fluctuations. Specifically, these patients are experiencing intolerable "off" periods when untreated parkinsonian signs are readily apparent and at other times significant drug-induced dyskinesia. Advanced age had been a relative contraindication, but one series indicated similar efficacy and safety in elderly versus younger patients undergoing unilateral, MR-microelectrode guided pallidotomy.[55] Results of pallidotomy done for atypical parkinsonism have not been encouraging, and therefore a responsiveness to levodopa should be demonstrated. Occasionally, patients with parkinsonism caused by other insults, such as hypoxic encephalopathy, have received benefit from pallidotomy.[56] In a survey of 28 centers who have performed 1219 pallidotomies for Parkinson's disease in 1015 patients, the best indication for pallidotomy was dyskinesia; good indications were listed as "on"/"off" fluctuations, dystonia, rigidity, and bradykinesis; and fair indications as freezing, tremor, and gait disturbance.[47] Speech disorders and postural instability typically do not respond to surgery and should not be thought of as indicators for surgery. Most institutions report that bilateral pallidotomy (and bilateral thalamotomy) should be avoided because of the risk of producing severe dysphonia. Pallidotomy has also been occasionally performed for treatment of pain associated with parkinsonism.[57,58]

Thalamotomy (ventral intermedial nucleus of the thalamus) should be considered in patients with severe unilateral or markedly asymmetric essential parkinsonian, or cerebellar tremor resulting in serious disability that is unresponsive to adequate trials of medications.[23,37] Similar to traditional thalamotomy, treatment with gamma knife lesioning has been performed for patients with activation tremor and tremor due to PD who are unable to tolerate standard neurosurgical procedures.[51–53]

Subthalamotomy is also reported to produce benefit in PD patients with minimal risk for hemiballismus. This treatment has been generally tried in patients in whom deep brain stimulation is not an option.[59]

As with any elective surgical procedure, significant medical and psychiatric illness is usually a contraindication to the surgical treatment of movement disorders. (Selected medically brittle patients may undergo gamma knife operations despite their higher risk for postoperative sequelae from slightly misplaced lesions.) Previous stroke or extensive intracranial lesions are a relative contraindication to pallidotomy, thalamotomy, transplantation, and thalamic stimulation, because of the difficulty in accurately determining the site of the lesion.[29] Dementia is considered a contraindication to these procedures at most centers, and preoperative neuropsychometric testing should be done.[60] Pallidotomy and thalamotomy can result in postoperative dysarthria and dysphagia, especially when performed bilaterally. Therefore, significant abnormalities of speech and swallowing are relative contraindications, although specific guidelines may vary between centers.[29]

OUTCOMES FOLLOWING ABLATIVE SURGERY

How does ablative surgery for Parkinson's disease compare with other surgical or medical treatment options? This is a difficult question to address because of a paucity of long-term data concerning any form of therapy, much less randomized comparisons between different modalities. There are no long-term randomized trials of surgical versus medical treatments, or surgery X versus surgery Y treatment. Surgical series are also particularly prone to problematic interpretation because of selection and follow-up bias. Both selection and follow-up may be more easily attained in patients who are doing well or require further manipulations in treatment. Because of the difficulties in assessing potential selection bias for both inclusion and ongoing data collection, it is difficult to interpret the true long-term efficacy of this therapy.

In considering the results of studies relating to the surgical treatment of movement disorders, it is important to keep in mind that most are not blinded or controlled, nor do they have the benefit of long follow-up. Patients are often highly selected and outcome measures are not standardized. Some reports use vague terms such as "improved," "excellent," or "good," which do not always give a clear indication of outcome and do not allow for clear comparison of outcome between studies.

Pallidotomy

Pallidotomy appears to be an effective treatment, but not a cure, for Parkinson's disease. A number of well-documented, systematic series have reported efficacy of pallidotomy in improving motor functioning.[55,61–64] Contralateral tremor, rigidity, and bradykinesia are all improved significantly in the "off" state, typically on the order of 25–35% reductions in standard motor functioning scales (Unified Parkinson's Disease Rating Scale). In general, parkinsonian signs that do not respond beneficially to levodopa also fail to improve significantly with pallidotomy. A recently published randomized study also reported that positive effects of unilateral pallidotomy were stable up to 1 year after surgery and patients taking lower amounts of daily levodopa were most likely to improve.[64]

The most striking functional improvements for patients are related to increases in time spent during the day with good motor function, usually because of pronounced reductions in levodopa-induced dyskinesia.[65] Motor, physical, and social functioning and vitality measures on the Medical Outcome scale all improved in a 15-patient series with 1-year follow-up.[61] Comparison at 1-year follow-up between groups who did and did not (for financial reasons) have pallidotomy show significant benefit for surgical patients in motor status.[66] Some have found that pallidotomy also improves balance and ambulation, [67] but these improvements are far from universally observed.[68] Pallidotomy may not be as effective for the relief of tremor as thalamotomy but does affect that symptom to some degree.[26] In 44 patients with parkinsonian tremor treated with pallidotomy, two-thirds of those with severe tremor had at least 50% improvement, and better tremor control was found when tremor synchronous cells, as noted on microelectrode recording, were included in the lesion.[69] Pallidotomy may also significantly improve quality-of-life measures in PD patients.[70]

Bilateral pallidotomy is associated with abolition of dyskinesias, reduced "off" time, and improved activities in daily living one[71] and two[72] years postoperatively. It may also be associated with an increase in walking speed postoperatively.[73]

A recent review of 263 articles regarding radiofrequency pallidotomy in 1959 PD patients treated at 40 centers in 12 countries concluded that there were consistent benefits for "off" period motor function and "on" period, drug-induced dyskinesias. The magnitude of benefit was generally a 45% improvement in UPDRS motor scoring during "off" periods and 85% improvement in contralateral dyskinesia during "on" periods. The overall mortality rate was 0.4%, with major adverse events occurring in 5% of patients reported.[74] Long-term (3–5 years) follow-up after pallidotomy discloses persistent improvements in "off" state contralateral signs and "on" period contralateral dystonia.[75]

Some studies evaluating size and location of pallidal (and thalamic) lesions produced at surgery indicate that akinetic effects correlated with larger lesion volumes while antidyskinetic/dystonic and tremor effects were pronounced and unrelated to size of lesion. The average lesion size varies between 100 and 200 cubic millimeters when measured on MRI within the first week after surgery. The most posterior ventral pallidal lesions had the greatest positive effects on akinesia,[76] while anteromedial and central lesions were more predictably associated with improvements in postural instability, gait, and reduced dyskinesia.[77] Variability in lesion location speaks to the importance of clinical and physiological corroboration for correct lesion placement.[77]

While most centers do not routinely perform bilateral pallidotomy for PD, one report of 11 patients indicated that walking speed improved by 2-fold with bilateral surgery.[73] Antiparkinsonian medication requirements are generally not changed (with some patients taking more levodopa postoperatively because of ablation of levodopa-induced dyskinesia). The effect of levodopa on parkinsonian signs is maintained in most patients following pallidotomy,[78] and most patients experience a widening in the therapeutic window associated with this medication due to reduction of levodopa-induced dyskinesia.[79] The beneficial effect of levodopa on cognitive "on"/"off" fluctuations may be curtailed following pallidotomy.[80] Finally, studies have demonstrated weight gain following pallidotomy, with findings suggesting changes in underlying homeostasis associated with Parkinson's disease rather than secondary changes.[81]

A study of quality-of-life measures concerning ablative surgery (unilateral thalamotomy, unilateral or bilateral pallidotomy, and subthalamotomy) has been performed. This study suggested that quality-of-life measures improve significantly, particularly in those patients with unilateral[82] and bilateral[83] pallidotomy.

Thalamotomy

Thalamotomy provides relief of rest tremor in about 80–90% of patients treated for Parkinson's disease.[27,60] Kelly and colleagues found complete abolition of contralateral upper-extremity rest tremor in 10 of 12 patients with PD treated with thalamotomy.[37] Recent series report complete or nearly complete resolution of tremor in over 70% of patients undergoing VIM thalamotomy.[84,85] The procedure is not without risk; one recent thalamotomy series reported permanent hemiparesis and speech difficulties in 6 of 37 patients.[84] Pollack and colleagues reported improvement of disability due to tremor in five PD patients and two patients with tremor due to other causes and state that the improvement is comparable to that reported in other forms of surgery for these disorders.[53] PET studies following thalamotomy for tremor-predominant PD have shown decreased activation of the left sensorimotor cortex, lateral premotor cortex, and parietal area 7 on hand movement, in conjunction with tremor relief.[86]

Lesioning volumes for thalamotomy and pallidotomy have been measured with MRI and found to be smaller in thalamotomies when measured with T1-weighted images and similar when comparisons were based on T2-weighted images. However, different techniques were used in separating discrete lesions along lesioning tracts between the two procedures.[87] Effective lesion volumes appear to be smaller in thalamotomy than pallidotomy. However, some have reported that the effects of thalamotomy are unrelated to lesion volume.[76]

Ohye and colleagues performed gamma knife thalamotomy on six patients with tremor secondary to PD, one patient with intention tremor not otherwise specified by the authors, and one patient with essential tremor.[51] Over a period of 5 months to 1 year, tremor improved.[51] Pan and colleagues performed gamma knife thalamotomy on a total of eight patients with medically refractory parkinsonian tremor.[52] They found that in the six patients available for follow-up at a mean of 4.5 months, tremor disappeared in three and improved in the other three, while rigidity improved in four cases. Unilateral subthalamotomy carried out with semimicroelectrode recordings may produce significant motor benefit without dyskinesia or hemiballismus.[59]

ADVERSE EFFECTS

Overall mortality with thalamotomy has been reported at 0.3% or less when performed for essential tremor.[23] There is an associated 1% mortality, 25% transient morbidity, and 8% permanent morbidity when the procedure is undertaken for Parkinson's disease.[60] Mortality typically is due to hemorrhage at the thalamotomy site.[29] Potential morbidity includes intellectual deficits, hemiparesis, seizures, other involuntary movements, and deterioration of speech, especially with bilateral thalamotomy.[24, 88] With bilateral thalamotomy, there is an estimated risk of 20% or more of severe speech impairment.[88] In a study of eight patients who underwent nine thalamotomies, patients who experienced persistent deficits were older that 65 years, or had undergone bilateral thalamotomies.[85] Kelly and colleagues found no persistent major deficits in 12 patients who underwent thalamotomy, although one was confused for several weeks postoperatively, two had mild cognitive deficits on neuropsychometric testing postoperatively, and one had mild hyperreflexia and distal extensor weakness contralateral to thalamotomy.[37] Two of 12 patients had complications related to ventriculography done for preoperative evaluation, a seizure in one, and dysphasia and confusion for several weeks in another.[37]

Pallidotomy appears to be similar in risk to other stereotactic intracranial procedures. In a review of 259 cases of unilateral pallidotomy, bilateral pallidotomy, or pallidotomy combined with thalamotomy, the most common complication was scotoma in the visual field, contralateral to the procedure, occurring in 4% of patients.[2] Studies employing Goldmann visual testing in patients who had microelectrode-guided pallidotomy detect visual field defects in approximately 7.5% of patients.[89] Other complications included dysphagia, stroke, seizure secondary to edema, and foot apraxia.[2] A separate study described no significant perioperative morbidity or mortality in 18 PD patients who underwent ventral pallidotomy; however, one patient was sexually disinhibited for 24 hours after surgery, and another patient suffered a stroke 7 months after the procedure.[26]

However, significant variability in adverse events has been reported with pallidotomy. Shannon and colleagues reported one death and seven other serious complications in 26 patients.[90] Samuel and colleagues reported two deaths and four major complications in 26 patients.[63] Hariz and De Salles reported no deaths and only six major complications in 152 consecutive pallidotomies.[91] Iacono and colleagues described an overall complication rate of 6.3% and a permanent complication rate of 3.2% in 126 patients treated for PD with unilateral or bilateral pallidotomy.[39] Complications included both permanent and transient hemianopsia, transient hemiparesis unrelated to hemorrhage, intracranial abscess, subcortical hematoma, and intrapallidal hemorrhage. Curiously, there was not a significant increased complication rate among those who underwent bilateral rather than unilateral procedures.[39] One center has reported delayed (10–117 days following surgery) internal capsule infarctions following pallidotomy; MR studies in these individuals showed lesions extended into the posterior limb of the internal capsule ipsilateral to the pallidotomy.[92]

Neuropsychological measures remain largely unchanged following unilateral pallidotomy or pallidal stimulation, apart from mild reductions in verbal fluency in dominant-hemisphere operations.[55,93–98] Mild impairments in speech intelligibility also occur in 30% of patients undergoing unilateral pallidotomy,[99] although some studies suggest that occasional patients may demonstrate some improvements in acoustic measures.[100] While pallidotomy generally improves motor function in PD, eye movements, specifically internally mediated saccades, tend to be more impaired, albeit subclinically, following surgery.[101]

No adverse effects were noted in eight patients who underwent gamma knife thalamotomy in one series,[51] and other series also report good safety and long-term efficacy.[102,103] However, in a separate series, one patient out of six available for follow-up at a mean of 4.5 months following gamma knife thalamotomy suffered contralateral hemiparesis and was noted to have a larger lesion than intended and edema in the thalamus.[52] There have been other reports of gamma knife pallidotomy resulting in permanent contralateral homonymous hemianopsia.[104]

PROGNOSIS FOLLOWING ABLATIVE SURGERY

Because poorer surgical outcomes may be more likely lost to follow-up and consequently are less likely to be reported, it is worthwhile to maintain a somewhat cautious view of long-term follow-up data of the surgical treatment of movement disorders. Furthermore, adequately controlled trials are lacking regarding most of these treatments, and most studies cited have been retrospective.

It is debated whether or not stereotactic surgery can affect the course of Parkinson's disease. Some authors assert that pallidotomy slows the progression of PD.[2,105] However, a 10-year follow-up study by Kelly and Gillingham suggests that stereotactic surgical procedures do not slow the progression of the disease.[106] Studies of motor outcome 4–5 years following unilateral pallidotomy indicated that patients continued to have reduced levodopa-induced dyskinesia, contralateral to surgery, but that other improvements had returned to preoperative baseline.[75,107] Patient self-assessment surveys continued to suggest improved quality of life compared to preoperative status.[107] Prognosis following electrophysiologically guided versus non-microelectrode-guided unilateral pallidotomy appears to be similar.[108]

A follow-up series of PD patients at least 10 years following unilateral ventrolateral nucleus thalamotomy revealed no progression in 31 of 64 patients.[109] Of 22 patients who underwent bilateral surgery, 15 patients showed no progression.[109] That the benefit of thalamotomy can be sustained is further supported by a follow-up study 3.25–10 years after ventralis intermedius nucleus thalamotomy for PD or essential tremor.[110] It was found that in the patients with PD, 10 of 14 had complete abolition of the tremor, three had residual tremor, and one underwent reoperation.[110] In that same study, 6 of 11 essential tremor patients had complete relief of their tremor, four had slight residual tremors, and one underwent reoperation.[110] In another study, of 28 PD patients examined 2 years after intermedius nucleus thalamotomy, 85% had sustained improvement in contralateral tremor.[29] There was deterioration of speech and locomotion, but this may have been due to the natural progression of the disease.[29]

CONCLUSIONS

Ablative surgery for Parkinson's disease represents a surgical treatment that has a long history characterized by evolutions in technique, understanding, efficacy and safety. This type of surgery can produce immediate benefit in patients with PD. Whether other forms of surgery offer significant advantages over ablation remains an unanswered issue. At present, specific ablative surgical procedures continue to be viable considerations for selected patients with the disease.

REFERENCES

1. Gillingham FJ, Watson WS, Donaldson AA, Naughton JAL. The surgical treatment of Parkinsonism. Br Med J 1960;1395–1402.
2. Laitinen LV. Pallidotomy for Parkinson's disease. Neurosurg Clin N Am 1995;6:105–112.
3. Alexander GE, DeLong MR, Strick PL. Parallel organization of functionally segregated circuits linking basal ganglia and cortex. Annu Rev Neurosci 1986;9:357–381.
4. DeLong MR. Primate models of movement disorders of basal ganglia origin. Trends Neurosci 1990;13:281–285.
5. Guridi J, Luquin MR, Herrero MT, Obeso JA. The subthalamic nucleus: a possible target for stereotaxic surgery in Parkinson's disease. Mov Disord 1993;8:421–429.

6. Bakay RA, DeLong MR, Vitek JL. Posteroventral pallidotomy for Parkinson's disease [letter]. J Neurosurg 1992;77:487–488.
7. Lemstra AW, Verhagen Metman L, Lee JI, Dougherty PM, Lenz FA. Tremor-frequency (3–6 Hz) activity in the sensorimotor arm representation of the internal segment of the globus pallidus in patients with Parkinson's disease. Neurosci Lett 1999;267:129–132.
8. Krack P, Benazzouz A, Pollak P et al. Treatment of tremor in Parkinson's disease by subthalamic nucleus stimulation. Mov Disord 1998;13:907–914.
9. Guridi J, Obeso JA. The subthalamic nucleus, hemiballismus and Parkinson's disease: reappraisal of a neurosurgical dogma. Brain 2001;124:5–19.
10. Krack P, Pollak P, Limousin P et al. Subthalamic nucleus or internal pallidal stimulation in young onset Parkinson's disease. Brain 1998;121:451–457.
11. Yelnik J, Damier P, Bejjani BP et al. Functional mapping of the human globus pallidus: contrasting effect of stimulation in the internal and external pallidum in Parkinson's disease. Neuroscience 2000;101:77–87.
12. Uitti RJ, Obwegeser AA, Lucas JA et al. Pallidotomy location and correlations with motor, speech, and neuropsychological outcomes [abstract]. Mov Disord 2000;15:1039.
13. Jankovic J, Ben-Arie L, Schwartz K et al. Movement and reaction times and fine coordination tasks following pallidotomy. Mov Disord 1999;14:57–62.
14. Uitti RJ, Wharen RE, Duffy JR et al. Unilateral pallidotomy for Parkinson's disease: speech, motor, and neuropsychological outcome measurements. Parkinsonism Rel Disord 2000;6:133–143.
15. Eidelberg D, Moeller JR, Kazumata K et al. Metabolic correlates of pallidal neuronal activity in Parkinson's disease. Brain 1997;120:1315–1324.
16. Samuel M, Ceballos-Baumann AO, Turjanski N et al. Pallidotomy in Parkinson's disease increases supplementary motor area and prefrontal activation during performance of volitional movements an $H_2(15)O$ PET study. Brain 1997;120:1301–1313.
17. Fukuda M, Mentis MJ, Ma Y et al. Networks mediating the clinical effects of pallidal brain stimulation for Parkinson's disease: a PET study of resting-state glucose metabolism. Brain 2001;124:1601–1609.
18. Fukuda M, Mentis M, Ghilardi MF et al. Functional correlates of pallidal stimulation for Parkinson's disease. Ann Neurol 2001;49:155–164.
19. Lozano AM, Lang AE, Levy R, Hutchison W, Dostrovsky J. Neuronal recordings in Parkinson's disease patients with dyskinesias induced by apomorphine. Ann Neurol 2000;47:s141–146.
20. Bergman H, Wichmann T, DeLong MR. Reversal of experimental parkinsonism by lesions of the subthalamic nucleus. Science 1990;249:1436–1438.
21. Limousin P, Pollak P, Benazzouz A et al. Effect of parkinsonian signs and symptoms of bilateral subthalamic nucleus stimulation. Lancet 1995;345:91–95.
22. Zincone A, Landi A, Piolti R et al. Physiologic study of the subthalamic volume. Neurol Sci 2001;22:111–112.
23. Elble RJ, Koller WC. Tremor. Baltimore: Johns Hopkins University Press, 1990.
24. Narabayashi H. Stereotaxic Vim thalamotomy for treatment of tremor. Eur Neurol 1989;29:29–32.
25. Marsden CD, Obeso JA. The functions of the basal ganglia and the paradox of stereotaxic surgery in Parkinson's disease. Brain 1994;117:877–897.
26. Dogali M, Fazzini E, Kolodny E et al. Stereotactic ventral pallidotomy for Parkinson's disease. Neurology 1995;45:753–761.
27. Andrew J. Surgical treatment of tremor. In: Findley LJ, Capildeo R (eds), Movement Disorders: Tremor. New York: Oxford University Press, 1984, pp. 339–351.
28. Zonenshayn M, Rezai AR, Mogilner AY et al. Comparison of anatomic and neurophysiological methods for subthalamic nucleus targeting. Neurosurgery 2000;47:282–292; discussion 292–284.
29. Tasker RR. Thalamotomy. Neurosurg Clin N Am 1990;1:841–864.
30. Honey CR, Nugent RA. A prospective randomized comparison of CT and MRI pre-operative localization for pallidotomy. Can J Neurol Sci 2000;27:236–240.
31. Holtzheimer PE, Roberts DW, Darcey TM. Magnetic resonance imaging versus computed tomography for target localization in functional stereotactic neurosurgery. Neurosurgery 1999;45:290–297.
32. Meneses MS, Arruda WO, Hunhevicz SC et al. Comparison of MRI-guided and ventriculography-based stereotactic surgery for Parkinson's disease. Arq Neuropsiquiatr 1997;55:547–552.
33. Vitek JL, Bakay RA, Hashimoto T et al. Microelectrode-guided pallidotomy: technical approach and its application in medically intractable Parkinson's disease. J Neurosurg 1998;88:1027–1043.
34. Guridi J, Gorospe A, Ramos E et al. Stereotactic targeting of the globus pallidus internus in Parkinson's disease: imaging versus electrophysiological mapping. Neurosurgery 1999;45:278–287.

35. Alterman RL, Sterio D, Beric A, Kelly PJ. Microelectrode recording during posteroventral pallidotomy: impact on target selection and complications. Neurosurgery 1999;44:315–321.
36. Oh MY, Hodaie M, Kim SH et al. Deep brain stimulator electrodes used for lesioning: proof of principle. Neurosurgery 2001;49:363–367; discussion 367–369.
37. Kelly PJ, Ahlskog JE, Goerss SJ et al. Computer-assisted stereotactic ventralis lateralis thalamotomy with microelectrode recording control in patients with Parkinson's disease. Mayo Clin Proc 1987;62:655–664.
38. Anagnostou E, Sporer B, Steude U et al. Contraversive eye deviation during deep brain stimulation of the globus pallidus internus. Neurology 2001;56:1396–1399.
39. Iacono RP, Shima F, Lonser RR et al. The results, indications, and physiology of posteroventral pallidotomy for patients with Parkinson's disease. Neurosurgery 1995;36:1118–1125; discussion 1125–1117.
40. Yokoyama T, Sugiyama K, Nishizawa S et al. Visual evoked potential guidance for posteroventral pallidotomy in Parkinson's disease. Neurol Med Chir (Tokyo) 1997;37:257–263; discussion 263–264.
41. Guridi J, Rodriguez-Oroz MC, Lozano AM et al. Targeting the basal ganglia for deep brain stimulation in Parkinson's disease. Neurology 2000;55:s21–28.
42. Bronstein JM, DeSalles A, DeLong MR. Stereotactic pallidotomy in the treatment of Parkinson disease: an expert opinion. Arch Neurol 1999;56:1064–1069.
43. Rodriguez-Oroz MC, Rodriguez M, Guridi J et al. The subthalamic nucleus in Parkinson's disease: somatotopic organization and physiological characteristics. Brain 2001;124:1777–1790.
44. Kishore A, Turnbull IM, Snow BJ et al. Efficacy, stability and predictors of outcome of pallidotomy for Parkinson's disease: six-month follow-up with additional 1-year observations. Brain 1997;120:729–737.
45. Giller CA, Dewey RB, Ginsburg MI, Mendelsohn DB, Berk AM. Stereotactic pallidotomy and thalamotomy using individual variations of anatomic landmarks for localization. Neurosurgery 1998;42:56–62; discussion 62–55.
46. Eskandar EN, Shinobu LA, Penney JB, Cosgrove GR, Counihan TJ. Stereotactic pallidotomy performed without using microelectrode guidance in patients with Parkinson's disease: surgical technique and 2-year results. J Neurosurg 2000;92:375–383.
47. Favre J, Taha JM, Nguyen TT, Gildenberg PL, Burchiel KJ. Pallidotomy: a survey of current practice in North America. Neurosurgery 1996;39:883–890; discussion 890–892.
48. Milligan BD, Wilkinson S, Overman J et al. Magnitude of microelectrode refinement in pallidotomy and thalamotomy(1). Stereotact Funct Neurosurg 2001;76:2–18.
49. Kamiryo T, Laws ER. Identification and localization of intracerebral vessels by microvascular doppler in stereotactic pallidotomy and thalamotomy: technical note. Neurosurgery 1997;40:877–878; discussion 878–879.
50. Fukuda M, Kameyama S, Noguchi R, Tanaka R. Intraoperative monitoring for functional neurosurgery during intravenous anesthesia with propofol. No Shinkei Geka 1997;25:231–237.
51. Ohye C, Shibazaki T, Hirato M, Inoue H, Andou Y. Gamma thalamotomy for parkinsonian and other kinds of tremor. Stereotact Funct Neurosurg 1996;66:333–342.
52. Pan L, Dai JZ, Wang BJ et al. Stereotactic gamma thalamotomy for the treatment of parkinsonism. Stereotact Funct Neurosurg 1996;66:329–332.
53. Pollak P, Benabid AL, Limousin P, Krack P. Treatment of Parkinson's disease: new surgical treatment strategies. Eur Neurol 1996;36:400–404.
54. Niranjan A, Kondziolka D, Baser S, Heyman R, Lunsford LD. Functional outcomes after gamma knife thalamotomy for essential tremor and MS-related tremor. Neurology 2000;55:443–446.
55. Uitti RJ, Wharen RE, Turk MF et al. Unilateral pallidotomy for Parkinson's disease: comparison of outcome in younger versus elderly patients. Neurology 1997;49:1072–1077.
56. Goto S, Kunitoku N, Soyama N et al. Posteroventral pallidotomy in a patient with parkinsonism caused by hypoxic encephalopathy. Neurology 1997;49:707–710.
57. Ghika J, Ghika-Schmid F, Fankhauser H et al. Bilateral contemporaneous posteroventral pallidotomy for the treatment of Parkinson's disease: neuropsychological and neurological side effects. Report of four cases and review of the literature. J Neurosurg 1999;91:313–321.
58. Honey CR, Stoessl AJ, Tsui JK, Schulzer M, Calne DB. Unilateral pallidotomy for reduction of parkinsonian pain. J Neurosurg 1999;91:198–201.
59. Alvarez L, Macias R, Guridi J et al. Dorsal subthalamotomy for Parkinson's disease. Mov Disord 2001;16:72–78.

60. Tasker RR, Siqueira J, Hawrylyshyn P, Organ LW. What happened to VIM thalamotomy for Parkinson's disease? Appl Neurophysiol 1983;46:68–83.
61. Baron MS, Vitek JL, Bakay RA et al. Treatment of advanced Parkinson's disease by posterior GPi pallidotomy: 1-year results of a pilot study. Ann Neurol 1996;40:355–366.
62. Lang AE, Lozano AM, Montgomery E et al. Posteroventral medial pallidotomy in advanced Parkinson's disease. N Engl J Med 1997;337:1036–1042.
63. Samuel M, Caputo E, Brooks DJ et al. A study of medial pallidotomy for Parkinson's disease: clinical outcome, MRI location and complications. Brain 1998;121:59–75.
64. de Bie RM, Schuurman PR, Bosch DA et al. Outcome of unilateral pallidotomy in advanced Parkinson's disease: cohort study of 32 patients. J Neurol Neurosurg Psychiatry 2001;71:375–382.
65. Lai EC, Jankovic J, Krauss JK, Ondo WG, Grossman RG. Long-term efficacy of posteroventral pallidotomy in the treatment of Parkinson's disease. Neurology 2000;55:1218–1222.
66. Merello M, Nouzeilles MI, Kuzis G et al. Unilateral radiofrequency lesion versus electrostimulation of posteroventral pallidum: a prospective randomized comparison. Mov Disord 1999;14:50–56.
67. Roberts-Warrior D, Overby A, Jankovic J et al. Postural control in Parkinson's disease after unilateral posteroventral pallidotomy. Brain 2000;123:2141–2149.
68. Melnick ME, Dowling GA, Aminoff MJ, Barbaro NM. Effect of pallidotomy on postural control and motor function in Parkinson disease. Arch Neurol 1999;56:1361–1365.
69. Taha JM, Favre J, Baumann TK, Burchiel KJ. Tremor control after pallidotomy in patients with Parkinson's disease: correlation with microrecording findings. J Neurosurg 1997;86:642–647.
70. Martinez-Martin P, Valldeoriola F, Molinuevo JL et al. Pallidotomy and quality of life in patients with Parkinson's disease: an early study. Mov Disord 2000;15:65–70.
71. Counihan TJ, Shinobu LA, Eskandar EN, Cosgrove GR, Penney JB. Outcomes following staged bilateral pallidotomy in advanced Parkinson's disease. Neurology 2001;56:799–802.
72. Favre J, Burchiel KJ, Taha JM, Hammerstad J. Outcome of unilateral and bilateral pallidotomy for Parkinson's disease: patient assessment. Neurosurgery 2000;46:344–353; discussion 353–355.
73. Siegel KL, Metman LV. Effects of bilateral posteroventral pallidotomy on gait of subjects with Parkinson disease. Arch Neurol 2000;57:198–204.
74. Alkhani A, Lozano AM. Pallidotomy for parkinson disease: a review of contemporary literature. J Neurosurg 2001;94:43–49.
75. Fine J, Duff J, Chen R et al. Long-term follow-up of unilateral pallidotomy in advanced Parkinson's disease. N Engl J Med 2000;342:1708–1714.
76. Hariz MI, Hirabayashi H. Is there a relationship between size and site of the stereotactic lesion and symptomatic results of pallidotomy and thalamotomy? Stereotact Funct Neurosurg 1997;69:28–45.
77. Gross RE, Lombardi WJ, Hutchison WD et al. Variability in lesion location after microelectrode-guided pallidotomy for Parkinson's disease: anatomical, physiological, and technical factors that determine lesion distribution. J Neurosurg 1999;90:468–477.
78. Uitti RJ, Wharen RE, Turk MF. Efficacy of levodopa therapy on motor function after posteroventral pallidotomy for Parkinson's disease. Neurology 1998;51:1755–1757.
79. Skalabrin EJ, Laws ER, Bennett JP. Pallidotomy improves motor responses and widens the levodopa therapeutic window in Parkinson's disease. Mov Disord 1998;13:775–781.
80. Alegret M, Vendrell P, Junque C et al. Effects of unilateral posteroventral pallidotomy on "on-off" cognitive fluctuations in Parkinson's disease. Neuropsychologia 2000;38:628–633.
81. Ondo WG, Ben-Aire L, Jankovic J et al. Weight gain following unilateral pallidotomy in Parkinson's disease. Acta Neurol Scand 2000;101:79–84.
82. Ahmad SO, Mu K, Scott SA. Meta-analysis of functional outcome in Parkinson patients treated with unilateral pallidotomy. Neurosci Lett 2001;312:153–156.
83. Gray A, McNamara I, Aziz T et al. Quality of life outcomes following surgical treatment of Parkinson's disease. Mov Disord 2002;17:68–75.
84. Akbostanci MC, Slavin KV, Burchiel KJ. Stereotactic ventral intermedial thalamotomy for the treatment of essential tremor: results of a series of 37 patients. Stereotact Funct Neurosurg 1999;72:174–177.
85. Goldman MS, Ahlskog JE, Kelly PJ. The symptomatic and functional outcome of stereotactic thalamotomy for medically intractable essential tremor. J Neurosurg 1992;76:924–928.
86. Boecker H, Wills AJ, Ceballos-Baumann A et al. Stereotactic thalamotomy in tremor-dominant Parkinson's disease: an $H_2(15)O$ PET motor activation study. Ann Neurol 1997;41:108–111.
87. Tollefson TT, Burns J, Wilkinson S et al. Comparative magnetic resonance image-based evaluation of thalamotomy and pallidotomy lesion volumes. Stereotact Funct Neurosurg 1998;71:131–144.

88. Marsden CD, Fahn S. Movement disorders. London: Butterworth Scientific, 1982.
89. Biousse V, Newman NJ, Carroll C et al. Visual fields in patients with posterior GPi pallidotomy. Neurology 1998;50:258–265.
90. Shannon KM, Penn RD, Kroin JS et al. Stereotactic pallidotomy for the treatment of Parkinson's disease: efficacy and adverse effects at 6 months in 26 patients. Neurology 1998;50:434–438.
91. Hariz MI, De Salles AA. The side-effects and complications of posteroventral pallidotomy. Acta Neurochir Suppl 1997;68:42–48.
92. Lim JY, De Salles AA, Bronstein J, Masterman DL, Saver JL. Delayed internal capsule infarctions following radiofrequency pallidotomy: report of three cases. J Neurosurg 1997;87:955–960.
93. Troster AI, Fields JA, Wilkinson SB et al. Unilateral pallidal stimulation for Parkinson's disease: neurobehavioral functioning before and 3 months after electrode implantation. Neurology 1997;49:1078–1083.
94. Scott R, Gregory R, Hines N et al. Neuropsychological, neurological and functional outcome following pallidotomy for Parkinson's disease: a consecutive series of eight simultaneous bilateral and twelve unilateral procedures. Brain 1998;121:659–675.
95. Junque C, Alegret M, Nobbe FA et al. Cognitive and behavioral changes after unilateral posteroventral pallidotomy: relationship with lesional data from MRI. Mov Disord 1999;14:780–789.
96. Yokoyama T, Imamura Y, Sugiyama K et al. Prefrontal dysfunction following unilateral posteroventral pallidotomy in Parkinson's disease. J Neurosurg 1999;90:1005–1010.
97. Obwegeser AA, Uitti RJ, Lucas JA et al. Predictors of neuropsychological outcome in patients following microelectrode-guided pallidotomy for Parkinson's disease. J Neurosurg 2000;93:410–420.
98. Stebbins GT, Gabrieli JD, Shannon KM, Penn RD, Goetz CG. Impaired frontostriatal cognitive functioning following posteroventral pallidotomy in advanced Parkinson's disease. Brain Cogn 2000;42:348–363.
99. Uitti RJ. Surgical treatments for Parkinson's disease. Can Fam Physician 2000;46:368–373.
100. Schulz GM, Greer M, Friedman W. Changes in vocal intensity in Parkinson's disease following pallidotomy surgery. J Voice 2000;14:589–606.
101. Blekher T, Siemers E, Abel LA, Yee RD. Eye movements in Parkinson's disease: before and after pallidotomy. Invest Ophthalmol Vis Sci 2000;41:2177–2183.
102. Young RF, Shumway-Cook A, Vermeulen SS et al. Gamma knife radiosurgery as a lesioning technique in movement disorder surgery. J Neurosurg 1998;89:183–193.
103. Duma CM, Jacques DB, Kopyov OV et al. Gamma knife radiosurgery for thalamotomy in parkinsonian tremor: a five-year experience. J Neurosurg 1998;88:1044–1049.
104. Bonnen JG, Iacono RP, Lulu B et al. Gamma knife pallidotomy: case report. Acta Neurochir (Wien) 1997;139:442–445.
105. Hariz MI, Bergenheim AT. A 10-year follow-up review of patients who underwent Leksell's posteroventral pallidotomy for Parkinson disease. J Neurosurg 2001;94:552–558.
106. Kelly PJ, Gillingham FJ. The long-term results of stereotaxic surgery and L-dopa therapy in patients with Parkinson's disease: a 10-year follow-up study. J Neurosurg 1980;53:332–337.
107. Baron MS, Vitek JL, Bakay RA et al. Treatment of advanced Parkinson's disease by unilateral posterior GPi pallidotomy: 4-year results of a pilot study. Mov Disord 2000;15:230–237.
108. Samii A, Turnbull IM, Kishore A et al. Reassessment of unilateral pallidotomy in Parkinson's disease: a 2-year follow-up study. Brain 1999;122:417–425.
109. Matsumoto K, Shichijo F, Fukami T. Long-term follow-up review of cases of Parkinson's disease after unilateral or bilateral thalamotomy. J Neurosurg 1984;60:1033–1044.
110. Nagaseki Y, Shibazaki T, Hirai T et al. Long-term follow-up results of selective VIM-thalamotomy. J Neurosurg 1986;65:296–302.

8

Deep Brain Stimulation for Parkinson's Disease

A. L. Benabid, J. F. Le Bas, S. Grand, P. Krack, S. Chabardès, V. Fraix, B. A. Wallace, C. Ardouin, and P. Pollak

INTRODUCTION

Movement disorders deserve a special place in the field of functional neurosurgery given the severity of the patient's deficits requiring treatment. The elucidation of numerous physiological and biochemical aspects of the basal ganglia have led to an increased understanding of the mechanisms underlying Parkinson's disease (PD) and have established the basis of a therapeutic approach. This approach, however, was primarily based on an empirical process, largely derived from anatomical considerations.[1]

Through a relatively random process, the ventrointermediate nucleus (VIM) was found to be the most effective target for the tremor component of PD. This nucleus was the primary target of functional neurosurgery for decades, and improved the understanding of both the pathophysiology of the disease as well as the physiology of motor function. The discovery of levodopa and its lack of immediate side-effects rendered the neurosurgical treatment of parkinsonian tremor temporarily obsolete. However, after 5 to 10 years of use, levodopa-induced dyskinesias develop and these are often as disabling as the disease itself.

Levodopa side-effects revived the need for a surgical intervention that was efficient, yet free of side-effects and permanent deficits. High-frequency stimulation (HFS) provided such a new surgical method. As deep brain stimulation (DBS) had been used since the 1950s for pain, it was readily adaptable to become an alternative to ablative methods and/or inadequate medical management. Since 1987,[2–4] HFS has proven to be a safe, efficient, and stable method to produce neural inhibition in areas of the brain where lesions were previously made. These areas include the thalamus and the pallidum, but also now include targets previously considered dangerous, such as the subthalamic nucleus (STN), or corpus Luysii.

Currently, there are three commonly used surgical targets for the treatment of PD:

- the thalamic ventrointermediate nucleus and additionally the centromedial and parafascicularis complex (CM–Pf)[5]
- the internal pallidum or globus pallidus internus (GPi)[6,7]
- the subthalamic nucleus (STN).

Both HFS and ablation (thalamotomy) of the VIM are uniquely efficacious on tremor, providing very little significant improvement of the other parkinsonian symptoms.[8–25] There is still a controversy about the relative efficacies of bilateral DBS of the GPi versus the STN. The major difference is the ability to decrease significantly, or even suspend, the replacement dopaminergic treatment in STN-stimulated patients. This reduction in dopamine medication may explain the occasionally observed postoperative depression in patients who have been implanted in the STN. In contrast to the empirical approach that identified VIM as a target for tremor, the use of STN as a human therapeutic target[26–29] was based on experimental evidence from rodents and monkeys that identified it as a key structure in the functional organization of basal ganglia.[30–36] We abandoned the GPi as a target for PD, given the difference in outcome we observed between these two targets. This disparity in efficacy has been further demonstrated in other studies.[37]

GENERAL PRINCIPLES

The basic approach for stereotactic targeting of basal ganglia structures is the same for the STN, GPi, and VIM, with the only difference being their coordinates. There is evidence that the quality of symptom alleviation depends on the precision of the implantation. Each radiological modality has drawbacks: ventriculography is the most precise method, but is more invasive than magnetic resonance (MR) imaging. MRI is the best method for visualization of the STN, but suffers from distortions.

The surgical implantation of electrodes can be done in one session or can be divided into five steps on different days: ventriculography and implantation of titanium skull screws for repositioning; MRI; implantation of electrodes; postoperative MRI; and implantation of the intermittent pulse generator.[25]

Ventriculography is, in our opinion, the gold standard. A diagram which allows pre-targeting of all targets can be superimposed on the lateral and anteroposterior views. MRI may be used in conjunction with ventriculography, but it is intraoperative electrophysiology (microelectrode recording, MER) and microstimulation that identify the final, correct location.[38–41] In our opinion, atlases[42,43] can be misleading.

VENTRICULOGRAPHY

Positive-contrast ventriculography is performed under biorthogonal teleradiological conditions (3.5 m between x-ray tube and film, average magnification coefficient of 1.05). Injection of 6.5 mL of Iopamiron 200 (Schering) at precise landmarks, and an air bubble test, prevent any of the reported complications.[44,45] Ventriculography provides a very precise delineation of the midline of the third ventricle and of the anterior (AC) and posterior (PC) commissures. A Guiot's scheme[46] may then be superimposed for use as a template in final targeting. The average dimensions of the third ventricle (V3) are: AC–PC length 24.63 ± 1.64 mm (n = 153, extrema: 21.21–27.59); height of thalamus (HT) 16.62 ± 1.47 mm (n = 153, extrema: 12.57–19.95); width of V3 5.22 ± 1.64 mm (n = 153, extrema: 1.52–19.46).

In order to eliminate the individual variations, coordinates are normalized using the length of the AC–PC and height of the thalamus, which are divided into 12 and 8 parts, respectively. On the AP view, the laterality, which has no good normalization method, remains expressed in unmodified millimeters from the midline. The coordinates of the various nuclei are given below.

MAGNETIC RESONANCE IMAGING

MRI is used, but spatial distortion – which depends on the sequence and on the presence of metallic implants in patients – must be carefully controlled.

Sequences

Stereotactic MRI is performed in a 1.5-tesla Philips Gyroscan before (for targeting purposes) and after electrode implantation (to define the position of the implanted electrodes, although they create a strong artifact). Preoperative MRI also defines the cortical sulci, helping to avoid the F1/F2 sulcus.

Target Visibility

T2-weighted MRI is the key imaging modality for the STN, where it is visible as a small, almond-shaped, hypointense structure, situated 1–2 mm anterior to the red nucleus, 2–3 mm superior and slightly lateral to the substantia nigra reticulata (SNr). Externally, the STN is limited by the internal capsule (IC), and posterior to the mamillary bodies.

The VIM is not visible on MRI; but on T1 (and particularly on IR–TSE sequences), its lateral border corresponds to the external limit of the thalamus, at one-fourth of the AC–PC length, anterior to PC, in the AC–PC horizontal plane, and its medial limit is separated by a slight change in density from the intralaminar nuclei. On the sagittal sections, the somatosensory thalamus is visible, limited anteriorly by the oblique IC, and posteriorly by the hypointensity of the pulvinar.

The GPi is visible on IR–TSE and on T2-weighted sequences as a strong hypointense signal. The putamen is even more hypointense than the pallidum on IR–TSE images, precisely marking the external limit of the pallidum. This is of special importance in the posterior part of the pallidum where the optimal target is situated. Fibers located medial and inferior to the pallidum include the internal capsule and the optic tract (OT), which are visible on coronal as well as sagittal T1 and T2 sections.

Fusion with CT

Computed tomography (CT) imaging has made tremendous progress, and is capable of providing high-quality three-dimensional reconstructions with no spatial deformation. However, it does not match the quality of MRI. CT–MRI fusion may circumvent these errors, provided that the fusion process reformats the MRI data in the non-deformed space defined by the CT scan.

FINAL COORDINATES OF THE THEORETICAL TARGET

Atlases and Targets

Atlases[47–61] can be misleading when targeting a nucleus, as matching of the three planes is rarely achieved. However, due to the high topographical stability of the brain, they have great value for pre-targeting of the basal ganglia, provided that the coordinates of the target refer to anatomical landmarks visible on the radiographical images (ventriculography, CT scan, or MRI).

Each of the three targets currently used can be defined by the conjunction of data based on:

- geometrical landmarks obtained from ventriculography (which provides a preliminary statistical estimation of the target position), using the modified proportional geometric scheme of Guiot based on the AC–PC line
- MRI data (which may help adjust the coordinates for each patient, particularly for laterality which is the only non-normalized coordinate).

On this basis, the stereotactic parameters (x,y,z coordinates of the target point and of the entry point) are calculated, which will guide the trajectories aiming at the target point with microelectrodes. The final site for implantation of the chronic tetrapolar electrodes is determined by the data obtained from the electrophysiology and intraoperative stimulation. Contacts responsible for the best improvement of symptoms are identified by the clinicians in the postoperative period. The average coordinates of these "clinically validated targets" are determined for the entire series of patients. Table 8.1 shows numerical values for the target coordinates.

IMPLANTATION OF ELECTRODES

Placement

VIM and GPi are consistently implanted parallel to the midline plane. The first 50 STN patients were also implanted parallel to the midline plane, but the risk of disrupting a vessel, such as a branch of the pericallosal artery producing a supraventricular hematoma, was too high. The theoretical STN target is currently approached in double obliquity, and parallel to the anterior border of the VIM. The average coronal angle is 13.1 ± 7.4 degrees. The average sagittal angle on the AC–PC plane is theoretically, from the Guiot scheme, 63.6 ± 2.4

TABLE 8.1 Numerical values for the target coordinates (mm)

	STN coordinates[a]	*VIM coordinates*	*GPi coordinates*
AP	5.28±0.5 1/12th of AC–PC length Extrema: 2.88–7.08	3.53±0.91 1/12th of AC–PC length Extrema: 1.43–5.98	8.4±1.2 1/12th of AC–PC length Extrema: 6.6–9.9
Vertical	1.22±0.65 1/8th of HT Extrema: −3.29–0.19	1.15±1.18 1/8th of HT Extrema: −2.37–4.26	−0.7±0.8 1/8th of HT Extrema: −1.7–0.3
Lateral	12.14±2.05 from midline Extrema: 9–15.2[b]	15.36±1.61 from midline Extrema: 12.27–19.22[c]	19.1±2.9 from midline Extrema: 16.0–23.2

[a]200 bilaterally implanted patients.

[b]Corrected from x-ray magnification.

[c]To compensate for changes in third ventricular width (which affects directly the position of the VIM which is lateral to V3 and not of the STN which is below V3), one may use the "rule of Tasker" where the laterality for the VIM is 11.5 mm + (V3 width)/2.

degrees; the actual angle is 59.5±17.4 degrees, the difference being due to adjustment of the entry point on the MRI to avoid cortical veins, the F1/F2 sulcus, and the lateral ventricle.

We use a five-channel guide system ("Ben Gun", ISS, France), which allows the insertion of five guide tubes separated by 2 mm, and which encompasses a 4-mm diameter area centered on the theoretical target. The trajectory in which the best recording and stimulation data are obtained is used for final insertion of the chronic electrode.

Electrophysiology (stimulation and recording performed along 10–15 mm of the trajectory encompassing the theoretical target) provides the functional signature of the target, and compensates for individual variations in the average coordinates of the theoretical target which can differ significantly from the final target. The final identification of the target is based on both microrecordings of the specific activity of target neurons, and observation of the clinical effects (best alleviation of symptoms with the least side-effects) of HFS in cooperation with the neurologist.

Microrecording

During the past several years, the development of this field of functional neurosurgery has enticed companies to design systems equipped with a microdrive and technological features to help neurosurgical teams perform electrophysiological investigation in the operating room (stimulation, simultaneous recording of several electrodes, data processing). Spontaneous and evoked neuronal activities are considered to be the signatures of the explored structure. They depend on the nucleus being investigated and on the type of electrode used. Furthermore, neuronal activity varies along the track and can provide information about the boundaries of the different nuclei. White matter bundles are usually silent and have a low neural noise.[62,63] Neural noise is high in the VIM and diminishes markedly when the electrode enters the internal capsule. Similar patterns are observed in the STN and Gpi.[64] The exact position of each stimulating and/or recording site is verified by x-rays and mapped on to the final operating diagram.

VIM

Neuronal activity can be recorded along tracks in both the VIM and the VPL. In VIM, cells fire in bursts of 5–10 large spikes. Some cells have spontaneous bursting activity independent of any peripheral stimulation or muscular activity. Others fire in bursts synchronously with the tremor, and respond to passive movements of the limbs. Thalamotomy, as well as HFS, of this nucleus provide very good results.[41,46,65] VPL cells respond to superficial stimulation of the skin (touch, pressure).

GPi

The GPi is a larger structure than the VIM or STN, but its functional spatial distribution is not as clear, making electrode placement difficult. Electrophysiological recording, depending on the obliquity of the trajectory, provides characteristic firing patterns, originally described by Hutchinson.[64] In the GPe, two types of cells are recorded: low-frequency burst neurons (LFB: 10.6 ± 8.9 Hz), and higher-frequency neurons (60 ± 36 Hz) with an irregular pattern and pauses in activity. In the GPi, neurons fire at a high rate with a very irregular firing pattern, at 55 ± 27 Hz in the external part, and at 82 ± 32 Hz in the medial part. These three subnuclei are also separated by border cells with a regular firing pattern of about 30 Hz. Below the GPi, the optic tract runs obliquely parallel to the main axis of GPi. Flashing a light into the patient's eyes may induce evoked potentials and stimulation may induce phosphenes.

STN

Electrophysiology helps precise identification of the STN. Recordings show an increase in neuronal firing rate in the STN relative to the surrounding area, particularly at the site where the best effects on rigidity and akinesia are obtained. STN cells produce large, asymmetrical spikes with a high-frequency (35.2 ± 8.8 Hz) bursting firing rate, as well as biphasic spikes at a lower rate (11.1 ± 2.3 Hz) that are responsive to passive movements and to tremor. Below the plane of the STN, the SNr is encountered with even larger, very symmetrical spikes which also have a lower, irregular firing rate and are unresponsive to stimuli. Further below this area, neuronal silence is characteristic of the IC and provides the inferior limit for electrode positioning.[66]

Microstimulation

Shifts of several millimeters between the theoretical (MRI- and/or ventriculography-based) and the corrected (electrophysiology-based) targets may be observed, confirming the necessity for electrophysiological studies for target localization, although this is still a matter of controversy.[67] However, these shifts are rather small, and the first localization of the target using ventriculography is nearly always correct (average distance from the active contact to the theoretical target = 2.1 ± 0.9 mm for STN).

Notably, the benefits of ventriculography are a matter of controversy.[68] Stimulation may identify surrounding structures but, most importantly, identify the efficacy of stimulation by showing to what extent symptoms are suppressed by intraoperative stimulation and where this can be achieved. Contrary to popular belief, efficient microstimulation can be routinely and safely performed, provided that trains of stimulation are kept shorter than 10 seconds. This has the advantage of comparing the data from recording and the effects of stimulation at the same site. The exact position of each stimulating and/or recording site is confirmed using x-rays. This provides a set of data for the exact location of the nucleus into which the chronic DBS electrode will be implanted. Test stimulation is performed using a pulse width of 60 μs, a frequency of 130 Hz, and a current intensity of 0.1–10 mA.

VIM

The effect of stimulation on tremor can be quantified using an accelerometer attached to the patient's finger. VIM HFS-induced tremor suppression using the lowest current strength (0.2–2 mA) is the major criterion in choosing the final placement. For each track, a comparison between motor and sensory thresholds helps to determine the optimal electrode placement. In the VIM nucleus, stimulation with currents as low as 0.2 mA induces immediate suppression of the tremor, in a manner dependent on current intensity. If stimulation is truly effective, the tremor disappears at the onset of the current, with no more than 1 or 2 seconds of delay, and recurs almost immediately when the current is turned off. After-effects, when observed, do not last more than 10–20 seconds. During electrode progression towards the final target, a decrease in spontaneous tremor intensity is often observed, along with increased post-stimulation effects and difficulty in reinducing the tremor. This is considered as a minor equivalent of the thalamotomy-like effect which is classically observed when entering the thalamic target with a large electrode.

GPi

Stimulation of the GPi produces a clear decrease in rigidity, or even in akinesia and tremor in some areas. This is used to guide the correct electrode placement, although the major indication is a reduction in levodopa-induced dyskinesias or abnormal involuntary movements (LIDs or AIMs) which cannot be tested in the operating room.

STN

During STN stimulation, continuous monitoring by the neurologist of passive wrist rigidity is the most reliable test. Motor performance scores are significantly improved, although the reproducibility of this type of assessment is limited due to patient fatigue.

When the symptoms (tremor or bradykinesia) are bilateral, the contralateral side is implanted during the same session.

Introduction and Fixation of the Chronic DBS Electrode and Implantation of the Implantable Programmable Generator

At the time of writing, a total of 545 electrodes have been implanted in 305 patients: 121 in the VIM (64 bilateral), 12 in the GPi (8 bilateral), and 172 in the STN (4 unilateral: a total of 340 STN tetrapolar electrodes have been implanted in 172 patients, parallel to the mid-sagittal plane in 54 patients (99 electrodes), and 251 others in double obliquity).

The first 108 electrodes were monopolar (Medtronic SP.5535, currently DBS 3388) with an insulated tip, 1.27 mm in diameter and 3.5 mm long. The remaining 437 were tetrapolar (Medtronic 3387 or 3389) with four contacts, 1.27 mm in diameter and 1.5 mm long, each separated by 1.5 mm or 0.5 mm, respectively. The electrode is fixed to the skull by a suture anchored in the skull and then embedded using dental cement. Several days after surgery (or the same day for some teams), the programmable stimulators (Medtronic Soletra or Kinetra) are implanted in the subclavicular area.

TARGETS AVAILABLE

The three classical targets

Experimental data gathered fairly recently have led to the concept of the parallel processing model, which, if not accurate, has enormous didactical value and provides a practical basis for reasoning. According to this concept,[30,31,35] the degeneration of dopaminergic neurons of the substantia nigra pars compacta (SNc) denervate the striatum (putamen and caudate nucleus) from the regulatory neurotransmitter, dopamine. The D1 and D2 receptors of the striatum are then deprived and undergo a process of deafferentation supersensitivity, while the two output GABAergic pathways originating from them become unbalanced. The direct pathway projects to the GPi and SNr, while the indirect pathway projects to the GPe, which in turn exerts its GABAergic influence on the subthalamic nucleus. The STN is a glutamatergic nucleus which sends excitatory axons to the complex SNr–GPi. SNr and GPi are thus placed in the same functional "black box," which sends globally inhibitory GABAergic output on to the motor thalamic nuclei. This has been proposed as the basis of the akinesia of Parkinson's disease. Obviously, certain aspects of the model are oversimplified as it explains neither the pathophysiology of tremor, nor the effect of destruction or inhibition of the STN, GPi, VIM or CM–Pf on tremor.

The STN receives GABAergic input from the GPe, but also glutamatergic inputs from the cortex and the CM–Pf. Contrary to what the model suggests, the SNr does not have the same therapeutic properties when stimulated as the GPi in Parkinson's disease. According to this concept, the decrease in striatal dopamine levels induces a hyperactivity of the STN, as well as of the GPi and SNr. Neuronal firing in the ventrolateral motor thalamus and the cortex are reduced. Accordingly, one might expect that destruction of the STN or GPi would improve symptoms by eliminating abnormal neuronal activity in these two nuclei, which is coherent with the clinical observations following subthalamotomy and pallidotomy, or neuroinhibition of these structures by high-frequency stimulation.

Putative and Theoretical Targets

Substantia Nigra Pars Reticulata

According to the current concepts of basal ganglia organization, the GPi and SNr have equivalent properties and share common features and roles in the control of motricity. Therefore, the SNr should also have the same properties as the GPi and be equally considered as a functional target. Its position just below the STN makes it easy to explore as well as to stimulate with the lower contacts of the electrode used for STN stimulation.

Unfortunately, as could have been predicted from the different electrophysiological properties of the SNr, the neuronal firing does not change in response to stimulus, and stimulation of the SNr has no effect on parkinsonian symptoms, regardless of frequency. Further studies are needed to better evaluate the absence of effects of SNr stimulation, such as that on oculomotricity given the existence of projections from the SNr to the superior colliculus as this pathway might be effective in treating epilepsy.[69–71]

Globus Pallidus Externus

In theory, the GPe is a potent GABAergic structure, which exerts a strong inhibitory influence on both the STN and GPi. However, this has never been directly observed as no definite attempts have been made to explore its properties.

Cortex

Motor cortex stimulation is being investigated and seems to be effective for some forms of intractable pain. It has been reported that intraoperative cortex stimulation might stop parkinsonian tremor, and that chronic stimulation could alleviate action tremor.[72,73]

Pedunculopontine Nucleus

From animal experiments and basic neurophysiology, there is enough evidence that the pedunculopontine nucleus (PPN) might play an important role in the control of motor function. However, the PPN is subject to degeneration in Parkinson's disease and early attempts to lesion or stimulate it in animal models have yet to demonstrate any clear benefit.[74] Furthermore, the PPN is more difficult to access safely and might not be a practical target in human patients.

CM–Pf

High-frequency stimulation of the centromedial and parafascicularis complex has been shown to alleviate parkinsonian tremor, as well as levodopa-induced dyskinesias. This might be related to the strong pallido-CM–Pf projections.[5]

RESULTS

The surgical treatment of PD is not a first-line, stand-alone therapy. It is part of a treatment strategy that is appropriate only after medical management fails. Current selection criteria include severe disability with a preserved response to levodopa treatment, and the absence of dementia.

Patient Selection

A total of 305 patients (545 sides) were operated on for movement disorders in the three primary targets: thalamus, subthalamus, and pallidum.

VIM cases: Sixty-one patients were implanted in the VIM using the monopolar electrode SP-5535 or -3388. Sixty patients were implanted using the DBS-3387[75] or -3389[25] electrodes.

STN cases: Since 1993, 172 PD patients (114 males, 58 females; age 56.2±8.3 years, min. 32.8, max. 77.2; age of onset 41.2±8.0 years, min. 27, max. 62) have been implanted, 168 of them bilaterally (340 electrodes, 162 patients during the same session).

GPi cases: Only 12 patients were implanted in the GPi for PD, mainly for levodopa-induced dyskinesias. The results appeared to be significantly less satisfactory than those produced by STN HFS, and the target was abandoned for the treatment of PD early in our DBS experience. Thirteen patients were operated in the GPi for dystonia. The GPi appears to be the most effective target to date for dystonia.

Indications According to Symptoms

Patients were deemed appropriate DBS candidates when the following conditions were met:

- existence of "on"/"off" periods, levodopa-induced dyskinesias (LIDs), and periods of severe akinesia despite high doses of levodopa
- medical management is efficient but not tolerated at doses required for a satisfactory functional result, such as disabling LIDs
- the remaining disability is high enough to significantly disturb the patient's activities of daily living
- there are no general contraindications for surgery, no significant alteration of mental functions, and no psychiatric or severely depressive states.

The Triad of PD Symptoms

PD is by far the best indication for high-frequency stimulation (HFS) of deep brain targets. Categorically, tremor is controlled by VIM HFS, levodopa-induced dyskinesias by GPi HFS, and akinesia and rigidity by STN HFS. Notably, GPi HFS is also efficient on tremor, akinesia, and rigidity, as previously reported for pallidotomies. Moreover, STN HFS is able to completely control tremor, akinesia, and rigidity when electrode placement is correct, and allows for a significant decrease of the drug dosage, which in turn suppresses the levodopa-induced dyskinesias. The superior results consistently obtained with the STN have led us to choose it as the unique target for HFS in PD patients.

The response to a levodopa test is a good predictive index,[76] with the effect of STN HFS being similar to the best "on" rating using levodopa. Multiple-system atrophy and other atypical parkinsonian syndromes are currently not considered appropriate for DBS treatment.

Dyskinesias

LIDs are poorly controlled by VIM HFS, directly suppressed by GPi HFS, and indirectly suppressed by STN HFS through the decrease in drug dosage allowed by the striking improvement of akinesia and rigidity. LIDs do respond well to CM–Pf stimulation.[5]

Results: Thalamus

High-frequency stimulation of the VIM is effective on parkinsonian rest tremor.[4] There is almost no change in bradykinesia or any other PD symptom. Unilateral pain, however, which accompanied severe tremor and rigidity in many cases was greatly reduced. The effect on tremor was scored independently by the neurologist using a 5-point scale. Immediately after surgery, a microthalamotomy-like effect is responsible for transitory tremor suppression for a few days – 22 (20.5%) out of 107 patients, 23 (15%) out of 153 electrodes. A very good result (scores 3 and 4) was obtained in 71% of the operated sides. Resting tremor was better controlled than action tremor, distal limb tremor better than proximal or axial tremor, and upper-limb better than lower-limb tremor. In all cases the effect was strictly coincident with stimulation, without significant delay at the onset or cessation of stimulation. Thirty-nine of 80 PD patients (48.7%) had their levodopa dosage decreased by 20% at 3-month follow-up.

There were only 12 patients (15%) at the last follow-up, due to progression of the disease. Caparros-Lefebvre et al.[77] have reported much better results in five patients with levodopa-induced, choreic dyskinesias and ballistic dyskinesias which were clearly improved by thalamic stimulation. However, these patients may have possibly been implanted in the CM–Pf.[5]

Results: Pallidum

Pallidal DBS is a safe and effective procedure for the treatment of advanced PD. Bilateral DBS results in a reduction of about 34% in the activities of daily living scores during the "off" period and of about 35–40% improvement of motor scores in the "off" period. In addition, there are significant improvements in patients' symptoms during the "on" period and in "on"/"off" motor fluctuations. Compared to STN stimulation, levodopa-induced dyskinesias were directly diminished even when the drug dosage was not decreased. In fact, GPi stimulation does not allow for a significant decrease in drug dosage (+10% at 6 months, –15% at 36 months).

Results: Subthalamus

Dyskinesias

The improvement of levodopa-induced dyskinesias following STN stimulation is due to the significant improvement of akinesia and rigidity,[75,78] allowing an approximately 55% reduction in the amount of drugs used by patients. Subsequently, dyskinesias are eliminated. Approximately 10% of our patients have completely stopped pharmacological therapy. In fact, stimulating the patient at levels higher than needed to control the parkinsonian symptoms, one can induce dyskinesias, which could be described as a ballismus or choreoballic dyskinesias.[75] Over time, levodopa challenges induce decreasing LIDs. Similarly, STN HFS-induced dyskinesias are also more difficult to induce over time. This raises the question of whether postsynaptic desensitization is also observed during long-term apomorphine administration.

The improvement is also visible on midline symptoms such as gait, standing from recumbency, and stability. Speech is also improved, although not to the same extent as the others. One of the most spectacular effects was that on "off" dystonia, which was significantly improved in 16 of our 20 patients who had it in this survey. When the stimulator is turned on, dystonia disappears within seconds; when the stimulator is turned off again, it reappears equally as quickly. This is, of course, also true for akinesia and rigidity.

Hypophonia

Hypophonia should not be considered as a complication of surgery as it may respond to increased doses of levodopa or even to stimulation. However, in these patients, the reduction in voice volume may be disabling as the patient may be barely understandable. The current hypothesis to explain this phenomenon is centered on a somatotopic organization of the subthalamic nucleus. The current functional method of targeting is based on the reduction of rigidity assessed by the passive mobilization of the wrist, which may not be as good an indicator for the orofacial activity as it is for the limbs. If midline functions, such as the voice, are located in a different part of the subthalamic nucleus, we might consistently miss it using the method employed. Therefore, during chronic stimulation, the patient with significant improvements in rigidity and akinesia of the limbs is deprived of levodopa as it is no longer useful and may precipitate dyskinesias. As a consequence the patient, in terms of hypophonia, is medically untreated given the significant reduction of drug doses, and is not surgically treated as the placement of the electrode in the STN does not include the area corresponding to voice control. Although merely speculative, this raises the issue of the need for developing intraoperative methods for voice exploration which would allow us to target better this symptom.

Cognitive Functions and Quality of Life (QoL)

Overstimulation may be responsible for the spreading of current into immediately adjacent structures, resulting in side-effects related to these abnormally stimulated structures. This could be manifested as strong depressive stages, or as irrepressible laughter, as we have observed in one patient. Neuropsychological testing has not shown any change after long-term stimulation in the STN.

At 12-months follow-up, bilateral STN stimulation greatly improves motor symptoms (UPDRS III −55%) and activities of daily living (UPDRS II −45%, Schwab and England Scale +142%) in the "off" drug condition, as well as dyskinesias in the "on" drug condition (−90%). Dopaminergic treatment (levodopa equivalent dose) was decreased by 50%. Patients were only mildly depressed before surgery (Beck Depression Inventory 10.45±6.6) and there was a very mild but significant improvement of mood after surgery (Beck Depression Inventory 8.5±4.1). No significant differences were found in the "on" drug condition for motor score, activities of daily living, or mentation and behavior as assessed by UPDRS I. There were five transient psychiatric complications (1 mania, 1 paranoia, 3 depressions, including one suicide and two suicide attempts).

The PDQL (Parkinson's Disease Quality of Life) total score improved from 90.3 to 129 (the maximum is 185); parkinsonian symptoms increased from 33.2 to 49.1 (max. 70); systemic symptoms increased from 17.3 to 23.1 (max. 35); emotional functioning increased from 24.2 to 31.2 (max. 45); and social functioning increased from 15.7 to 25.6 (max. 35).

The improvement of the score of the UPDRS III was significantly correlated with the improvement of the total PDQL score. We found an improvement of health-related quality of life with bilateral STN stimulation.[79,80] Bilateral STN stimulation improves all aspects of health-related QoL in Parkinson's disease including emotional and social functioning. The QoL did not fully normalize, but rather improved to the level of a large population of PD patients with less advanced disease. This finding is not surprising as bilateral STN stimulation only improves the motor symptoms in the off-drug condition and dyskinesias in the on-drug condition. "On"-period symptoms, as well as cognitive symptoms, showed little or no improvement. A significant decrease in PD patient social isolation is the real success of STN stimulation. Therefore, in selected, highly levodopa-sensitive patients, suffering from motor complications of dopaminergic treatment, and without severe depression, the motor complications seem to be the main determinant of quality of life.

Side-effects related to surgery, stimulation, or changes in medication are likely to influence QoL. However, the overall study tends to confirm that the benefit of motor improvement largely supersedes the impact of side-effects on quality of life and that it is worth taking the relatively small risk, and operating on patients before their quality of life becomes too low.

Rigidity, Akinesia, and Tremor[26–28,80]

The clinical changes, as well as improvement in quantitative testing, are strongly evident when stimulation is turned on and off. Moreover, surface EMG recordings of agonist and antagonist muscles of the forearm during passive wrist manipulation show that reflex hyperactivity of the stretched antagonist muscle, which is typical of extrapyramidal rigidity, is almost completely suppressed during STN stimulation, in a way very similar to that observed after apomorphine injection or levodopa administration. The continuous follow-up of these patients[26] shows an increasing improvement of about 60% in all symptoms evaluated using the corresponding scales, and a decrease in drug dosage in the range 30–100% (mean 50%), resulting in the disappearance of LIDs. Patients who have LIDs before surgery exhibit similar complications using STN stimulation and their regular drug regimen concurrently. This diminishes over time, as long as drug dosages are progressively decreased.[74] Tremor is abolished by STN HFS comparable to that by VIM HFS. As a general rule, it may be said that STN HFS provides the patient with a permanent level of improvement equal to his or her best status during "on" periods, and that all levodopa-sensitive parkinsonian symptoms were similarly improved.

Complications: the Overall Picture

Some side-effects are not related to the stimulation of the target nucleus and occur as a consequence of the procedure or the general condition of the patient. Observation of complications in patients treated in the VIM or GPi at our center may help define the specific morbidity of STN implantation versus the non-specific complications of deep brain stimulation in general.

Of 197 patients operated on 316 sides, including all three primary targets, we observed:

- one large supraventricular hematoma (0.5% of patients, 0.3% of operated sides)
- three micro hematomas with transient or slight permanent symptoms (1.7%/0.95%)
- three asymptomatic micro hematomas (1.7%/0.95%)
- two subdural hematomas (1.01%/0.6%; one was surgically explored)
- three electrode tracks surrounded by hyperintense signals on the MRI (1.7%/0.95%)
- three asymptomatic intraventricular hemorrhages related to the transventricular approach to the target (1.7%/0.95%)
- seven late local infections, erosion, or granuloma of the external leads (3.5%/2.2%)
- one local hematoma in the stimulator subcutaneous pocket (0.5%/0.3%)
- four ruptures of the external extension needing replacement (2%/1.3%)
- three repositionings of the stimulator because of patient discomfort (1.7%/0.95%)
- three cases of thrombophlebitis with two pulmonary emboli ending with good resolution (1.7%/0.95%)
- 17 cases of postoperative confusion often related to the previous general status of the patient (8.6%/5.4%).

Apraxia of eyelid opening (5.6%/3.5%) was observed in 11 out of 51 STN patients (six of whom needed botulin toxin injection) and lasted more than

6 months in three of them (21.6%/11.6%) and in one GPi patient. Four patients who had previous demented states were not improved and had their mental status impaired permanently. These complications can be also analyzed for each target.

The Thalamus as Target

For VIM implantations (134 patients, 202 implanted sides)[4] there were four intracranial micro hematomas which induced a long-term thalamotomy-like effect or slight motor neglect which recovered over several weeks. Three others were detected only on routine postoperative CT scan. In this series, no epileptic seizures were induced by thalamic kindling. Five patients were confused and disoriented for several days postoperatively. There were no complications related to ventriculography. All adverse effects of stimulation – contralateral paresthesias (9%), limb dystonia (9%), dysequilibrium (7.6%) and dysarthria – were mild and tolerated by the patients and disappeared immediately when stimulation was decreased or stopped. Dysarthria more often affected patients who had a previous contralateral thalamotomy (12 of 23 patients = 51.7%) than those who were bilaterally stimulated (10 of 66 patients = 15%), suggesting that the morbidity rate from dysarthria for VIM stimulation is lower than that for thalamotomy.

Switching the stimulator off induced transient rebound tremor in about half of the patients without clinical implications. However, continuous stimulation in some patients (7 of 20), mainly those with action tremor, induced a tolerance phenomenon causing a progressive loss of stimulation efficacy over time.

The Pallidum as Target

Our experience with GPi is too small to be significant. However, we had to withdraw by 2 mm an electrode the tip of which was against the optic tract and induced visual flashes which disappeared thereafter.

The Subthalamus as Target

Complications and side-effects have not been frequent. We, unfortunately, had two hematomas out of 100 patients: one in the supraventricular area from a pericallosal branch injured by the exploratory electrode (the patient died 3 years later), and one in the thalamus. We have had no hematomas in the subthalamic nucleus itself. We had three asymptomatic brain contusions along electrode tracks, five postoperative or late infections, three patients had asymptomatic intraventricular blood on the routine postoperative MRI, which was attributable to a transventricular approach. One patient had a secondary scalp ulceration over the electrode-to-extension connection. Permanent hemiballism has never been observed during clinical follow-up. However, acute and transient hemiballism, which resolved within 24 hours, was observed in one case at the time of permanent 3389 electrode implantation. In several cases, various degrees of peripheral limb dyskinesias and involuntary movements, which we considered as symptoms of STN penetration, were induced during advancement of the recording electrodes and, in five cases, during insertion of chronic electrodes.

In three cases, a lesioning DC current leak from a defective test generator resulted in hemiballism. It was transient in all patients but one, who at 6 months after surgery still experienced a major resolution of the PD symptoms with no deficit, making stimulation useless. Seven patients were confused and disoriented for several days to 3 months postoperatively, which was likely related to the age of the patient. The severity of transient confusion depends on the preoperative clinical state of the patient, and the age, with younger patients having less severe episodes. As described above, we have observed the appearance of eyelid apraxia in about 20% of the cases; 11 patients exhibited transient eyelid opening apraxia, which in four cases needed botulinum toxin injection in the eyelids. Eyelid opening apraxia is known to happen in parkinsonian patients and the pathophysiology is unknown. It could be related to the proximity of the SNr which projects on to the colliculus superior which is related to the vertical oculomotricity, including extrinsic motricity of the eyelids. Hypophonia which was previously discussed is observed in about 20% of the patients. Worsening of motor performance is extremely rare and is possibly due to abnormally induced dyskinesias in a manner similar to the LIDs that are actually part of the physiology of the STN. Most of the patients had weight gain related to recovery of normal behavior and the loss of dyskinesias. Weight gain does not appear to be related to hypothalamic-like hormonal disturbances, as it has also been observed after pallidotomy.[81]

The average follow-up period was 87.4±13.9 months (min. 61, max. 123).

Mortality and Morbidity

There has been no operative mortality. One patient (VIM-implanted) died suddenly on the eleventh postoperative day from pulmonary embolism due to a pre-existing cardiovascular problem. Notably, he had recovered from stereotaxy and was ambulating in the neurosurgery department. Seven others died from various non-neurological diseases at 3, 6, 7, 10, 11, 23, and 116 months. Due to the long-distance referral of many patients, postmortem pathological examinations were not available.

Immediate postoperative morbidity has been higher in STN patients than VIM patients. This may be due to the fact that the patient populations are different. Patients implanted in the STN are in a more advanced stage of Parkinson's disease than are VIM-implanted patients who are of a similar age (VIM: 59.3±11.4 years, n =118; STN: 56.6±7.6 years, n = 60), but are most often only disabled by their tremor and are in a better general clinical state. Alternatively, this could also be due to the target itself and to the trajectory of the stereotactic approach. The target itself does not seem to be responsible for the observed side-effects as they were not always present. The trajectory, however, was closer to the midline, and may have involved at the upper level the white matter of the supplementary motor area or the thalamocortical frontal projections. Another possibility is that the caudate nucleus was damaged by the central portion of the five tubes. It is clear that confusion occurs, most often during the second side. More specifically, the onset of confusion seemed to coincide with the introduction of the guide tubes, but not the electrodes which corresponds to the upper border of the ventricle where the caudate is located. This correlates with the three different approaches used: a transventricular approach parallel to the midline, an oblique approach close to the lateral ventricle and caudate, and finally a more lateral approach in the internal capsule where less confusion seemed to occur, despite the occasional presence of edema on postoperative MRIs.

Complications According to the Method

We carefully reviewed 166 patients operated in the STN for complications of all types:

- 88 (54%) were complication-free
- 75 (46%) had at least one complication – 11 (6.7%) after the initial ventriculographic step, 52 (31.9%) after electrode implantation, and 12 (7.4%) after the IPG implant.

Ventriculography

Twelve complications were observed (7.4%) in 11 patients (6.7%). There was one case of edema, two asymptomatic concussions, two asymptomatic epidural hematomas which were associated with the frame pins, one seizure, one transitory deficit, three infections (one primary and two revisions of surgical wounds) which were treated with local wound care and a short course of antibiotics, and two miscellaneous complications (one pneumopathy, one delirious episode).

Electrode Implantation

Of 166 patients, 79 (48.4%) complications after implantation of the IPG and connexion to the electrode were observed in 55 patients (33.7%): 40 patients were confused (25 isolated, 15 with positive MRI), 11 had cortical contusions, nine had hematomas (regardless of the size and symptomaticity), two had bleeding along the track, eight had intraventricular bleeding, six had deficits (three permanent, three transient including two monoballisms), two had infections, and seven had miscellaneous complications.

Bleeding (hemorrhage, concussion, or hypersignal) was asymptomatic in nine patients (5.5%), and symptomatic in 20 (12.3%).

IPG Implantation and Hardware

Twenty-seven complications (16.6%) were observed in 22 patients (13.5%): three primary and two secondary infections, one rupture of the extension, and 16 miscellaneous benign lesions. These complications in STN are comparable to other recent series.[82]

Side-effects of Stimulation

Chronic use of DBS was associated with six cases of hypophonia, 22 cases of blepharospasm (12 requiring botulinum toxin injections), and 26 psychic manifestations.

The incidence during the immediate postoperative period and at 12 months was respectively 2% and 11% for apathy, 11% and 7% for depression, and 6% and 8% for apathy associated with depression. One patient committed suicide and three attempted suicide. The causes of the depression and suicide were multifactorial, involving primarily the withdrawal of levodopa or a significant decrease of dose, as well as the important changes in social and familial context for these patients on whom they were dependent for 10–15 years. This stresses the importance of a careful preoperative neuropsychological evaluation, and of postoperative psychological support. Additionally a cautious and slow withdrawal of levodopa or agonists is warranted.

Depression or apathy may be reversible after increasing dopaminergic treatment. This was sometimes more effective than treatment using antidepressants. This suggests that the changes produced by STN stimulation do not completely mimic the effects of levodopa. This is based on the previous observation that improvement of motor symptoms by STN stimulation allows a decrease in dopaminergic drugs, and provides some dopaminergic-type deficit in symptomatology, such as mood changes. A similar observation can be made with other symptoms such as speech.

Acute reversible neuropsychological side-effects, such as acute depression or laughter, were reported, which might be related to stimulation of the vicinity of the STN rather than within the nucleus itself.[83,84]

DISCUSSION

Comparison with Other Ablative Methods

The data presented above demonstrate that STN HFS relieves parkinsonian tremor, rigidity, akinesia, and levodopa-induced dyskinesias, has no significant routine complications, and has no specific side-effects. Ventroposterolateral pallidotomy,[81,85–89] however, has been recently reintroduced and is under investigation in several centers. The results reported are in the same range as those of STN HFS and it has been claimed that pallidotomy relieves all the motor symptoms of Parkinson's disease, especially LIDs. However, bilateral procedures have been reported to produce cognitive dysfunction. Moreover, experience recently acquired by several teams with pallidal HFS[80,90,91] suggests that the need for pallidal inhibition could be equally addressed using HFS rather than by destruction, as bilateral procedures using HFS offer less morbidity.

Our experience with both STN and GPi HFS allowed us to compare the methods in two matched series of young-onset parkinsonian patients. Our conclusions definitely favor STN HFS which has become our primary DBS target for akinetic/rigid as well as tremor-dominant PD.[75,78,90] We have shown[78,90] that STN improves all the UPDRS items by more than 60% whereas they are improved by less than 60% in GPi-stimulated patients, in the medication "off" situation. When in the medication "on" situation, another specificity of GPi stimulation appears as a loss of sensitivity to levodopa treatment which has to be increased.[81,92]

Costs

Deep brain stimulation is more expensive than ablative procedures. In addition to the stereotaxic procedure, which is nearly identical for the two methods, stimulation requires electrodes, extension leads, and stimulators.

At the time of writing, since May 1989 we have implanted 208 Itrel II stimulators at all three targets. Due to the high frequency at which they are used (130–185 Hz), battery life is relatively short. Replacement of Itrel I stimulators was performed in 18 out of 20 patients after 38.7±23.5 months (range 17–109 months). The lifetime of the 90 Itrel IIs that have not yet been changed in the STN averages 87 months. However, the significant decrease in drug dosage which is currently observed in our STN patients leads to a reduction in the overall cost of the procedure, which must be further evaluated, so the procedure could be competitive with medical treatment.

CONCLUSIONS

Because of its total and immediate reversibility, high-frequency stimulation has been used in parkinsonian patients without the drawbacks of lesions. HFS has been used in the VIM for tremor, in the GPi to treat levodopa-induced dyskinesias, and in the STN to treat rigidity, bradykinesia, and tremor. Bilateral implants of all three nuclei can be performed in the same session, due to the low morbidity of the procedure, and without producing the classic side-effects of bilateral ablative surgeries.

The effects of high-frequency stimulation of the STN are stable in patients now operated on 10 years ago. Some of these patients are now completely off pharmacological treatment.

The major advantages of DBS are its reversibility (particularly of side-effects in cases where incorrect implantation of the electrode can be changed or replaced); adaptability of the parameters (to fit the patient's clinical status and follow the evolution of its disease); the possibility of performing bilateral implantation in one session (which is most often needed); and the absence of significant permanent neuropsychological side-effects (not possible to achieve by ablative methods). Levodopa doses can be reduced which as a consequence decreases dyskinesias and may afford a potentially neuroprotective effect.

STN high-frequency stimulation is, in our experience, a remarkable therapy effective against all symptoms of Parkinson's disease. It is currently the treatment of choice to be proposed systematically as a first choice when evolution of the disease and failure of medical management occurs. The excellent results obtained by DBS justify its use as first-line treatment of parkinsonian symptoms. Moreover, this procedure would not exclude the patient from consideration for alternative treatments in the future, such as fetal transplant. As electrical stimulation is reversible, not only are its effects on symptoms more easily observable, but this method provides a privileged scientific opportunity to better understand the underlying mechanisms of PD, of tremor, and of other movement disorders, as well as of normal motor control in humans.

REFERENCES

1. Benabid AL, Benazzouz A, Hoffmann D et al. Long term electrical inhibition of deep brain targets in movement disorders. Mov Disord 1998;13:119–125.
2. Benabid AL, Pollak P, Louveau A, Henry S, de Rougemont J. Combined (thalamotomy and stimulation) stereotactic surgery of the Vim thalamic nucleus for bilateral Parkinson's disease. Appl Neurophysiol 1987;50:344–346.
3. Benabid AL, Pollak P, Gervason C et al. Long-term suppression of tremor by chronic stimulation of the ventral intermediate thalamic nucleus. Lancet 1991;337:403–406.
4. Benabid AL, Pollak P, Gao D et al. Chronic electrical stimulation of the ventralis intermedius nucleus of the thalamus as a treatment of movement disorders. J Neurosurg 1996;84:203–214.
5. Caparros-Lefebvre D, Blond S, Feltin MP, Pollak P, Benabid AL. Improvement of levodopa induced dyskinesias by thalamic deep brain stimulation is related to slight variation in electrode placement: possible involvement of the centro-median and parafascicularis complex. J Neurol Neurosurg Psychiatry 1999;67:306–314.
6. Laitinen L, Bergenheim AT, Hariz MI. Leksell's posteroventral pallidotomy in the treatment of Parkinson's disease. J Neurosurg 1992;76:53–61.
7. Svennilson E, Torvik A, Lowe R, Leksell L. Treatment of parkinsonism by stereotactic thermolesions in the pallidal region: a clinical evaluation of 81 cases. Acta Psychiatr Neurol Scand 1960;35:358–377.
8. Derome PJ, Jedynak CP, Visot A, Delalande O. Traitement des mouvements anormaux par lésions thalamiques. Rev Neurol (Paris) 1986;142:391–397.
9. Fox MW, Ahlskog JE, Kelly PJ. Stereotactic ventrolateralis thalamotomy for medically refractory tremor in post-levodopa era Parkinson's disease patients. J Neurosurg 1991;75:723–730.
10. Goldman MS, Ahlskog JE, Kelly PJ. The symptomatic and functional outcome of stereotactic thalamotomy for medically intractable essential tremor. J Neurosurg 1992;76:924–928.
11. Hirai T, Miyazaki M, Nakajima H, Shibazaki T, Ohye C. The correlation between tremor characteristics and the predicted volume of effective lesions in stereotaxic nucleus ventralis intermedius thalamotomy. Brain 1983;106:1001–1018.
12. Kelly P, Derome P, Guiot G. Thalamic spatial variability and the surgical results of lesions placed with neurophysiological control. Surg Neurol 1978;9:307–315.
13. Matsumoto K, Asano T, Baba T, Miyamoto T, Ohmoto T. Long-term follow-up review of cases of Parkinson's disease after unilateral or bilateral thalamotomy. Appl Neurophysiol 1976/77;39:257–260.
14. Matsumoto K, Shichijo F, Fukami T. Long-term follow-up review of cases of Parkinson's disease after unilateral or bilateral thalamotomy. J Neurosurg 1984;60:1033–1044.
15. Nagaseki Y, Shibazaki T, Hirai T et al. Long term follow-up of selective Vim-thalamotomy. J Neurosurg 1986;65:296–302.
16. Narabayashi H. Stereotaxic Vim thalamotomy for treatment of tremor. Eur Neurol 1989;29:29–32.
17. Ohye C, Maeda T, Narabayashi H. Physiologically defined Vim nucleus: its special reference to control of tremor. Appl Neurophysiol 1977;39:285–295.
18. Ohye C, Hirai T, Miyazaki M, Shibazaki T, Nakajima H. VIM thalamotomy for the treatment of various kinds of tremor. Appl Neurophysiol 1982;45:275–280.
19. Ohye C. Rôle des noyaux thalamiques dans l'hypertonie et le tremblement de la maladie de Parkinson. Rev Neurol (Paris) 1986;142:362–367.
20. Stellar S, Cooper IS. Mortality and morbidity in cryothalamectomy for Parkinson's disease: a statistical study of 2868 consecutive operations. J Neurosurg 1968;28:459–467.
21. Talairach J, Hecaen H, David M, Monnier M., de Ajuriaguerra J. Recherches sur la coagulation thérapeutique des structures sous-corticales chez l'homme. Rev Neurol (Paris) 1949;81:4–24.
22. Taren J, Guiot G, Derome P, Trigo JC. Hazards of stereotaxic thalamotomy: added safety factors in corroborating X-ray target localization with neurophysiological methods. J Neurosurg 1968;29:173–182.
23. Tasker RR, Organ LW, Hawrylyshyn PA. Investigation of the surgical target for alleviation of involuntary movement disorders. Appl Neurophysiol 1982;45:261–274.
24. Tasker RR, Siquiera J, Hawrylyshyn P, Organ LW. What happened to Vim thalamotomy for Parkinson's disease? Appl Neurophysiol 1983;46:68–83.
25. Benabid AL, Benazzouz A, Gao DM et al. Chronic electrical stimulation of the ventralis intermedius nucleus of the thalamus and of other nuclei as a treatment for Parkinson's disease. Techn Neurosurg 1999;5(1):5–30.

26. Limousin P, Pollak P, Benazzouz A et al. Effect of parkinsonian signs and symptoms of bilateral subthalamic nucleus stimulation. Lancet 1995;345:91–95.
27. Limousin P, Pollak P, Benazzouz A et al. Bilateral subthalamic nucleus stimulation for severe Parkinson's disease. Mov Disord 1995;10:672–674.
28. Limousin P, Krack P, Pollak P et al. Electrical stimulation of the subthalamic nucleus in advanced Parkinson's disease. N Engl J Med 1998;339:1105–1111.
29. Pollak P, Benabid AL, Gross C et al. Effets de la stimulation du noyau sous-thalamique dans la maladie de Parkinson. Rev Neurol (Paris) 1993;149:175–176.
30. Albin RL, Young AB, Penney JB. The functional anatomy of basal ganglia disorders. Trends Neurosci 1989;12:365–375.
31. Alexander GE, Crutcher MD. Functional architecture of basal ganglia circuits: neural substrates of parallel processing. Trends Neurosci 1990;13:266–271.
32. Aziz TZ, Peggs D, Sambrook MA, Crossman AR. Lesion of the subthalamic nucleus for the alleviation of 1-methyl-4-phenyl-1,2,3,6-tetrahydro-pyridine (MPTP)-induced parkinsonism in the primate. Mov Disord 1991;6:288–292.
33. Benazzouz A, Gross C, Feger J, Boraud T, Bioulac B. Reversal of rigidity and improvement in motor performance by subthalamic high-frequency stimulation in MPTP-treated monkeys. Eur J Neurosci 1993;5:382–389.
34. Bergman H, Wichmann T, DeLong MR. Reversal of experimental parkinsonism by lesions of the subthalamic nucleus. Science 1990;249:1346–1348.
35. DeLong M. Primate models of movement disorders of basal ganglia origin. Trends Neurosci 1990;13:281–285.
36. Feger J, Robledo P. The effects of activation or inhibition of the subthalamic nucleus on the metabolic and electrophysiological activities within the pallidal complex and substantia nigra in the rat. Eur J Neurosci 1991;3:947–952.
37. The Deep-Brain Stimulation for Parkinson's Disease Study Group. Deep-brain stimulation of the subthalamic nucleus or the pars interna of the globus pallidus in Parkinson's disease. N Engl J Med 2001;345:956–963.
38. Albe-Fessard D, Arfel G, Guiot G et al. Identification et délimitation précise de certaines structures sous-corticales de l'homme par l'électrophysiologie: son interêt dans la chirurgie stéreotaxique des dyskinesies. CR Acad Sci (Paris) 1961;253:2412–2414.
39. Albe-Fessard D, Arfel G, Guiot G et al. Dérivations d'activités spontanées et évoquées dans les structures cérébrales profondes de l'homme. Rev Neurol (Paris) 1962;106:89–105.
40. Albe-Fessard D, Arfel G, Guiot G. Activités électriques caractéristiques de quelques structures cérébrales chez l'homme. Ann Chir 1963;17:1185–1214.
41. Guiot G, Derome P, Arfel G, Walter S. Electrophysiological recordings in stereotaxic thalamotomy for parkinsonism. Prog Neurol Surg 1973;5:189–221.
42. Schaltenbrand G, Wahren W. Atlas for Stereotaxy of the Human Brain, 2nd edn. Stuttgart: Georg Thieme Verlag, 1977.
43. Talairach J, David M, Tournoux P, Corredor H, Kvasina T. Atlas d'anatomie stéreotaxique des noyaux gris centraux. Paris: Masson, 1957.
44. Cheshire WP, Ehle AL. Hemi-parkinsonism as a complication of an Ommaya reservoir. J Neurosurg 1990;73:774–776.
45. Marks PV, Wild AM, Gleave JRW. Long-term abolition of parkinsonian tremor following attempted ventriculography. Brit J Neurosurg 1991;5:505–508.
46. Guiot G, Arfel G, Derôme P. La chirurgie stéreotaxique des tremblements de repos et d'attitude. Gaz Med France 1968;75:4029–4056.
47. Alesch F, Koos WT. Computer-assisted multidimensional atlas for functional stereotaxy. Acta Neurochir (Wien) 1995;133(3/4):153–156.
48. Benabid AL, Hoffmann D, Ashraf A et al. [The robotization of neurosurgery: state of the art and future outlook]. Bull Acad Natl Med 1997;181:1625–1636.
49. Berks G, Pohl G, Keyserlingk DG. 3D-VIEWER: an atlas-based system for individual and statistical investigations of the human brain. Methods Inf Med 2001;40(3):170–177.
50. Gybels J, Suetens P. [Image-guided surgery]. Verh K Acad Geneeskd Belg 1997;59(1):35–57.
51. Hardy TL, Smith JR, Brynildson LR et al. Magnetic resonance imaging and anatomic atlas mapping for thalamotomy. Stereotact Funct Neurosurg 1992;58(1–4):30–32.
52. Nowinski WL, Fang A, Nguyen BT et al. Multiple brain atlas database and atlas-based neuroimaging system. Comput Aided Surg 1997;2(1):42–66.

53. Nowinski WL, Yeo TT, Thirunavuukarasuu A. Microelectrode-guided functional neurosurgery assisted by Electronic Clinical Brain Atlas CD-ROM. Comput Aided Surg 1998;3(3):115–122.
54. Nowinski WL, Yang GL, Yeo TT. Computer-aided stereotactic functional neurosurgery enhanced by the use of the multiple brain atlas database. IEEE Trans Med Imaging 2000;19:62–69.
55. diPierro CG, Francel PC, Jackson TR, Kamiryo T, Laws ER. Optimizing accuracy in magnetic resonance imaging-guided stereotaxis: a technique with validation based on the anterior commissure–posterior commissure line. J Neurosurg 1999;90:94–100.
56. Serra L, Nowinski WL, Poston T et al. The Brain Bench: virtual tools for stereotactic frame neurosurgery. Med Image Anal 1997;1:317–329.
57. Shabalov VA, Kazarnovskaya MI, Borodkin SM et al. Functional neurosurgery using 3-D computer stereotactic atlas. Acta Neurochir Suppl (Wien) 1993;58:65–67.
58. Vannier MW, Marsh JL. Three-dimensional imaging, surgical planning, and image-guided therapy. Radiol Clin N Am 1996;34:545–563.
59. Vayssiere N, Hemm S, Cif L et al. Comparison of atlas- and magnetic resonance imaging-based stereotactic targeting of the globus pallidus internus in the performance of deep brain stimulation for treatment of dystonia. J Neurosurg 2002;96:673–679.
60. Yeo TT, Nowinski WL. Functional neurosurgery aided by use of an electronic brain atlas. Acta Neurochir Suppl 1997;68:93–99.
61. Zincone A, Landi A, Piolti R et al. Physiologic study of the subthalamic volume. Neurol Sci 2001;22:111–112.
62. Ohye C, Narabayashi H. Physiological study of presumed ventralis intermedius neurons in the human thalamus. J Neurosurg 1979;50:290–297.
63. Ohye C, Shibazaki T, Hirai T et al. Further physiological observations on the ventralis intermedius neurons in the human thalamus. J Neurophysiol 1989;61:488–500.
64. Hutchinson WD, Lozano AM, Davis KD et al. Differential neuronal activity in segments of globus pallidus in Parkinson's disease patients. Neuroreport 1994;5:1533–1537.
65. Guiot G, Derome P, Trigo JC. Le tremblement d'attitude: indication la meilleure de la chirurgie stéreotaxique. Presse Med 1967;75:2513–2518.
66. Bejjani BP, Dormont D, Pidoux B et al. Bilateral subthalamic stimulation for Parkinson's disease by using three-dimensional stereotactic magnetic resonance imaging and electrophysiological guidance. J Neurosurg 2000;92:615–625.
67. Hariz MI, Fodstad H. Do microelectrode techniques increase accuracy or decrease risks in pallidotomy and deep brain stimulation? A critical review of the literature. Stereotact Funct Neurosurg 1999;72:157–169.
68. Alterman RL, Kall BA, Cohen H, Kelly PJ. Stereotactic ventrolateral thalamotomy: is ventriculography necessary? Neurosurgery 1995;37:717–722.
69. Benabid AL, Minotti L, Koudsie A, De Saint Martin A, Hirsch E. Antiepileptic effect of high-frequency stimulation of the subthalamic nucleus (corpus Luysii) in a case of medically intractable epilepsy caused by focal dysplasia: a 30-month follow-up. Neurosurgery 2002;50:1385–1392.
70. Depaulis A. The inhibitory control of the substantia nigra over generalized non-convulsive seizures in the rat. J Neural Transm Suppl 1992;35:125–139.
71. Iadarola MJ, Gale K. Substantia nigra: site of anticonvulsant activity mediated by gamma-aminobutyric acid. Science 1982;218:1237–1240.
72. Nguyen JP, Pollin B, Feve A, Geny C, Cesaro P. Improvement of action tremor by chronic cortical stimulation. Mov Disord 1998;13:84–88.
73. Woolsey CN, Erickson TC, Gilson WE. Localization in somatic sensory and motor areas of human cerebral cortex as determined by direct recording of evoked potentials and electrical stimulation. J Neurosurg 1979;51:476–506.
74. Nandi D, Liu X, Winter JL, Aziz TZ, Stein JF. Deep brain stimulation of the pedunculopontine region in the normal non-human primate. J Clin Neurosci 2002;9(2):170–174.
75. Krack P, Pollak P, Limousin P et al. From off-period dystonia to peak-dose chorea: the clinical spectrum of varying subthalamic nucleus activity. Brain 1999;122:1133–1146.
76. Charles PD, Van Blercom N, Krack P et al. Predictors of effective bilateral subthalamic nucleus stimulation for PD. Neurology 2002;59:932–934.
77. Caparros-Lefebvre D, Blond S, Vermersch P et al. Chronic thalamic stimulation improves tremor and levodopa induced dyskinesias in Parkinson's disease. J Neurol Neurosurg Psychiatry 1993;56:268–273.
78. Krack P, Limousin P, Benabid AL, Pollak P. Chronic stimulation of the subthalamic nucleus improves levodopa-induced dyskinesias in Parkinson's disease. Lancet 1997;350:1676.

79. Lagrange E, Krack P, Moro E et al. Bilateral subthalamic nucleus stimulation improves health-related quality of life in PD. Neurology 2002;59:1976–1978.
80. Lozano AM, Lang AM, Galvez-Jimenez N et al. Effect of GPi pallidotomy on motor function in Parkinson's disease. Lancet 1995;346:1383–1387.
81. Lang AE, Lozano A, Tasker R et al. Neuropsychological and behavioral changes and weight gain after medial pallidotomy. Ann Neurol 1997;41:834–836.
82. Oh MY, Abosch A, Kim SH, Lang AE, Lozano AM. Long-term hardware-related complications of deep brain stimulation. Neurosurgery 2002;50:1268–1274.
83. Bejjani BP, Damier P, Arnulf I et al. Transient acute depression induced by high-frequency deep-brain stimulation. N Engl J Med 1999;340:1476–1480.
84. Kumar R, Krack P, Pollak P. Transient acute depression induced by high-frequency deep-brain stimulation. N Engl J Med 1999;341:1003–1004.
85. Baron MS, Vitek JL, Bakay RA et al. Treatment of advanced Parkinson's disease by posterior GPi pallidotomy: 1-year results of a pilot study. Ann Neurol 1996;40:355–366.
86. Dogali M, Fazzini E, Kolodny E et al. Stereotactic ventral pallidotomy for Parkinson's disease. Neurology 1995;45:753–761.
87. Eskandar EN, Cosgrove GR, Shinobu LA, Penney JB. The importance of accurate lesion placement in posteroventral pallidotomy. J Neurosurg 1998;89:630–634.
88. Lang AE, Lozano AM, Montgomery E et al. Posteroventral medial pallidotomy in advanced Parkinson's disease. N Engl J Med 1997;337:1036–1042.
89. Tronnier VM, Fogel W, Kronenbuerger M, Steinvorth S. Pallidal stimulation: an alternative to pallidotomy? J Neurosurg 1997;87:700–705.
90. Krack P, Pollak P, Limousin P et al. Opposite effects of pallidal stimulation in Parkinson's disease. Ann Neurol 1998;43:180–192.
91. Siegfried J, Lippitz B. Bilateral chronic electrostimulation of ventroposterolateral pallidum: a new therapeutic approach for alleviating all parkinsonian symptoms. J Neurosurg 1994;35:1126–1130.
92. Verhagen L, Mouradian M, Chase T. Altered levodopa dose-response profile after pallidotomy [abstract]. Neurology 1996;46:A416–417.

9

Gene Therapy for Parkinson's Disease

Biplob Dass and Jeffrey H. Kordower

INTRODUCTION

Parkinson's disease (PD) is a neurodegenerative disorder of the basal ganglia, featuring a slow progressive loss of the neurons that project from the substantia nigra pars compacta to the striatum.[1] Currently, no available treatment can either halt or reverse the progression of the disease, although recently a phase 1 clinical trial of coenzyme Q_{10} showed some efficacy.[2] Although levodopa therapy can reverse the motor disabilities associated with PD, the therapeutic window shrinks to a point where efficacy cannot be sustained without unacceptable side-effects, such as dyskinesia and dystonia.[3] Thus, there is a strong desire to discover alternative therapies.

One such strategy is to deliver therapeutic genes utilizing viral vectors. The delivery of genes can theoretically result in the expression of therapeutic proteins for many years, and has the immediate advantage of offering a means of long-term therapy with no further intervention. In contrast, current methods of delivering putative protective or restorative molecules may require multiple surgical administrations, or infusions via pumps and indwelling cannulae, which can have biological (e.g., infection) or technical (e.g., blockage) problems. In addition, production of a therapeutic molecule might also be a difficult and expensive problem. Viral vector delivery of neuroprotective or restorative treatments can circumvent all of these issues. Gene delivery can also result in the expression of functional enzymes within cells, which may be capable of optimizing symptomatic therapies for PD, and so offers alternative therapeutic strategies for investigation.

Four viral vectors are commonly employed in studies that are attempting to achieve therapeutic gene delivery in models of neurodegenerative diseases. They are adenoviruses, herpes simplex viruses, adeno-associated viruses, and lentiviruses. Each of these will be reviewed here.

ADENOVIRUS

Adenovirus (Ad) is one of the best characterized viral vectors and was one of the first to be considered for use in animal models of PD.[4] This family of viruses was first identified in the 1950s and currently more than 50 members have been identified.[5] In humans it is associated with the common cold and intestinal and eye infections.[6] It possesses a simple structure of approximately 70–90 nm,[7] consisting of double-stranded DNA surrounded by a capsid, and from these 12 fibers project outwards. These fibers end in a globular knob which mediates attachment and entry into a cell. Variations of the fiber length and knob end account for the differences between adenoviral serotypes.[7]

Expression of a transgene, following transfection into a cell by adenovirus, does not require any incorporation of the viral DNA into the host genome.[8] Instead, the virus transfers its DNA, via cellular endosomes, into the cell nucleus, where cellular transcription promoters activate encoded genes.[8] (Also see reference 6 for a review.) Thus, the construction of the vector and the specificity of the viral promoter are extremely important for the subsequent expression of the transgene, or other viral genes.

In 1993, four groups separately reported transfection of the β-galactosidase gene (β-Gal) into the brain parenchyma of rats or mice following the administration of a replication-deficient adenovirus encoding that gene sequence.[9–12] The locations of administration included the striatum, globus pallidus, substantia nigra, hippocampus, or lateral ventricle, and resulted in the expression and detection of β-Gal activity in these discreet areas. Histochemical examination with X-Gal of the tissues revealed that neurons, myelinated axons, astrocytes, microglia, and oligodendrocytes all contained blue reaction product, indicative of successful transduction. Relevant to PD, immunohistochemical double labeling of the substantia nigra with tyrosine hydroxylase (TH) antibodies and X-Gal showed that approximately 50% of the TH-immunoreactive (TH-IR) neurons were also β-Gal positive.[9]

At lower titers of approximately 10^5–10^7 plaque forming units, there was no associated cytopathology associated with the injection of the adenovirus.[9,10] However, Akli and colleagues reported seeing cell death, gliosis, inflammatory responses, and tissue loss around the site of injection of 10^8 viral particles in the rat thalamus.[11] Following this, Byrnes and colleagues reported that a type-5 E1-deleted adenovirus activated both innate and adaptive immune responses and that this was due primarily to the viral particle itself, rather than to any transgene expression.[13]

Using the same virus in a follow-up study, a second peripheral administration of adenovirus 2 months after an injection into the caudate caused a greater inflammatory response in the rat brain than in control animals.[14] Microglial activation and demyelination occurred within 2 weeks of the second injection of adenovirus, and the level of transgene expression was reduced severely. If animals were immunized peripherally, prior to the administration of adenovirus in the brain parenchyma, expression of β-Gal in the striatum was reduced within 2 weeks.[15] However, if the animals were challenged with an adenovirus that had been gutted of most viral genes, transgene expression was maintained over 60 days, although this was reduced when compared to non-immunized controls.[15]

Therefore, using this "second-generation" adenovirus reduces inflammation but also decreases transgene expression compared to the unaltered vector.[15]

The first use of an adenovirus in a model of PD utilized the vector to transfect human tyrosine hydroxylase into the striatum of rats with an established 6-hydroxydopamine (6-OHDA) lesion.[4] In these animals, TH transfection resulted in a small decrease in apomorphine-induced rotational behavior (20–30%), but the expression of the gene seemed to be greater in reactive astrocytes than neurons. Inflammatory responses and gliosis were also noted around the site of injection of the adenovirus, and the expression of the transgene was monitored for only 2 weeks.[16]

Following this, another group injected Ad–TH into the striatum of 6-OHDA lesioned rats at either one, four, or eight sites, and found that apomorphine-induced rotational behavior had a linear relationship to the number of transfected TH-IR cell bodies in the striatum.[17] Four weeks after viral administration, rotational behavior was lost completely, as apomorphine-induced circling returned in these animals.

To provide control of expression of the transgene, Corti and colleagues created an Ad–TH virus that used a tetracycline-sensitive negative control system to modulate the expression of TH, and injected this into the striatum of 6-OHDA lesioned rats.[18] They tested whether TH expression could be turned off and on by the administration of doxycycline. In animals treated initially with the suppressive antibiotic and then switched to water, transgene expression recovered to 40% level compared to animals undergoing no suppression of expression. For rats initially treated with water, TH expression was entirely lost within 2 weeks of subsequent doxycycline administration. Thus, this adenovirus construct offered a mechanism of control of expression, and could therefore provide a means of titrating the availability of the transgene, and this method could also be used for the transfection of other genes.

In-vivo glial-cell-line-derived neurotrophic factor (GDNF) gene transfection by adenovirus in rodents was reported by four groups in 1997.[19–22] In Choi-Lundberg's study, supranigral administration of Ad–GDNF seven days before the initiation of a striatal 6-OHDA lesion in rats resulted in a 75% protection of nigral fluorogold-positive dopaminergic neurons, compared to 25% survival in animals treated with a control vector. However, no reduction in the size of the lesion was observed in the striatum of these animals, compared to controls. No behavioral effects were examined by this study.

In contrast to the Choi-Lundberg study, Horellou's group injected Ad–GDNF into the rat striatum, six days before the initiation of a striatal 6-OHDA partial lesion.[20] The number of TH-IR cells in the substantia nigra was significantly greater than in control animals, although again complete protection of the nigra was not achieved. Interestingly in the striatum, a qualitative analysis showed that TH immunoreactivity was increased following striatal Ad–GDNF administration compared to vehicle or Ad–β-Gal treatment. Also, amphetamine-induced rotational asymmetry was attenuated by treatment with striatal Ad–GDNF. Thus, the site of administration of GNDF is critical to the protection of the nigrostriatal pathway following a neurotoxic insult. Using GDNF protein, similar results have been obtained when comparing the protective effects of intra-striatal, intra-nigral, or intra-ventricular administration.[23]

Accordingly, GDNF was able to protect the anatomy and function of the nigrostriatal pathway only following an intra-striatal injection of Ad–GDNF; so if Ad–GDNF were considered for use in PD patients, it is more likely to be efficacious to administer the vector into the caudate and putamen.

In the studies by Choi-Lundberg and Bilang-Bleuel, both groups reported adverse cellular reactions to the administration of "first-generation" adenovirus, regardless of the particular gene sequence transfected by the vector.[19,20] Choi-Lundberg reported that 12 out of 14 rats injected with adenovirus possessed a mild to moderate reaction in the nigra, whilst Bilang-Bleuel and colleagues found that the size of the striatum was reduced and that Ad–β-Gal administration alone reduced the number of TH-IR cells by 37%. Therefore it is likely that the actions of transfected GDNF not only protect cells from 6-OHDA mediated cell death but also from the toxicity induced by the adenovirus itself.

In a follow-up study, Choi-Lundberg and colleagues repeated the administration of Ad–GDNF, but chose to inject the vector into the striatum before initiating a 6-OHDA partial lesion.[24] Upon careful examination, it was observed that Ad–GDNF did not actually protect or improve the density of TH-IR fibers in the striatum. However, behavioral asymmetry was reduced in these rats compared to vehicle-treated or Ad–β-Gal treated animals, and nigral TH-IR cell numbers were protected. This could be explained by the retrograde transport of GDNF or Ad–GDNF into the substantia nigra, and the subsequent trophic support that GDNF could provide to the functionality of the cell body.

They found that GDNF was detectable at nanogram levels in the striatum and at picogram levels in the nigra. Since GDNF can undergo retrograde transportation along the nigrostriatal tract, it was unclear if this finding was as a result of the actions on GDNF or a function of the adenovirus.[22,25,26] However, transgene GDNF mRNA was also detectable in the substantai nigra, although the level of amplification through PCR (polymerase chain reaction) required for the detection of a GDNF transcript was much greater than in the striatum. This indicated that the level transport of the adenoviral vector was moderate, but if used clinically, this feature of adenovirus could be advantageous in allowing the entire nigrostriatal pathway to be treated with GDNF following a single administration.

In their initial study, Choi-Lundberg and colleagues analyzed the levels of transfected GDNF protein, mRNA, and DNA and found that in the period of one to four weeks after administration, protein and mRNA levels decreased, whilst the GDNF DNA was unaffected by time.[19] This would indicate that the Rous sarcoma virus promoter may not have suitably maintained expression of the transgene, and similar results were found when β-Gal levels were examined following Ad–β-Gal injections. In their subsequent study, histochemical X-Gal visualization in the nigra of animals, one week after the administration of Ad–lacZ in the striatum, showed the presence of a small number of blue nucleated cells.[24] However, the expression in these cells was almost lost completely when the rats were examined 7 weeks after transfection. Also in the striatum, the intensity of blue reaction product in β-Gal positive cells was reduced in animals sacrificed 7 weeks after transfection compared to those analyzed after one week, again indicating a reduction in the expression of transgene over time. This therefore would be a significant drawback to clinical Ad–GDNF treatment, since the duration of the effect of Ad–GDNF would be minute compared to the course of PD.

Lapchak and colleagues attempted to use Ad–GDNF to restore the dopaminergic function of the nigrostriatal pathway of rats with an established 6-OHDA lesion.[22] Their 6-OHDA administration paradigm resulted in a 73% loss of dopamine in the substantia nigra and a 99% reduction in the striatum. In animals injected into the substantia nigra with Ad–GDNF, the nigral dopamine content was elevated to 44% of the levels on the intact side, while dopamine levels in the striatum were increased to 4% of the contralateral side. These neurochemical improvements in the nigrostriatal system were reflected in a moderate reduction in apomorphine-induced asymmetry, and an improvement in locomotor activity.

These behavioral changes lasted for only two weeks, but no conclusions could be drawn as to whether the short duration of the effects was due to a function of the CMV promoter, a reduction in transcription or translation of the transgene, an immune response resulting in the removal of transfected cells, or because there was a diminished number of target cells available for Ad–GDNF to infect, as no investigation of expression of GDNF over time was performed. However, the experiment did show that adenoviral transfection of GDNF could moderately improve nigrostriatal function after the degeneration of most of the pathway, offering the possibility that this treatment could be effective many years after the diagnosis of PD in humans.

Connor and colleagues pretreated aged rats with Ad–GDNF before initiating a striatal 6-OHDA lesion and found differences in TH immunoreactivity in the striatum, relative to previous experiments performed in the same laboratory.[24,27] Previously Choi-Lundberg et al. had shown that striatal treatment with Ad–GDNF in young rats prevented the behavioral asymmetries following 6-OHDA lesioning, but striatal TH-IR nerve fiber density was unaltered by Ad–GDNF pretreatment. In contrast, Connor et al. found that, in older animals, the administration of Ad–GDNF increased the number of TH-IR fibers in the striatum. The explanation for this difference between the two experiments remains unclear, but it may be due to the ability of the surviving neurons in the younger animals to undergo spontaneous recovery, thus masking the effect of GDNF, which might not occur in aged rats. Therefore, the administration of Ad–GDNF and 6-OHDA to aged rats should more accurately model the degenerative/regenerative situation seen in idiopathic PD.

Ad–GDNF has also been utilized in mice treated with 1-methyl-4-phenyl-1,2,3,6-tetrahydropyridine (MPTP).[21] In this experiment, mice were injected in the striatum with Ad–GDNF, two days prior to the administration of MPTP. Striatal dopamine levels were reduced in control MPTP lesioned animals, but were elevated in mice treated with Ad–GDNF, although striatal dopamine content was still severely reduced compared to naive animals. Unfortunately no evidence of in-vivo transfection of GDNF was shown in this study, and no conclusions could be drawn about the long-term expression and effects of Ad–GDNF.

In a very interesting study, Ad–GDNF was administered with an adenovirus encoding the protein caspase inhibitor, X-chromosome-linked inhibitor of apoptosis (XIAP).[28] The transfection of Ad–XIAP into the striata of mice resulted in the protection of TH-positive cells in the substantia nigra pars compacta following MPTP treatment, but striatal dopamine, DOPAC, and HVA contents were still reduced. Treatment of the mice with Ad–GDNF, followed by a chronic lesioning paradigm with MPTP injections over 5 days, resulted in no protection of TH-IR neurons in the substantia nigra, and no elevation of striatal dopamine, DOPAC, or HVA levels. However, when Ad–XIAP and Ad–GDNF treatments were administered in combination, both nigral TH-IR cell numbers and the catecholamine content of the striatum were protected from MPTP treatment. The actions of the trophic factor and the apoptosis inhibitor also appeared to be synergistic as the elevation of dopamine content and its metabolites were higher than might have been estimated by the additive effects of each vector alone. This would indicate that transfecting multiple molecules for protection or restoration could be a more potent than simply increasing the titer of a single vector, and that this can be achieved when using adenovirus.[28]

Another inhibitor of apoptosis is JNK interacting protein 1 (JIP-1), which binds to and blocks the actions of c-Jun N-terminal kinases (JNKs).[29] Expression of the JNK binding domain (JBD) of JIP-1 by an adenovirus can prevent apoptosis in PC12 cells and TH-IR cell loss in the mouse striatum following exposure to MPTP.[30] Thus, after the administration of Ad–JBD into the mouse striatum, dopaminergic cells in the substantia nigra expressed Flag-tagged JBD, showing that the adenovirus could undergo retrograde transportation in the mouse nigrostriatal pathway. The administration of (+)-amphetamine resulted in rotational behavior in the Ad–JBD treated MPTP-lesioned mice and the transfection protected the levels of striatal catecholamines and the number of TH-IR cells in the substantia nigra. The mechanism of protection may be due to the prevention of MPTP administration-induced caspase-3 activation, as in Ad–JBD treated animals no activated caspase-3 was observed, in contrast to MPTP-lesioned mice transfected with control virus.

ADENO-ASSOCIATED VIRUSES

Adeno-associated viruses (AAVs) were discovered approximately 40 years ago as a contaminant of a clinical sample of adenovirus.[31] However, AAVs are entirely unrelated to adenoviruses, and belong to the class of parvoviridae viruses. The AAV itself is a small organism, its total genome being approximately 5 kb, and it possesses a simple viral coat, made from only four different molecules.[31] Currently eight serotypes of AAV have been characterized and cloned, with types 2 and 5 being the most commonly employed for gene therapy.[32]

The advantage of using adeno-associated viruses as a vector for delivering therapeutic genes relies on the properties they exhibit in gene transduction. They are able to infect a wide variety of cells, including non-dividing cells like neurons, and can achieve longlasting expression of selected genes of up to 4.7 kbp in length.[33,34] Interestingly, serotype-2 AAV preferentially infects neurons, type 4 shows greater transfection in ependymal cells, while type 5 has no preference between neurons and astrocytes.[35,36] However, the administration of either type 4 or type 5 results in a ten-fold greater level of transfection compared to type-2 AAV injections.[36] The possible hosts for transfection comprise many species, including mice, rats, and primates.

The genome of an AAV is single-stranded, and wild-type viral DNA integrates specifically at chromosome 19 in humans. However, when modified for use as a vector, integration occurs randomly.[37] Once the DNA has entered the host genome, the synthesis of the complementary second strand must occur before transgene transcription and expression can take place, and thus a delay of weeks may be found before the transgene levels are maximal.[38] Alternatively, the virus can exist latently within a cell as an episome, and integrate into the nucleus at a later stage.[39–41]

Perhaps most important is the characteristic that AAVs, when used as viral vectors, have very minimal inflammatory properties and are non-pathogenic in humans. This is due to the fact that almost all of the viral gene sequences are deleted, with only two short stretches of AAV DNA, containing self-complementary stretches of DNA (termed "inverted terminal repeats"), remaining in the vector.[31] In the brain, direct administration of AAV capsid proteins only transiently resulted in the production of antibodies, and a re-injection of AAV–β-Gal two months later caused expression of the transgene.[33] Finally, in rodents, two groups have proved that expression of a transgene following a single administration of an AAV can last for 12–15 months, which is a marked contrast to experiments with adenovirus.[33,42]

A serotype-2 virus encoding tyrosine hydroxylase was the first AAV to be utilized in an animal model of PD. In that study, tyrosine hydroxylase immunoreactivity was detectable in the striata of 6-OHDA lesioned rats transfected with AAV–TH up to 4 months after vector administration.[43] This also resulted in a persistent reduction of apomorphine-induced rotational behavior in the lesioned animals for the duration of the experiment.

Following this, combinations of genes involved in the synthesis of levodopa have been transfected into the denervated striata of rats using separate AAVs. Thus, double or triple transfection of tyrosine hydroxylase, aromatic acid decarboxylase (AADC), and GTP-cyclohydrolase-1 (GCH-1) have been found to be extremely effective at producing levodopa in the 6-OHDA lesioned striatum, as measured by microdialysis.[42,44,45] In fully lesioned animals transfected with TH and GCH-1, apomorphine-induced rotational behavior was not attenuated, but rats with a partially preserved nigrostriatal pathway did exhibit reductions.[45] Behavioral recovery, as measured by apomorphine-induced rotational behavior, was also observed in fully lesioned rats transfected with all three genes using separate viruses in a 1:1:1 ratio. Although the increase in striatal dopamine content was modest in these animals, the effects of AAV transfection lasted for 12 months.[44] Expression of the transgenes was mainly neuronal, since serotype-2 AAV was used in these studies. Similar experiments performed using adenovirus, which predominately transfected astrocytes, resulted in inflammation and a loss of effectiveness.[4]

When administered in MPTP-treated primates, expression of genes following striatal transfection by an AAV encoding tyrosine hydroxylase and aromatic acid decarboxylase was observed for 10 weeks.[46] No inflammation or other adverse effects were noted after AAV administration. However, no behavioral recovery was observed in the monkeys. In contrast, triple transfection in the putamen of tyrosine hydroxylase, aromatic acid decarboxylase, and GTP-cyclohydrolase did result in behavioral recovery in four MPTP-treated primates, and this lasted for 10 months.[47] The animals exhibited an improvement in primate parkinsonian rating scale scores of 40–60%, and two animals tested for dexterity required less time to retrieve raisins using the hand contralateral to AAV treatment. Dopamine synthesis in the striatum was also increased approximately five-fold.

AAVs have also been used to transfect the DNA for two trophic factors in 6-OHDA lesioned rats.[48,49] BDNF was delivered into the substantia nigra pars compacta (SNpc) of rats by a recombinant AAV, which also encoded green fluorescent protein.[48] Expression of the green fluorescent protein was observed at 9 months after the administration of the viral vector. Six months after gene transfection, the animals were partially lesioned with 6-OHDA and rotational behavior in response to amphetamine was reduced in the AAV–BDNF treated animals in comparison to controls. However, no protection from 6-OHDA induced dopaminergic cell death in the SNpc was found.

GDNF, when expressed following transfection by an AAV, has been very successful at preventing dopaminergic cell death in the SNpc and reducing behavioral deficits in 6-OHDA lesioned rats.[49–51] Expression of GDNF was found to be stable for over 6 months, but no protection of the striatal dopaminergic immunoreactive terminals was observed and behavioral recovery did not occur following striatal 6-OHDA treatment.[50] In contrast, when AAV–GDNF was administered into the striatum of rats prior to a 6-OHDA lesion, the dopaminergic nigrostriatal pathway was completely protected and this was accompanied by a reduction in (+)-amphetamine-induced asymmetry.[50] To complement this study, another group investigated the effect of administration of AAV–GDNF after the initiation of a striatal 6-OHDA partial lesion in rats. Delayed delivery of the AAV also prevented nigral cell death, when administered 4 weeks following 6-OHDA lesioning. Behavioral recovery, assessed by apomorphine-induced rotations and contralateral limb use, was also improved following AAV–GDNF treatment, and these changes were maintained for 20 weeks.[51] Thus, AAVs offer a mechanism for the expression of molecules in the striatum over a long period of time, while inducing minimal side-effects, such as inflammation, and so could be used to achieve a long-term administration of trophic factors.

Intracerebral GDNF protein administration reversed motor disability and nigrostriatal function in rhesus monkeys and marmosets with established lesions of the dopaminergic system.[52,53] However, examining the neuroprotective ability of AAV–GDNF has difficulties, when lesions are initiated by treatment with MPTP, since animals possess varying susceptibilities to the neurotoxin. To circumvent this problem, AAV–GDNF was administered into the striatum and substantia nigra of marmosets, before a stereotaxic injection of 6-OHDA into the medial forebrain bundle (MFB) to create a lesion of the nigrostriatal tract.[54] Treatment with the AAV–GDNF only provided a modest protection of dopaminergic cells in the substantia nigra, although some TH immunoreactive fibers were observed in the striatum. However, modified clinical rating of the animals found that at 5 weeks after 6-OHDA treatment, motor function was reversed to pre-lesion levels. Also, (+)-amphetamine-induced rotational behavior and head positional bias were attenuated at all time points after lesioning, indicating that AAV transfected GDNF protected motor function in the primates. This study was the first to transfect a trophic factor into the primate brain by utilizing an AAV, but it failed to investigate if any inflammatory reaction occurred in response to the administration of the vector. It should be noted, however, that the total titer injected was of the same order of magnitude as used in rats and the transfection of TH in primates, where no inflammation was observed.[45,46,54]

Currently, a phase 1 clinical trial utilizing an AAV expressing the GAD gene in PD patients is underway in New York.[55] The rationale behind this study is that the overactivity of the excitatory subthalamic nucleus (STN) in PD patients might be reduced by the transfer of the GAD gene into this nucleus, and so provide relief from thalamic inhibition. Previously, this group had shown that AAV–GAD transfection into the STN of fully 6-OHDA lesioned rats could induce a phenotypic change in these nuclei, causing them to release the neurotransmitter GABA in addition to glutamate.[56] Injection of an AAV–GAD65 vector, 3 weeks before lesioning, also resulted in a 35% protection of nigral TH-positive cells, and decreased rotational behavior and behavioral asymmetries. As with other studies utilizing AAVs, no inflammation was found 4–5 months after administration, and no antibodies against the viral capsid were detected in the sera of these animals.[56] Thus, the basis for further studies utilizing AAV–GAD has been set, but currently no results from non-human primate experiments have been published.

HERPES SIMPLEX VIRUS

Knowledge of herpes simplex virus (HSV) dates back to the time of Hippocrates, who first described the problems of infectious lytic skin infections. HSV is an interesting tool for use in gene therapy as it has specificity for infecting neuronal cells, and has a larger capacity for transfecting foreign genes than adenovirus or adeno-associated virus.[57] Thus, the complete wild-type genome of HSV has 80 genes within 152 kb of double-stranded DNA, of which 30–150 kb can be replaced for the transfection of other genes.[58,59] In contrast, Ad and AAV wild-type DNA sequences are 36 or 5 kb, respectively, and can be used only to transfect genes that are a maximum of 7.5 or 4.5 kb in size. Following the infection of a cell, HSV DNA does not integrate with the host genome, and exists as an episome in the nucleus.[60] The life-cycle of HSV either results in the production of more viral particles and cell lysis following the expression of all its genes, or the virus can enter into a latency phase.[61] In this situation only a few viral genes, termed "latency-associated transcripts," are activated and so can be replaced to induce the transcription of exogenously introduced sequences.

HSV can be utilized in two ways to transfect cells. By deleting the immediate early genes that are essential for the viral cycle (and hence lytic infections) a replication-deficient recombinant vector can be created.[57,62] Five immediate early genes are present in the wild-type HSV genome, and deletion of some of these can reduce the cytotoxicity of infection, while removing all of them completely abolishes the deleterious effects of the virus. However, the downside of this strategy is that transgene expression is dramatically and quickly reduced, and so makes the modified vector unsuitable for long-term gene therapy in PD.

An alternative strategy to utilizing a recombinant virus is to use the HSV virion containing an *E. coli* origin of replication sequence, HSV origin of replication, and HSV packaging signals, and a transgene or transgenes of interest in a plasmid. The plasmid can be constructed and amplified in bacteria and finally packaged into an HSV particle using a defective HSV helper virus.[63] The resultant particle is termed an "HSV-packaged amplicon" and has the ability of HSV to transfer its DNA into the nucleus of a cell. However, two major problems exist with this system. First, the infectious particle titers that can be harvested are fairly low, usually in the region of 10^4 particles. Second, the repeated incubation of defective HSV helper virus with the amplicon can create wild-type HSV, and previously this was attributed to the death of approximately 10% of rats transfected with HSV-packaged amplicons.[64]

Despite the problems with HSV as a vector for gene therapy, some groups have utilized the virus to express genes in animal models of PD. The first strategy to utilize an HSV vector incorporated the tyrosine hydroxylase gene using an amplicon system.[64] This was used to transfect the gene into the partially denervated striatum of a 6-OHDA treated rat. Apomorphine-induced rotations were reduced over one year of behavioral testing, while levodopa levels and dopamine levels in the striatum were increased compared to lesioned animals transfected with a control vector. However, these characteristics were not greatly reversed compared to naive animals. The number of TH-immunopositive cells found in the striatum was also low, ranging from 5–10 to 200–300 neurons, and this did not correlate with the observed rotational behavior. Isacson later argued that the HSV construct could have induced further cell loss in the striatum, and that modulated the apomorphine-induced rotational behavior.[65] However, no changes in rotational behavior were seen in animals treated with an HSV–lacZ control vector, so the issue remains unclear. This vector system can result in the production and administration of wild-type virus, and 10% of the animals administered with the HSV amplicon died, possibly because of cytotoxic effects associated with this.

Using a replication-defective HSV vector, Yamada and colleagues transfected the anti-apoptotoic gene Bcl-2 into primary cortical neurons and survival of these cells was monitored for 3 weeks.[66] Expression of Bcl-2 reduced the number of cells that died, and TUNEL staining suggested that the transgene expression also reduced the number of apoptotic nuclei.

Injection of HSV–Bcl-2 into the rat striatum, one week before the initiation of a striatal 6-OHDA lesion, also prevented cell death.[66] Thus, both fluorogold- and TH-positive nigral cell counts were doubled in HSV–Bcl-2 treated animals compared to animals administered with a control vector; however, this protection was not complete as only 50% of the neurons survived in comparison to the intact untreated hemisphere. Animals in this study were followed for only 3 weeks after the injection of the HSV vector, and so long-term in-vivo expression of the transgene could not be confirmed. Most importantly, administration of either HSV–Bcl-2 or a control virus resulted in a 40% reduction in fluorogold- and TH-positive cells, in the absence of 6-OHDA lesioning. Although the authors noted that there was no inflammation using hematoxylin and eosin staining 3 weeks after the injection of the vector, it is likely that the cell loss observed was caused by HSV and this could have a significant impact on the use of this virus for transgene expression in higher species.

In an extension of the previous study, the same group transfected cells in the rat striatum with two HSV vectors, one encoding Bcl-2 and the other GDNF.[67] Amphetamine-induced rotational behavior was significantly reduced by the administration of either vector 2 weeks after a striatal injection of 6-OHDA, and this was also observed with the co-administration of both vectors. Again, both fluorogold- and TH-positive nigral cell counts were doubled in HSV–Bcl-2 treated animals compared to animals administered with a control vector, and similar results were observed in HSV–GDNF administered rats. Co-administration of HSV–Bcl-2 and HSV–GDNF resulted in a greater protection of nigral neurons, with fluorogold-positive cell levels being 75% of the intact side and TH-positive cell numbers were 90% of the untreated hemisphere. However, this study failed to examine any cytotoxic effects of recombinant HSV administration, and looked only for transgene expression at one week after transfection; so conclusions about the suitability of HSV for further gene therapy experiments could not be drawn.

LENTIVIRUS

Lentiviruses are small collections of retroviruses that have been derived from human immunodeficiency virus type 1 (HIV-1),[68] or non-human equivalents, such as equine infectious anemia virus (EIAV),[69,70] or feline immunodeficiency virus (FIV).[71] Typically retroviruses are incapable of infecting and causing the expression of foreign genes in non-dividing cells as they require the breakdown of the membrane of the nucleus for genomic insertion of DNA.[72] However, HIV is capable of integrating its DNA into the genome of a host cell, thanks to a pair of proteins called Vpr and matrix which transfer the viral particle into the nucleus.[68,73]

HIV is a cytotoxic virus. To circumvent the problem of cell death following its administration *in vivo*, Naldini and colleagues created a form of the virus which lacked most of the genes required for the replication of the virus.[68] To produce the vector, 293T human kidney cells were transfected by three plasmids each of which possessed some HIV genes to create replication-deficient particles. Thus, one plasmid would be responsible for the creation of the viral protein envelope, and a packaging plasmid would express proteins to help insert the genes of the transfer plasmid into the particle. This system should make it unlikely that recombination into a pathogenic HIV particle can occur. Another advantage of this method is that titers of 10^8–10^9 viral particles per milliliter can be generated, which is greater than for HSV. The transgene capacity of lentivirus is approximately 9 kb and so is larger than adeno-associated virus but smaller than HSV.

In initial studies, lentiviruses were created to express β-Gal, and this was examined in the striatum and hippocampus of rats.[68] At either 7 or 30 days after transfection of the lenti–β-Gal vector, the regions around the injection sites exhibited very little inflammation, while β-Gal-positive neurons, astrocytes, and oligodendrocytes were all observed.

In an expansion of this study, the same group examined lentivirally mediated β-Gal expression in the striatum and hippocampus over 6 months and compared this to the actions of second-generation adenovirus, adeno-associated virus type 2, and murine leukemia virus, which acted as a control.[73] Lentivirus administration achieved a denser infection of cells compared to all other vectors over the 6 months of the study. The percentage of neurons transfected by lentivirus was also higher than was observed following AAV treatment, and the expression of the transgene was very stable over the 6 months. In contrast to adenovirus, lentivirus did not induce any inflammation, as shown by immunofluorescent histochemistry for CD4 helper T-cell precursors, OX8-positive T-cytotoxic precursor lymphocytes, or ED1 positive macrophages.

Following this, our group, in collaboration with Patrick Aebischer, injected lenti–β-Gal into the striatum of three rhesus monkeys.[74] Two monkeys that were sacrificed one month after vector administration possessed approximately 10^6 β-Gal-positive cells and exhibited minimal inflammation in the striatum, although there was some minor perivascular cuffing around some blood vessels. In the animal sacrificed 3 months after injection of lenti–β-Gal, approximately 1.5×10^6 cells were infected by the virus, and again there was little inflammation observed. This monkey also received a lenti–β-Gal administration in the substantia nigra and here 2×10^5 cells were positively transfected, and no inflammation or perivascular cuffing was observed, indicating that lentivirus could be safely and reliably used in primates over long periods.

Following that study, this collaborative group generated a GDNF expressing lentivirus and injected it into the striatum and nigra of young adult rhesus monkeys one week after MPTP lesioning or unlesioned aged monkeys.[75] In all monkeys, strong GDNF immunoreactivity was observed and this was coupled with increased striatal fluorodopa uptake, TH immunoreactivity, dopamine and HVA content. Interestingly, GDNF immunoreactivity was also observed in the globus pallidus and substantia nigra pars reticulata (SNpr), indicating anterograde transport of the transgene.

MPTP-lesioned animals before lenti–GDNF or lenti–β-Gal administration displayed clear motor disability, as measured by a clinical rating scale. After injections of the virus, lenti–β-Gal-treated animals exhibited no improvements in motor disability, whilst lenti–GDNF administration resulted in a reduction over the following 3 months. Dexterity, as measured by a hand-reach task, was also improved in lenti–GDNF administered monkeys compared to the lenti–β-Gal-treated animals. PET scans taken at 3 months after vector injection showed that lenti–GDNF-treated animals had a 300% increase in fluorodopa uptake compared to the control monkeys, although this was limited to the putamen only.

Lenti–GDNF treatment also enhanced the striatal TH immunoreactivity in a manner that correlated with the dexterity levels of each MPTP-lesioned monkey. Thus the animals that had the best scores on the hand-reach task also possessed the greatest intensity of TH-positive immunoreactivity. Overall, TH immunoreactivitity in the striatum was significantly greater in lenti–GDNF-treated monkeys compared to lenti–β-Gal-treated animals. In the substantia nigra, lenti–GDNF expression resulted in an increase in TH-positive cell numbers and cell density compared to the untreated hemisphere, while animals administered lenti–β-Gal had large decreases in cell counts and density on the MPTP-lesioned side. Immunohistochemistry for CD45, CD3, and CD8 resulted in negligible levels of positive cells, indicating that the lentivirus caused no immunogenicity.

Two young unlesioned rhesus monkeys were also administered with lenti–GDNF into the right caudate and putamen and left SNpc and examined 8 months later for gene expression. ELISA analysis found 2.5–3.5 ng/mg tissue of GDNF in the caudate and putamen, while in the nigra many GDNF immunoreactive cells were observed, proving long-term transgene expression.

In a subsequent study, the effect of lenti–GDNF was examined stereologically in the striatum of aged monkeys and unilaterally MPTP-lesioned monkeys.[76] MPTP treatment alone increased the numbers of intrinsic dopamine neurons in the striatum, and lenti–GDNF administration further increased the striatal TH-immunoreactive cell counts seven-fold. In aged monkeys, there was also a large increase in TH and DAT immunoreactivity in the striatum and this correlated with GDNF expression, indicating an autotrophic effect. The coupling of the two results suggests that lenti–GDNF is effective regardless of the level of down-regulation of the dopaminergic phenotype.

Lenti–GDNF has also been used to prevent 6-OHDA-induced degeneration in two other animal models of PD. In mice, lenti–GDNF was injected supranigrally, 2 weeks before a striatal administration of 6-OHDA.[77] In the nigra, the number of TH-positive cells was significantly higher in lenti–GNDF-treated mice compared to those administered with a control virus, and the total numbers of cells were only 25% below those of the intact side. However, striatal dopamine content was not protected at all by the supranigral administration of lenti–GDNF and all animals had 90% reductions compared to the intact hemisphere. Apomorphine-induced rotational behavior was also reduced following the expression of GDNF, although circling was not prevented. Similar to the studies performed in primates, nanogram quantities of GDNF were detected following vector administration, but the route of administration may have prevented greater benefits of lenti–GDNF administration from being observed.

In rats, two separate titers of lenti–GDNF were administered 3 weeks before a striatal injection of 6-OHDA.[78] Prior to lesioning, the animals were challenged with amphetamine and exhibited contralateral turning behavior correlated to the amount of vector received. After 6-OHDA treatment, TH-positive cell counts in the substantia nigra were increased compared to rats receiving a control vector. The cell numbers corresponded again to the titer of vector used, so that animals treated with a lower dose of vector had 65% of the neurons observable in the intact side, while animals administered with a higher concentration of lenti–GDNF had a 77% protection of TH-positive cells. Interestingly, intense sprouting of fibers was observed in the medial parts of the striatum, globus pallidus, and entopeduncular nucleus, and this corresponded to GDNF immunoreactivity, indicating that GDNF was transported and having effects away from the injection site.

The same group repeated this experiment with a single titer of vector, but administered the lenti–GDNF into the striatum.[79] As before, TH-positive cell numbers in the nigra were preserved by lenti–GDNF treatment and amphetamine-induced rotational behavior was reversed. Tracing the nigrostriatal pathway using fluorogold retrograde labeling from the striatum, or AAV–GFP anterograde marking from the nigra, showed that lenti–GDNF administration also protected the axonal projections of the SNpc into the striatum. However TH fiber immunoreactivity was down-regulated in the striatum, the authors speculating an effect of GDNF. Also, non-drug-induced motor asymmetry was unchanged by lenti–GDNF administration, and this was attributed to the aberrant sprouting of TH-positive fibers from the striatum projecting to the globus pallidus, entopenduncular nucleus, and the substantia nigra.

As an alternative strategy to transfecting GDNF, a lentivirus based on equine infectious anemia virus was used to transfect neurons with AADC, TH, and GTP cyclohydrolase.[80] The theory behind using a non-human lentivirus is that it is less likely to recombine and cause a detrimental condition if used clinically. However, there is currently no evidence that lentivirus could recombine to form a pathogenic HIV particle, and there is also no proof that non-human forms of HIV would pose a lesser risk. The vector used by Azzouz and colleagues also featured a self-inactivating version of lentivirus, which reduced the expression of non-transgene coded proteins and so increased the safety of using the viral construct.

The lentivirus also incorporated genes for all three enzymes, and so was different from previous experiments involving AAV, HSV, or Ad, where multiple vectors were used to transfect enzymes. Rats were lesioned by injection of 6-OHDA into the medial forebrain bundle, resulting in a complete loss of TH-positive cells in the substantia nigra, and 5 weeks later were injected into the striatum with the vector. Rotational behavior induced by apomorphine administration was partially reversed by treatment with the tricistronic vector, although turning behavior was still greater than 5 per minute in these rats. Striatal dopamine content was also partially elevated by treatment with the lentivirus, but levels were still less than 10% of the intact hemisphere. Five months after transfection of the three genes, TH, AADC, and GTP cyclohydrolase immunoreactivity was still observable and dual immunofluorescence showed co-expression of the transgenes within neurons. No inflammation or perivascular cuffing was observed in these animals also, highlighting the lack of immunogenicity elicited by lentiviral gene transfer.

CONCLUSIONS

This review has covered all of the current gene therapy strategies utilized for the treatment of the symptoms of PD. The issue of which vector is ideal for use in the treatment of the disease raises a problem, since each virus has strengths and drawbacks (Table 9.1).

Adenovirus and HSV administrations cause high immunogenic responses and are short-acting, so are non-starters for clinical application in PD. Adeno-associated virus has a low level of transgene expression and lentivirus has a fairly small capacity, and the stigma of being associated with HIV. However, these vectors currently represent the best vehicles for the introduction of novel

TABLE 9.1 Characteristics and uses of viral vectors in animal models of PD

Vector	*Neuronal preference*	*Size of insert*	*Strength of expression*	*Length of expression*	*Immunogenicity*	*Tested applications*
Adenovirus	+	7.5 kb	++	Weeks	+++	TH, GDNF, XIAP, JBD, calpastatin, Cu/Zn SOD,
Adeno-associated virus	++++ (type 2) + (type 5)	4 kb	+ (type 2) ++ (type 5)	>1 year	+	TH, AADC, GTP-cyclohydrolase, BDNF, GDNF, GAD
Herpes simplex virus	++++	30–150 kb	++	Weeks	+++	TH, Bcl-2, GDNF
Lentivirus	+++	9 kb	+++	>1 year +	+	GDNF, TH, AADC, GTP-cyclohydrolase

genes into the human brain. Currently the ease and overall safety of using AAV has made this vector the most popular for gene therapy, and use of multiple vectors to transfect cells can somewhat circumvent the limited capacity the virus has for transgenes.

The most important issue to be addressed, if gene therapy is to be utilized clinically, is safety. Previously in 2002, a gene therapy trial involving patients with severe combined immune deficiency using a retrovirus was halted after one out of the eleven trial subjects developed leukemia.[81] Analysis of this patient revealed that the retrovirus had integrated into the host genome at 40 different sites including one, LMO-2, which was related to oncogenesis and this contributed to the abnormal growth of a T-cell. Insertational mutagenesis is therefore a major concern with the use of integrating viral vectors, especially those such as serotype-5 AAV or lentivirus, which are capable of infecting glial cells. Also, Nakai and colleagues recently showed in mice that AAV serotype-2 integrates its DNA more frequently into active genes rather than quiescent ones.[82]

More seriously, the case of Jesse Gelsinger in 1999 showed the degree of care which needs to be taken before embarking on any gene therapy trial. This patient suffered from ornithine transcarbamylase (OTC) deficiency, and was infused into the right hepatic artery with an adenovirus encoding the human OTC gene, as part of a phase 1 trial.[83] Unfortunately, the patient suffered from a severe immune reaction to the adenovirus and died five days after treatment. The reason for this may have been that the patient was previously exposed to adenovirus, and this may have contributed towards an increased autoimmune response to the vector. Most of the other patients in this trial, who all received lower titers of adenovirus, also rapidly developed fever, supporting the theory that previous exposure to adenovirus followed by a second administration of the virus could cause greater inflammation. Therefore rigorous screening of patients must be conducted before the commencement of gene therapy.

The best site of administration of a viral vector also must be ascertained. AAV, but not lentivirus, has shown a capability for retrograde transport. Anterograde transport can occur with trophic factors such as GDNF also. This could cause problems of unwanted expression of transgenes in other areas of the brain if the site of administration was the striatum. Currently this is just a theoretical concept as no adverse reactions have been demonstrated as a result of such transport. Thus, while it would be favorable to have transport of a trophic factor or dopamine synthesizing enzyme into the substantia nigra pars compacta, it is unclear whether transport to the pallidum, thalamus, or the neocortex would be beneficial, harmful, or inconsequential. Diffusion, following an injection of a vector into the nigral region, equally could result in major problems with alterations in the firing of VTA neurons. Thus, the preferential site of injection and the expression level of transgenes away from the administration location needs to be fully investigated. One possibility to limit the expression of a transgene is to infect cells with a viral vector and then transplant them into the brain, but currently this strategy has had mixed results in promoting behavioral recovery in 6-OHDA-lesioned rats.[84,85]

The ideal candidate for gene therapy in PD is another question that needs more study. Here we have outlined trophic factors, anti-apoptotic genes, dopamine synthesizing enzymes, and basal ganglia modulation therapies. The trophic factor transfection approach offers the greatest possible benefit, in that it would prevent the progressive degeneration of the dopaminergic nigrostriatal system, and could also enhance the functioning of those remaining neurons to provide functional benefits. GDNF appears to be the most suitable trophic factor, based on long-term infusion studies of the protein into the putamen, which resulted in motor function improvements and increased fluorodopa uptake in the striata of PD patients.[86] Currently there are ongoing studies involving other possible trophic factors which may be as potent as GDNF, such as neurturin and sonic hedgehog.[87–89] These may prove to be better, due to greater specificity to act on dopaminergic neurons, or require less trophic factor expression to gain a response, and so reduce the titer of vector required to be administered. However, currently GDNF represents the best and most extensively characterized therapeutic trophic factor available. Other strategies for the treatment of PD may also provide benefit for patients, by reducing their levodopa requirements, and so ameliorate the development of levodopa-induced side-effects.

Currently one clinical trial has begun in New York, featuring the transfection of GAD into the STN using an adeno-associated virus. Thus far, no problems have been reported and it is hoped that this trial will prove that gene therapy can be safely conducted in the basal ganglia. If this study does prove successful, it will hopefully lead to more experiments utilizing viral vectors for the treatment of PD, including the expression of trophic factors which may be able to halt or reverse the course of the disease.

REFERENCES

1. Ehringer H, Hornykiewicz O. [Distribution of noradrenaline and dopamine (3-hydroxytyramine) in the human brain and their behavior in diseases of the extrapyramidal system.] Klin Wochenschr 1960;38:1236–1239 [in German].
2. Shults CW, Oakes D, Kieburtz K et al., Parkinson Study Group. Effects of coenzyme Q10 in early Parkinson disease: evidence of slowing of the functional decline. Arch Neurol 2002;59:1541–1550.
3. Marsden CD. Parkinson's disease. Lancet 1990;335:948–952.
4. Horellou P, Vigne E, Castel MN et al. Direct intracerebral gene transfer of an adenoviral vector expressing tyrosine hydroxylase in a rat model of Parkinson's disease. Neuroreport 1994;6(1):49–53.
5. De Jong JC, Wermenbol AG, Verweij-Uijterwaal MW et al. Adenoviruses from human immunodeficiency virus-infected individuals, including two strains that represent new candidate serotypes Ad50 and Ad51 of species B1 and D, respectively. J Clin Microbiol 1999;37:3940–3945.
6. Lai CM, Lai YK, Rakoczy PE. Adenovirus and adeno-associated virus vectors. DNA Cell Biol 2002;21:895–913.
7. Ginsberg HS, Pereira HG, Valentine RC, Wilcox WC. A proposed terminology for the adenovirus antigens and virion morphological subunits. Virology 1966;28:782–783.
8. Trotman LC, Mosberger N, Fornerod M, Stidwill RP, Greber UF. Import of adenovirus DNA involves the nuclear pore complex receptor CAN/Nup214 and histone H1. Nat Cell Biol 2001;3: 1092–1100.
9. Le Gal La Salle G, Robert JJ, Berrard S et al. An adenovirus vector for gene transfer into neurons and glia in the brain. Science 1993;259:988–990.
10. Davidson BL, Allen ED, Kozarsky KF, Wilson JM, Roessler BJ. A model system for in-vivo gene transfer into the central nervous system using an adenoviral vector. Nat Genet 1993;3:219–223.
11. Akli S, Caillaud C, Vigne E et al. Transfer of a foreign gene into the brain using adenovirus vectors. Nat Genet 1993;3:224–228.
12. Bajocchi G, Feldman SH, Crystal RG, Mastrangeli A. Direct in-vivo gene transfer to ependymal cells in the central nervous system using recombinant adenovirus vectors. Nat Genet 1993;3:229–234.

13. Byrnes AP, Rusby JE, Wood MJ, Charlton HM. Adenovirus gene transfer causes inflammation in the brain. Neuroscience 1995;66:1015–1024.
14. Byrnes AP, MacLaren RE, Charlton HM. Immunological instability of persistent adenovirus vectors in the brain: peripheral exposure to vector leads to renewed inflammation, reduced gene expression, and demyelination. J Neurosci 1996;16:3045–3055.
15. Thomas CE, Schiedner G, Kochanek S, Castro MG, Lowenstein PR. Preexisting antiadenoviral immunity is not a barrier to efficient and stable transduction of the brain, mediated by novel high-capacity adenovirus vectors. Hum Gene Ther 2001;12:839–846.
16. Horellou P, Sabate O, Buc-Caron MH, Mallet J. Adenovirus-mediated gene transfer to the central nervous system for Parkinson's disease. Exp Neurol 1997;144:131–138.
17. Leone P, McPhee SW, Janson CG et al. Multi-site partitioned delivery of human tyrosine hydroxylase gene with phenotypic recovery in parkinsonian rats. Neuroreport 2000;11:1145–1151.
18. Corti O, Sanchez-Capelo A, Colin P et al. Long-term doxycycline-controlled expression of human tyrosine hydroxylase after direct adenovirus-mediated gene transfer to a rat model of Parkinson's disease. Proc Natl Acad Sci USA 1999;96:12120–12125.
19. Choi-Lundberg DL, Lin Q, Chang YN et al. Dopaminergic neurons protected from degeneration by GDNF gene therapy. Science 1997;275:838–841.
20. Bilang-Bleuel A, Revah F, Colin P et al. Intrastriatal injection of an adenoviral vector expressing glial-cell-line-derived neurotrophic factor prevents dopaminergic neuron degeneration and behavioral impairment in a rat model of Parkinson disease. Proc Natl Acad Sci USA 1997;94:8818–8823.
21. Kojima H, Abiru Y, Sakajiri K et al. Adenovirus-mediated transduction with human glial cell line-derived neurotrophic factor gene prevents 1-methyl-4-phenyl-1,2,3,6-tetrahydropyridine-induced dopamine depletion in striatum of mouse brain. Biochem Biophys Res Commun 1997;238:569–573.
22. Lapchak PA, Araujo DM, Hilt DC, Sheng J, Jiao S. Adenoviral vector-mediated GDNF gene therapy in a rodent lesion model of late stage Parkinson's disease. Brain Res 1997;777:153–160.
23. Kirik D, Rosenblad C, Bjorklund A. Preservation of a functional nigrostriatal dopamine pathway by GDNF in the intrastriatal 6-OHDA lesion model depends on the site of administration of the trophic factor. Eur J Neurosci 2000;12:3871–3882.
24. Choi-Lundberg DL, Lin Q, Schallert T et al. Behavioral and cellular protection of rat dopaminergic neurons by an adenoviral vector encoding glial cell line-derived neurotrophic factor. Exp Neurol 1998;154:261–275.
25. Tomac A, Widenfalk J, Lin LF et al. Retrograde axonal transport of glial cell line-derived neurotrophic factor in the adult nigrostriatal system suggests a trophic role in the adult. Proc Natl Acad Sci USA 1995;92:8274–8278.
26. Mufson EJ, Kroin JS, Sendera TJ, Sobreviela T. Distribution and retrograde transport of trophic factors in the central nervous system: functional implications for the treatment of neurodegenerative diseases. Prog Neurobiol 1999;57:451–484.
27. Connor B, Kozlowski DA, Schallert T et al. Differential effects of glial cell line-derived neurotrophic factor (GDNF) in the striatum and substantia nigra of the aged Parkinsonian rat. Gene Ther 1999;6:1936–1951.
28. Eberhardt O, Coelln RV, Kugler S et al. Protection by synergistic effects of adenovirus-mediated X-chromosome-linked inhibitor of apoptosis and glial cell line-derived neurotrophic factor gene transfer in the 1-methyl-4-phenyl-1,2,3,6-tetrahydropyridine model of Parkinson's disease. J Neurosci 2000;20:9126–9134.
29. Dickens M, Rogers JS, Cavanagh J et al. A cytoplasmic inhibitor of the JNK signal transduction pathway. Science 1997;277:693–696.
30. Xia XG, Harding T, Weller M et al. Gene transfer of the JNK interacting protein-1 protects dopaminergic neurons in the MPTP model of Parkinson's disease. Proc Natl Acad Sci USA 2001;98:10433–10438.
31. Muzyczka N. Use of adeno-associated virus as a general transduction vector for mammalian cells. Curr Top Microbiol Immunol 1992;158:97–129.
32. Gao GP, Alvira MR, Wang L et al. Novel adeno-associated viruses from rhesus monkeys as vectors for human gene therapy. Proc Natl Acad Sci USA 2002;99:11854–11859.
33. Lo WD, Qu G, Sferra TJ et al. Adeno-associated virus-mediated gene transfer to the brain: duration and modulation of expression. Hum Gene Ther 1999;10:201–213.
34. Chamberlin NL, Du B, de Lacalle S, Saper CB. Recombinant adeno-associated virus vector: use for transgene expression and anterograde tract tracing in the CNS. Brain Res 1998;793(1/2):169–175.
35. Bartlett JS, Samulski RJ, McCown TJ. Selective and rapid uptake of adeno-associated virus type 2 in brain. Hum Gene Ther 1998;9:1181–1186.

36. Davidson BL, Stein CS, Heth JA et al. Recombinant adeno-associated virus type 2, 4, and 5 vectors: transduction of variant cell types and regions in the mammalian central nervous system. Proc Natl Acad Sci USA 2000;97:3428–3432.
37. Young SM, McCarty DM, Degtyareva N, Samulski RJ. Roles of adeno-associated virus Rep protein and human chromosome 19 in site-specific recombination. J Virol 2000;74:3953–3966.
38. Ferrari FK, Samulski T, Shenk T, Samulski RJ. Second-strand synthesis is a rate-limiting step for efficient transduction by recombinant adeno-associated virus vectors. J Virol 1996;70:3227–3234.
39. Afione SA, Conrad CK, Kearns WG et al. In-vivo model of adeno-associated virus vector persistence and rescue. J Virol 1996;70:3235–3241.
40. Wu P, Phillips MI, Bui J, Terwilliger EF. Adeno-associated virus vector-mediated transgene integration into neurons and other nondividing cell targets. J Virol 1998;72:5919–5926.
41. Duan D, Sharma P, Dudus L et al. Formation of adeno-associated virus circular genomes is differentially regulated by adenovirus E4 ORF6 and E2a gene expression. J Virol 1999;73:161–169.
42. Mandel RJ, Rendahl KG, Spratt SK et al. Characterization of intrastriatal recombinant adeno-associated virus-mediated gene transfer of human tyrosine hydroxylase and human GTP-cyclohydrolase I in a rat model of Parkinson's disease. J Neurosci 1998;18:4271–4284.
43. Kaplitt MG, Leone P, Samulski RJ et al. Long-term gene expression and phenotypic correction using adeno-associated virus vectors in the mammalian brain. Nat Genet 1994;8:148–154.
44. Shen Y, Muramatsu SI, Ikeguchi K et al. Triple transduction with adeno-associated virus vectors expressing tyrosine hydroxylase, aromatic-L-amino-acid decarboxylase, and GTP cyclohydrolase I for gene therapy of Parkinson's disease. Hum Gene Ther 2000;11:1509–1519.
45. Kirik D, Georgievska B, Burger C et al. Reversal of motor impairments in parkinsonian rats by continuous intrastriatal delivery of L-dopa using rAAV-mediated gene transfer. Proc Natl Acad Sci USA 2002;99:4708–4713.
46. During MJ, Samulski RJ, Elsworth JD et al. In-vivo expression of therapeutic human genes for dopamine production in the caudates of MPTP-treated monkeys using an AAV vector. Gene Ther 1998;5:820–827.
47. Muramatsu S, Fujimoto K, Ikeguchi K et al. Behavioral recovery in a primate model of Parkinson's disease by triple transduction of striatal cells with adeno-associated viral vectors expressing dopamine-synthesizing enzymes. Hum Gene Ther 2002;13:345–354.
48. Klein RL, Lewis MH, Muzyczka N, Meyer EM. Prevention of 6-hydroxydopamine-induced rotational behavior by BDNF somatic gene transfer. Brain Res 1999;847(2):314–320.
49. Mandel RJ, Spratt SK, Snyder RO, Leff SE. Midbrain injection of recombinant adeno-associated virus encoding rat glial cell line-derived neurotrophic factor protects nigral neurons in a progressive 6-hydroxydopamine-induced degeneration model of Parkinson's disease in rats. Proc Natl Acad Sci USA 1997;94:14083–14088.
50. Kirik D, Rosenblad C, Bjorklund A, Mandel RJ. Long-term rAAV-mediated gene transfer of GDNF in the rat Parkinson's model: intrastriatal but not intranigral transduction promotes functional regeneration in the lesioned nigrostriatal system. J Neurosci 2000;20:4686–4700.
51. Wang L, Muramatsu S, Lu Y et al. Delayed delivery of AAV-GDNF prevents nigral neurodegeneration and promotes functional recovery in a rat model of Parkinson's disease. Gene Ther 2002;9:381–389.
52. Gash DM, Zhang Z, Ovadia A et al. Functional recovery in parkinsonian monkeys treated with GDNF. Nature 1996;380:252–255.
53. Costa S, Iravani MM, Pearce RK, Jenner P. Glial cell line-derived neurotrophic factor concentration dependently improves disability and motor activity in MPTP-treated common marmosets. Eur J Pharmacol 2001;412(1):45–50.
54. Eslamboli A, Cummings RM, Ridley RM et al. Recombinant adeno-associated viral vector (rAAV) delivery of GDNF provides protection against 6-OHDA lesion in the common marmoset monkey *(Callithrix jacchus)*. Exp Neurol 2003;184:536–548.
55. During MJ, Kaplitt MG, Stern MB, Eidelberg D. Subthalamic GAD gene transfer in Parkinson disease patients who are candidates for deep brain stimulation. Hum Gene Ther 2001;12:1589–1591.
56. Luo J, Kaplitt MG, Fitzsimons HL et al. Subthalamic GAD gene therapy in a Parkinson's disease rat model. Science 2002;298:425–429.
57. Chiocca EA, Choi BB, Cai WZ et al. Transfer and expression of the lacZ gene in rat brain neurons mediated by herpes simplex virus mutants. New Biol 1990;2:739–746.
58. Wang X, Zhang GR, Yang T, Zhang W, Geller AI. Fifty-one kilobase HSV-1 plasmid vector can be packaged using a helper virus-free system and supports expression in the rat brain. Biotechniques 2000;28(1):102–107.

59. Wade-Martins R, Smith ER, Tyminski E, Chiocca EA, Saeki Y. An infectious transfer and expression system for genomic DNA loci in human and mouse cells. Nat Biotechnol 2001;19:1067–1070.
60. Fink DJ, Poliani PL, Oligino T et al. Development of an HSV-based vector for the treatment of Parkinson's disease [review]. Exp Neurol 1997;144:103–121.
61. Speck PG, Simmons A. Divergent molecular pathways of productive and latent infection with a virulent strain of herpes simplex virus type 1. J Virol 1991;65:4001–4005.
62. Johnson PA, Wang MJ, Friedmann T. Improved cell survival by the reduction of immediate-early gene expression in replication-defective mutants of herpes simplex virus type 1 but not by mutation of the virion host shutoff function. J Virol 1994;68:6347–6362.
63. Geller AI, Freese A. Infection of cultured central nervous system neurons with a defective herpes simplex virus 1 vector results in stable expression of *Escherichia coli* beta-galactosidase. Proc Natl Acad Sci USA 1990;87:1149–1153.
64. During MJ, Naegele JR, O'Malley KL, Geller AI. Long-term behavioral recovery in parkinsonian rats by an HSV vector expressing tyrosine hydroxylase. Science 1994;266:1399–1403.
65. Isacson O. Behavioral effects and gene delivery in a rat model of Parkinson's disease. Science 1995;269:856–857.
66. Yamada M, Oligino T, Mata M et al. Herpes simplex virus vector-mediated expression of Bcl-2 prevents 6-hydroxydopamine-induced degeneration of neurons in the substantia nigra in vivo. Proc Natl Acad Sci USA 1999;96:4078–4083.
67. Natsume A, Mata M, Goss J et al. Bcl-2 and GDNF delivered by HSV-mediated gene transfer act additively to protect dopaminergic neurons from 6-OHDA-induced degeneration. Exp Neurol 2001;169:231–238.
68. Naldini L, Blomer U, Gallay P et al. In-vivo gene delivery and stable transduction of nondividing cells by a lentiviral vector. Science 1996;272:263–267.
69. Mitrophanous K, Yoon S, Rohll J et al. Stable gene transfer to the nervous system using a non-primate lentiviral vector. Gene Ther 1999;6:1808–1818.
70. Azzouz M, Ralph S, Wong LF et al. Neuroprotection in a rat Parkinson model by GDNF gene therapy using EIAV vector. Neuroreport 2004;15:985–990.
71. Wang G, Slepushkin V, Zabner J et al. Feline immunodeficiency virus vectors persistently transduce nondividing airway epithelia and correct the cystic fibrosis defect. J Clin Invest 1999; 104(11):R55–62.
72. Miller DG, Adam MA, Miller AD. Gene transfer by retrovirus vectors occurs only in cells that are actively replicating at the time of infection. Mol Cell Biol 1990;10:4239–4242.
73. Blomer U, Naldini L, Kafri T et al. Highly efficient and sustained gene transfer in adult neurons with a lentivirus vector. J Virol 1997;71:6641–6649.
74. Kordower JH, Bloch J, Ma SY et al. Lentiviral gene transfer to the nonhuman primate brain. Exp Neurol 1999;160:1–16.
75. Kordower JH, Emborg ME, Bloch J et al. Neurodegeneration prevented by lentiviral vector delivery of GDNF in primate models of Parkinson's disease. Science 2000;290:767–773.
76. Palfi S, Leventhal L, Chu Y et al. Lentivirally delivered glial cell line-derived neurotrophic factor increases the number of striatal dopaminergic neurons in primate models of nigrostriatal degeneration. J Neurosci 2002;22:4942–4954.
77. Bensadoun JC, Deglon N, Tseng JL et al. Lentiviral vectors as a gene delivery system in the mouse midbrain: cellular and behavioral improvements in a 6-OHDA model of Parkinson's disease using GDNF. Exp Neurol 2000;164:15–24.
78. Georgievska B, Kirik D, Rosenblad C, Lundberg C, Bjorklund A. Neuroprotection in the rat Parkinson model by intrastriatal GDNF gene transfer using a lentiviral vector. Neuroreport 2002;13:75–82.
79. Georgievska B, Kirik D, Bjorklund A. Aberrant sprouting and downregulation of tyrosine hydroxylase in lesioned nigrostriatal dopamine neurons induced by long-lasting overexpression of glial cell line derived neurotrophic factor in the striatum by lentiviral gene transfer. Exp Neurol 2002;177:461–474.
80. Azzouz M, Martin-Rendon E, Barber RD et al. Multicistronic lentiviral vector-mediated striatal gene transfer of aromatic L-amino acid decarboxylase, tyrosine hydroxylase, and GTP cyclohydrolase I induces sustained transgene expression, dopamine production, and functional improvement in a rat model of Parkinson's disease. J Neurosci 2002;22:10302–10312.
81. Hacein-Bey-Abina S, von Kalle C, Schmidt M et al. A serious adverse event after successful gene therapy for X-linked severe combined immunodeficiency. N Engl J Med 2003;348:255–256.

82. Nakai H, Montini E, Fuess S et al. AAV serotype 2 vectors preferentially integrate into active genes in mice. Nat Genet 2003;34:297–302.
83. Raper SE, Chirmule N, Lee FS et al. Fatal systemic inflammatory response syndrome in a ornithine transcarbamylase deficient patient following adenoviral gene transfer. Mol Genet Metab 2003;80(1/2):148–158.
84. Park S, Kim EY, Ghil GS et al. Genetically modified human embryonic stem cells relieve symptomatic motor behavior in a rat model of Parkinson's disease. Neurosci Lett 2003;353:91–94.
85. Ostenfeld T, Tai YT, Martin P et al. Neurospheres modified to produce glial cell line-derived neurotrophic factor increase the survival of transplanted dopamine neurons. J Neurosci Res 2002;69:955–965.
86. Gill SS, Patel NK, Hotton GR et al. Direct brain infusion of glial cell line-derived neurotrophic factor in Parkinson disease. Nat Med 2003;9:589–595.
87. Horger BA, Nishimura MC, Armanini MP et al. Neurturin exerts potent actions on survival and function of midbrain dopaminergic neurons. J Neurosci 1998;18:4929–4937.
88. Tsuboi K, Shults CW. Intrastriatal injection of sonic hedgehog reduces behavioral impairment in a rat model of Parkinson's disease. Exp Neurol 2002;173:95–104.
89. Dass B, Iravani MM, Huang C et al. Sonic hedgehog delivered by an adeno-associated virus protects dopaminergic neurones against 6-OHDA toxicity in the rat. J Neural Transm 2005;112(6):763–778.

SECTION 4

OVERVIEW OF SURGICAL PARKINSON'S DISEASE

10

Surgical Approaches to the Treatment of Parkinson's Disease

C. Warren Olanow
and Anthony H. V. Schapira

INTRODUCTION

This chapter serves to integrate the various aspects of the surgical management of Parkinson's disease (PD) that have been detailed in other parts of the book. In particular, it is intended to provide the reader with a practical approach to the application of surgery to the treatment of PD, relevant to the various stages of the disease at which such intervention may be deemed appropriate. Reference is made to other chapters in the book for the reader to follow detailed analysis of neurophysiology, anatomy and the relevant surgical principles.

Surgical treatments for Parkinson's disease (PD) have been employed since the start of the twentieth century. Initial approaches were directed at the motor cortex and corticospinal tracts. They were reported to provide some benefit particularly with respect to tremor, but were complicated by motor paresis and were discarded. Meyers subsequently reported anti-parkinsonian benefits without paralysis after lesioning the globus pallidus and the ansa lenticularis.[1] Thalamotomy came into vogue based on the reports of Cooper, who noted prominent anti-tremor effects with reduced side-effects in comparison to pallidotomy.[2,3] The most striking anti-tremor effects were observed with lesions placed in the ventro intermediate medial (VIM) nucleus of the thalamus, and VIM thalamotomy was commonly performed during the 1950s and 60s.

With the introduction of levodopa, surgery for PD was largely relegated to patients with severe tremor that was refractory to medical treatment. In the past decade, however, several factors have led to a resurgence in the use of surgery as a treatment for PD. First, levodopa therapy is not a panacea, and long-term therapy is frequently complicated by potentially disabling motor complications (dyskinesia and motor fluctuations) that limit the utility of the drug.[4,5] In addition, advances in neuroimaging, neuroanesthesia, surgical techniques and the use of intraoperative microelectrode recordings permit more accurate target identification with reduced adversity. Most importantly, there has been an increase in our understanding of the organization of the basal ganglia that provide a rational basis for identifying brain targets and considering surgical interventions in PD.[6,7] Specifically, neurophysiological and metabolic studies demonstrate that there is increased firing of neurons in the subthalamic nucleus (STN) and globus pallidus pars interna (GPi) in PD,[8] suggesting that lesions in these targets might improve parkinsonian motor features. Indeed, lesions of the GPi and STN are associated with improvement in motor function in animal models of PD.[9,10] Finally, biological advances have led to studies exploring the possibility that transplantation of fetal nigral dopaminergic neurons or stem cells might replace degenerated dopamine cells or that gene therapies might deliver trophic factors or other critical proteins and thereby improve the features of PD. The surgical interventions that are currently being employed or tested in PD are illustrated in Table 10-1.

ABLATIVE LESIONS

In Chapter 7, Uitti, Putzke, and Wharen discuss the historical and present value of ablative lesions for the treatment of PD in detail. Historically, ablative lesions fell from common use with the advent of levodopa. In the modern era, they are still employed on occasion, but their use has once again been limited because of their potential to cause side-effects related to infarction, hemorrhage, and damage to neighboring structures. These are even more pronounced in the case of bilateral procedures where side-effects can include dysphagia, dysarthria, and cognitive deficits. As a consequence, ablative lesions have been largely replaced by high-frequency stimulation which avoids the need for destructive brain lesions. The strengths and weaknesses of these approaches and their current utility are reviewed below.

Thalamotomy (Table 10-2) was popularized by Cooper et al.[2,3] and shown to provide benefit for contralateral tremor, and possibly for dyskinesia.[11,12] The most effective anti-tremor results have been achieved with lesions in the VIM nucleus.[13] On the other hand, thalamotomy is not particularly helpful for the other more disabling features of PD and can be associated with morbidity related to the location of the lesion.[14] In the present era, thalamotomy has largely been replaced by medical therapies or deep brain stimulation (see below). Still, for an

TABLE 10-1 Summary of procedures

Ablative procedures	**Restorative procedures**
Thalamotomy	Cell-based therapies
Pallidotomy	Fetal human nigral cells
Subthalamotomy	Fetal porcine nigral cells
Deep brain stimulation	Retinal pigmented epithelial cells
VIM nucleus of thalamus	Stem cells
Globus pallidus pars interna (GPi)	Trophic factors
Subthalamic nucleus (STN)	Gene therapies

TABLE 10-2 Thalamotomy

Advantages
Marked anti-tremor effect
Possible anti-dyskinesia effect
Does not require long-term follow-up
Disadvantages
Does not improve the more disabling features of PD (e.g. rigidity, bradykinesia, gait and postural disturbances)
Necessitates making a destructive brain lesion (risk of damage to neighboring tissue)
Bilateral procedures are associated with increased risk (dysarthria, dysphagia, and cognitive impairment)

individual PD patient with severe unilateral tremor that is refractory to medical therapy and who lives in a region where there is no access to expert neurological follow-up care, thalamotomy might still be a consideration.

Pallidotomy (Table 10-3) initially fell from popularity with the advent of thalamotomy which was thought to be the safer procedure, and then with the development of levodopa. However, the pioneering work of Leksell demonstrated that improvement in tremor, rigidity and bradykinesia could be obtained with lesions placed in the posteroventral portion of the globus pallidus pars interna (GPi).[15,16] These results dovetailed with experiments in MPTP-lesioned monkeys demonstrating that neuronal firing rates and metabolic activity were abnormally increased in the GPi in PD.[17,18] Numerous clinical trials have now shown that posteroventral pallidotomy can provide long-lasting anti-parkinsonian benefits in PD patients.[19–22] Interestingly, the most striking benefit observed is a dramatic and consistent improvement in contralateral dyskinesia. This observation runs counter to predictions based on the classic model which suggest that reduced firing in GPi neurons following pallidotomy should be associated with an increase, rather than amelioration, of dyskinesia.[23] It is now appreciated that neuronal firing frequency is not the sole factor in transferring information from the basal ganglia to cortical and brainstem motor regions, and other physiological features that make up the neuronal firing pattern – including the number of pauses, bursts, degree of synchrony, inhibition etc. – are also important. Indeed, it now appears that it is the elimination of the abnormal firing pattern in basal ganglia outflow neurons that is responsible for the improvement in dyskinesia that is seen following pallidotomy.

TABLE 10-3 Pallidotomy

Advantages
Consistent and dramatic improvement in contralateral dyskinesia
Modest improvement in contralateral parkinsonian features
Does not require long-term follow-up
Disadvantages
Necessitates making a destructive brain lesion (risk of damage to neighboring tissue)
Bilateral procedures are associated with increased risk (dysarthria, dysphagia, and cognitive impairment)

TABLE 10-4 Subthalamotomy

Advantages
Improvement in parkinsonian features
Reduction in dyskinesia
Does not require long-term follow-up
Disadvantages
Necessitates making a destructive brain lesion (risk of damage to neighboring tissue)
Bilateral procedures are associated with increased risk (dysarthria, dysphagia, and cognitive impairment)
Risk of hemiballismus

Despite the benefits of pallidotomy, the potential for side-effects, particularly with bilateral pallidotomy, has limited its utility in the treatment of PD, and deep brain stimulation (DBS) has now become the preferred surgical procedure. As with thalamotomy, the procedure may still be of value for patients who suffer unilateral disabling dyskinesias, who lack access to continuing neurological follow-up, or who are for one reason or another not candidates for DBS.

Most centers use microelectrode recording to identify the target site and to minimize adversity, although there is still some debate with some centers arguing that this is not required and that the increased number of needle passes increases the risk of brain hemorrhage or trauma.[24]

Subthalamotomy (Table 10-4) is a logical procedure to consider as a treatment for PD based on the neurophysiological and metabolic evidence indicating that STN neurons are overactive in PD. Indeed, subthalamotomy has been shown to improve parkinsonian motor abnormalities in animal models[9,25,26] and in a small number of PD patients.[27–29] Anti-dyskinetic benefits have also been observed. As with other ablative procedures, there are complications particularly with bilateral procedures. In addition, lesions of the subthalamic nucleus have now been reported with postoperative dyskinesia and hemiballismus, which in a few cases have been permanent.[30,31] It is also theoretically possible that lesions of the STN might have neuroprotective effects by blocking glutamate-mediated excitotoxicity.[32] The STN uses glutamate as a transmitter and overactivity in PD could lead to excitotoxic damage in target neurons which include the GPi, the pedunculopontine nucleus (PPN), and the SNc. Indeed, lesions of the STN protect SNc dopamine neurons from 6-OHDA toxicity in rats.[33] Such a result has not, however, been demonstrated in PD patients.

The risk of hemiballismus as well as the side-effects associated with bilateral intracranial procedures will likely limit the utility of this procedure. It may prove to be of value in countries that do not have access to deep brain stimulation.

DEEP BRAIN STIMULATION

Deep brain stimulation (DBS; Table 10-5) is discussed in detail by Benabid and colleagues in Chapter 8. It was first proposed for use as a treatment in PD by Benabid based on his experience with high-frequency stimulation as a means of confirming the target site for an ablative lesion.[34] DBS has the advantage of

TABLE 10-5 Deep brain stimulation

Advantages
Does not necessitate making a destructive brain lesion
Can be performed bilaterally with relative safety in comparison to ablative lesions
Stimulation settings can be adjusted to maximize benefit and minimize adversity
Does not preclude future treatments that depend on the integrity of the basal ganglia
Disadvantages
Expensive
Adjustment of stimulation settings can be time-consuming and inconvenient
Risk of complications related to stimulation (dysarthria, eye-movement dysfunction) or the device (mechanical problems, lead breaks, infection)
Periodic need to replace battery

permitting bilateral procedures to be safely performed and enables targeting of brain regions that one might be unwilling to lesion, such as the subthalamic nucleus (STN). Other advantages include the ability to adjust the stimulator at any time in order to maximize benefits and minimize adversity. Further, the procedure does not prevent the later use of a more effective therapy that might require the integrity of the basal ganglia system. DBS simulates the effect of a lesion but avoids the need to make a destructive brain lesion. The precise mechanism of action is unknown, but possibilities include depolarization blockade, release of inhibitory neurotransmitters, backfiring, and/or jamming of abberant neuronal signals.[35]

Deep brain stimulation for PD was first tested in the VIM nucleus of the thalamus in patients with tremor-dominant symptoms who had undergone a previous thalamotomy, in order to diminish the risks associated with bilateral thalamic lesions.[36] Both open-label and double-blind studies demonstrate that DBS of the VIM dramatically ameliorates contralateral tremor.[37–39] Further, patients randomized to have DBS of the VIM were shown to have comparable benefits but fewer adverse events in comparison to patients randomized to receive a thalamotomy.[40] Benefits of DBS are long-lasting, and have been shown to persist for more than 10 years. For all of these reasons, DBS-VIM has largely replaced thalamotomy in the treatment of tremor-dominant PD patients. However, DBS-VIM, as is the case with thalamotomy, does not meaningfully affect the more disabling features of PD such as rigidity, bradykinesia, and levodopa-related motor complications. Accordingly, DBS-VIM is rarely performed today. Stimulation of the STN or GPi are associated with more general benefits (see below), and are preferred even in patients with tremor-dominant PD as they provide comparable anti-tremor effects and have the potential to influence other PD features should they develop later in the course of the disease.

Deep brain stimulation is most often employed in PD using stimulation of the GPi and STN, based on preclinical and clinical evidence indicating that stimulation of either of these targets can improve the entire constellation of parkinsonian motor dysfunction. Indeed, high-frequency stimulation of the STN has been shown to be well-tolerated and to provide marked behavioral improvement in MPTP-treated monkeys.[41]

The Grenoble group was the first to report on the results of DBS of the STN in PD. They noted improvement in all of the cardinal features of PD as well as in "off" time and dyskinesia.[42,43] These results have been reproduced by several groups who note comparable benefits with stimulation of either the STN or GPi.[44–48] A large multicenter study assessing the effects of bilateral DBS of the STN or GPi in 143 patients included a prospective randomized double-blind crossover component.[49] Stimulation of either target site in the medication "off" state resulted in significant motor benefits for each of the cardinal features of PD at each visit during the study. These benefits were confirmed in the double-blind crossover phase of the trial. There was also a dramatic and highly significant reduction in both "off" time and "on" time with dyskinesia. Thus patients who could not be further improved with medical therapies (typically because of motor complications) experienced a substantial reduction in disability following deep brain stimulation of the STN or GPi. The study was not designed to compare the results of stimulation of these two targets, but results seemed to be more impressive in the DBS-STN group and this procedure is presently the most widely used. Long-term studies demonstrate that benefits of DBS persist over more than 5 years of follow-up, although disability still progresses from year to year, possibly reflecting degeneration in non-dopaminergic sites.[50]

There has been interest in the potential of lesions or DBS of the STN to be neuroprotective, by preventing STN-mediated excitotoxic damage to target neurons.[51] Indeed, STN lesions reduce the extent of SNc neuronal degeneration following 6-OHDA lesions in rodents,[52] and lesions of the substantia nigra (equivalent of the globus pallidus pars externa in humans) which disinhibits the STN is associated with mild damage to the SNc, also in rodents.[53] However, these findings have not yet been replicated in patients with PD, where there is no evidence that the rate of deterioration in off-medication/off-stimulation UPDRS scores are different in patients who have undergone DBS of the STN and DBS of the GPi.[49]

Deep brain stimulation is associated with adverse events in relation to the intracranial procedure, the electrode system, and stimulation. The surgical procedure can be associated with hemorrhage, tissue damage, and infection. In the multicenter study, 7 of 143 patients experienced hemorrhage, and neurological deficits persisted in four patients.[49] Problems can also occur in relation to the device, including lead breaks, lead migration, infection, and skin erosion.[54] These occur in about 2–3% of cases and occasionally require replacement of the electrode. Side-effects related to stimulation such as muscle twitch, and paresthesiae, tend to be transient and can usually be attenuated by adjustment of stimulator settings. Others, such as dysarthria or eye-movement disorders, can be more problematic and emerge in association with stimulation that results in clinical benefits despite attempts to adjust stimulator settings. It is also noteworthy that stimulation within the same target site using different electrode combinations or stimulation settings can lead to either improvement or worsening of parkinsonian features and increases or amelioration of dyskinesia.[55–57] Profound mood alterations with severe depression and suicidal ideations or riotous laughing have been observed with stimulation of the STN,[59] suggesting that basal ganglia circuits are involved with higher cortical and/or limbic as well as motor functions. In general, clinical judgment must be used in determining the stimulator setting that provides the best patient control with the least intolerable side-effect. One DBS-treated patient who received diathermy suffered brain necrosis due to transmission of heat by the electrode.[59] Physicians should be aware of this potential complication and avoid diathermy or other situations that might lead to excess heat being conducted to the brain by the electrode wire.

Dyskinesia and hemiballismus have for the most part not been a problem even with stimulation of the STN, and transient ballism has been observed only in a small number of cases.[60] Interestingly, dyskinesia tends to diminish with chronic stimulation,[61] perhaps related to the reduction in levodopa dose which frequently accompanies DBS, although we have observed some patients who experience reduced dyskinesia despite constant doses of levodopa. It is possible that continuous stimulation stabilizes the basal ganglia and prevents the adverse consequences of changes in neuronal firing patterns associated with intermittent doses of levodopa and pulsatile stimulation of striatal dopamine receptors. Certainly, it is clear that dyskinesia is not a contraindication for DBS with either a GPi or STN target.

Cognitive function has for the most part not been impaired with stimulation of the STN or GPi,[62–64] although physicians should be aware of the fact that patients with underlying cognitive impairment may deteriorate with any intracranial neurosurgical procedure that involves cortical needle passes bilaterally. Hence, in our clinic, patients with existing cognitive impairment or significant changes on neuropsychological testing are generally not considered as candidates for surgery. Similarly, there is little evidence to suggest that non-dopaminergic features that are not controlled with levodopa are improved with DBS of the STN or GPi. Indeed, most studies indicate that stimulation provides no greater benefit than is obtained with levodopa, and that the major advantage of DBS is that it provides these benefits with reduced motor complications and with less adversity than with ablation procedures.

Other limitations of DBS include cost, the need for periodic battery replacement usually under general anesthesia, and the availability of a team with expertise in neurology, stereotactic surgery, and neurophysiology. Finally, adjustment of stimulation settings at postoperative visits requires expertise and can be time-consuming.

In summary, DBS of the STN or GPi has been established to provide advanced PD patients with reduced "off" time, reduced dyskinesia, and enhanced motor scores particularly during "off" stages. The optimal patient for DBS is one who is in good general health, has experienced a good response to levodopa, has motor complications that limit the ability to maximally utilize the drug, and is cognitively intact. The positive results obtained in many patients who could not be satisfactorily controlled with medical therapies and the relative reduction in serious adverse events have led to these procedures now being widely employed for patients with advanced PD. There is some debate in the literature as to the value of microelectrode recording in more precisely determining the target site. Most centers routinely employ this technique and find it useful for precisely identifying the brain target. Others have argued that the use of microelectrode recordings requires further needle passes with increased time of the procedure and increased risk of a neurological complication.[24] Indeed, there is a suggestion in the multicenter study of a correlation between the number of needle passes and the risk of hemorrhage.[49] There is also question as to whether the procedure should be performed bilaterally at a single sitting or in two separate procedures, as staged procedures are associated with reduced adversity but recent studies suggest that many patients are satisfactorily controlled with a unilateral procedure.[65]

The STN and GPi are the most widely employed targets for DBS, even for patients with tremor-dominant PD. It is, however, important to appreciate that DBS is of primary value for controlling levodopa-related motor complications and does not provide anti-parkinsonian benefits that are greater than can be obtained with levodopa. In addition, it should be appreciated as mentioned above that side-effects do occur, the procedure is expensive, and battery replacement will be required. Advances in medical therapy with the early use of dopamine agonists and the administration of levodopa in combination with a COMT inhibitor may substantially reduce the risk that PD patients will experience motor complications,[66] and it is possible that the role of DBS of the STN and GPi will diminish in the future. It is possible that stimulation of other brain targets such as the pedunculopontine nucleus (PPN), motor cortex, or supplementary motor area (SMA) may provide additional advantages; research targeting these areas continues.[67,68]

RESTORATIVE THERAPIES

Restorative interventions as a treatment for PD have been introduced in an effort to preserve and/or restore function to damaged dopamine neurons. Treatments have primarily been considered in patients with advanced disease, but such approaches might best be utilized at an earlier stage of the disease. Studies in the laboratory are proceeding apace based on the potential theoretical benefits of these approaches, and some clinical trials have already been carried out. These areas of research are extremely interesting and have caught the attention of the press and the lay public, but much work remains before any of these approaches can be recommended as a treatment for a PD patient. In addition, it is by no means clear that therapies directed exclusively at the dopamine system will benefit non-dopaminergic features such as freezing, postural instability, and dementia that can represent a major source of disability for levodopa-treated PD patients.

Cell-based therapies have been studied as possible therapies for PD based on their potential to restore anatomic and physiological dopaminergic innervation to the striatum. Experimentally, numerous types of implanted cells have been evaluated and shown to survive when implanted into the denervated striatum, but the best experimental results have been obtained with fetal nigral dopaminergic neurons which have been shown to reinnervate the striatum in an organotypic manner, manufacture and regulate the release of dopamine, and ameliorate motor features in rodent and non-human primate models of PD.[69–73] In initial trials in PD patients, clinical benefits were reported after transplantation of adrenal medullary cells into the caudate nucleus,[74] but these results were not replicated in other studies.[75–77] Fetal mesencephalic dopaminergic cells have been reported to provide significant clinical benefits and increases in striatal fluorodopa (FD) uptake on positron emission tomography (PET) in open-label studies.[78–85] Additionally, robust graft survival with reinnervation of the striatum in a patch matrix manner has been observed at postmortem.[86,87] However, comparable benefits were not observed in each of these studies, perhaps reflecting differences in the transplant variables employed, including donor age, method of tissue storage and preparation, target site, amount and distribution of implanted tissue, and use of immunosuppressants (see the review in reference 69).

Two double-blind, placebo-controlled trials of fetal nigral transplantation have recently been performed to better assess the value of this procedure in patients with advanced PD. The first study was a one-year trial in which 40 patients were randomized to receive a transplantation or placebo procedure.[88] Transplanted patients were bilaterally implanted with two donors per side into the caudate nucleus and putamen. Tissue was inserted as a solid graft (a "noodle") using two needle tracts per side. Placebo-treated patients received a sham procedure in which a burrhole was made, but needles were not inserted into the brain and no tissue was implanted. Immunosuppression was not employed and patients were followed for one year. A quality-of-life measure was used as the primary endpoint, and was not significantly improved in transplanted patients versus controls. Modest benefits of transplantation were observed in UPDRS scores of ADL and motor function in patients younger than 60 years. There was a significant increase in striatal FD uptake on PET, and there was modest survival of implanted cells at postmortem. The procedure was well tolerated, but approximately 15% of transplanted patients developed dyskinesias that persisted for days or weeks after levodopa was discontinued and were a source of major disability in some patients.[89]

The second double-blind trial of fetal nigral transplantation was a two-year study and used a slightly different treatment protocol.[90] Patients were randomized to three groups:

- Bilateral transplantation into the posterior putamen with four donors per side
- Bilateral transplantation into the posterior putamen with one donor per side
- Bilateral cosmetic placebo procedures in which patients received a partial burrhole but no needle was inserted or tissue implanted into the brain.

Patients who received transplantation had fetal nigral cells implanted diffusely throughout the target region so that tissue deposits were separated by no more than five millimeters in each of three dimensions. Patients were also given a 6-month course of cyclosporine. The primary endpoint was the change between baseline and final visit in UPDRS motor score in the practically defined "off" state (12 hours after the last evening dose of dopaminergic medication). Transplanted patients were not significantly improved in comparison to placebo patients, despite having significant increases in striatal fluorodopa uptake on PET and robust survival of implanted dopaminergic neurons at postmortem. Post-hoc analyses did not reveal an age effect, but did show that transplant provided significant benefits to patients with milder disease.

Fifty-six (56%) of transplanted patients in this study developed dyskinesia during the practically defined "off" state when they had been held off levodopa for more than 12 hours ("off-medication dyskinesia"). In three patients this was sufficiently severe to warrant a further surgical intervention. This phenomenon was not observed in non-transplanted patients. The precise mechanism responsible for off-medication dyskinesia remains unknown. Some authors suggest that this side-effect is due to regional graft overgrowth based on PET studies.[91] It has been suggested that off-medication relates to storage of tissue prior to implantation,[92] but we only implanted fresh tissue. Off-medication dyskinesias in our study were rhythmic, stereotyped movements of the lower extremities that occurred in association with parkinsonism in other body regions, suggestive of diphasic dyskinesia. This suggests that off-medication dyskinesia may relate to incomplete dopaminergic reinnervation of the striatum due either to transplant of an inadequate numbers of cells or to faulty synaptic connections. This hypothesis raises the possibility that increased numbers of surviving dopamine neurons or enhanced dopaminergic transmission might be associated with both a reduced risk of off-medication dyskinesia and enhanced antiparkinsonian effects.

One method of enhancing the number of surviving dopaminergic cells involves *co-administration of anti-oxidants, lazaroids, anti-apoptotic agents, or trophic factors*, and *implantation into multiple targets* such as the putamen, caudate, and SNc, but only a limited number of patients have been studied and there have been no double-blind trials.[92,93] Another approach involves alternate sources of dopaminergic tissue. *Transplantation of fetal nigral porcine cells* was reported to provide modest benefit to PD patients in an open-label study, although postmortem studies showed only minimal graft survival.[95] However, a double-blind controlled trial of transplantation with fetal porcine nigral cells showed no benefit (T. Freeman, personal communication). There was a major placebo effect in this study, emphasizing further the need for double-blind placebo-controlled trials. *Retinal pigmented epithelial cells* have the capacity to release levodopa and have been transplanted into PD patients attached to gelatin microcarriers (spheramine) to enhance their survival. It is postulated that these cells release levodopa into the striatum and provide a continuous source of dopamine to facilitate basal ganglia function in the PD patient. Open-label studies have reported benefits in UPDRS motor scores and in "off" time that persist for up to 2 years and off-medication dyskinesias were not encountered.[96] Double-blind controlled trials to better assess the benefits and side-effects of this therapy are currently under way.

Stem cells have attracted great interest because of their potential to provide an unlimited and readily available supply of dopaminergic neurons for transplantation in PD.[97] Interest has particularly focused on embryonic stem (ES) cells whose default pathway leads to neuronal differentiation, a small proportion of which stain for tyrosine hydroxylase (TH), aromatic amino acid decarboxylase (AADC), and the dopamine transporter, and are therefore presumably dopaminergic neurons.[98] Much attention is now being directed towards influencing the differentiation pathway so as to promote the formation of dopamine neurons using factors such as Nurr-1 and trophic factors.[99] It has now been shown that implanted ES cells can survive in the striatum of unilaterally lesioned 6-OHDA rodents and reduce abnormal circling behavior following a dopaminergic challenge.[98,100] Further, ES cells have recently been reported to improve motor function in the MPTP primate,[101] lending further credence to the potential value of stem cells in human PD patients. Stem cells can also be utilized to deliver specific proteins such as trophic factors to the PD brain. Adult-derived autologous stem cells are also being investigated.

Stem cells have not yet been tested in PD patients and many questions remain to be addressed. Can stem cells indeed yield a steady and predictable supply of dopaminergic neurons for transplantation? Will stem cells induce off-medication dyskinesia or other unanticipated side-effects related to unregulated growth? Can stem cells provide benefit that exceeds fetal nigral mesencephalic cells? To date, stem cells have not been demonstrated to provide anti-parkinsonian effects in animal models that equal, let alone exceed, that which can be obtained with fetal nigral cells which have not yet been confirmed to provide benefit in human trials. It is also important to consider that even complete restoration of the dopaminergic system may fail to correct disabling features of PD such as dementia and postural instability that are related to degeneration of non-dopaminergic neurons. Thus, while stem cells are theoretically interesting, success in PD is by no means guaranteed despite the excitement of the media and lay public, and there are many hurdles yet to be overcome.

In summary, cell-based therapies are a logical approach to the treatment of the dopaminergic defects in PD. However, double-blind trials have failed to show clinical benefits with fetal nigral transplantation and the majority of patients experienced potentially disabling off-medication dyskinesia. It is thus clear that cell-based therapies remain experimental and should not be recommended as a routine treatment for PD.

Trophic factors offer another opportunity to provide restorative effects in PD. Glial-derived neurotrophic factor (GDNF) has attracted considerable attention because of its capacity to protect or rescue dopaminergic neurons in tissue culture,[102] and in MPTP-treated monkeys.[103,104] Of particular note is the observation that benefits can be obtained with GDNF in the primate even when the trophic factor is administered days or weeks following MPTP administration.

A randomized double-blind controlled trial of GDNF administered through the ventricle did not provide benefit to PD patients,[105] but it is now appreciated that GDNF does not cross from the ventricle into the brain. Gill et al. used an infusion pump to directly administer GDNF into the striatum in five PD patients in an open-label study.[106] The study reported improvement in UPDRS motor scores during practically defined "off" as well as a slight increase in striatal FD uptake, primarily localized to the catheter tip. However, a double-blind trial comparing GDNF to placebo that has not yet been published did not show efficacy and was prematurely terminated (Tony Lang, personal communication). Further, several patients developed peripheral antibodies to GDNF and monkeys receiving long-term treatment developed cerebellar degeneration. For these reasons the company has stopped its GDNF program.

It is possible, however, that GDNF was not optimally tested. The dose employed was lower than that employed in the Gil et al. study and patients had advanced disease severity which may have precluded obtaining a beneficial effect. Patients also experienced complications associated with the chronic, indwelling hardware. The biggest concern, though, was that GDNF was delivered to a point source and may not have been adequately distributed throughout the striatum. Diffusion of the protein from a single point source is notoriously poor, and is typically limited to several millimeters from the point of distribution.[107]

Gene therapy, as discussed by Dass and Kordower in Chapter 9, represents a new and exciting way to deliver a protein diffusely to specific brain regions and cell types. Here, a viral vector is used to transfer the RNA of the desired protein into specific cells within a particular brain region (based on the site of injection and the specific promoter employed). The RNA is converted to DNA by a reverse transcriptase, incorporated into the cell's genome by an integrase, and the host cell now begins to manufacture the desired protein. In considering a gene therapy for PD, there are several factors that must be addressed:

1. What viral vector to employ – most studies have employed and adeno-associated virus (AAV) but retroviruses (e.g. lentivirus) can also be employed
2. What protein to select – e.g. a trophic factor to protect and restore function to dopamine neurons, aromatic amino acid decarboxylase (AADC) to promote the conversion of levodopa to dopamine, and glutamic acid decarboxylase (GAD) to inhibit overactive neurons
3. What promoter to use – e.g. TH to localize protein production to dopamine neurons or CMV to allow protein production by all nerve cells
4. Target site – e.g. striatum for trophic factors or AADC or the STN for GAD
5. Retrograde and/or anterograde transmission of the protein and in some instances the virus. This could be advantageous (e.g. retrograde transmission of trophic factor from striatum to SNc), but might also lead to unanticipated side-effects.
6. The possibility of immune reactions directed against either the virus or the new protein
7. Incorporation of a regulatory factor that can turn off DNA/protein production to protect against side-effects related to excess protein production. However, a regulatory agent has not yet been used in clinical trials and carries its own risks such as immunogenicity.

The first trials of gene therapy for PD have now been initiated using AAV delivery of GAD into the STN. This is designed to enhance inhibition of over-active STN neurons and to generate benefits similar to what have been obtained with subthalamotomy or DBS. There is the risk, though, that excessive inhibition of the STN could lead to hemiballismus. Gene therapy trials with AADC have shown benefit in the MPTP monkey, and clinical trials in PD patients have just begun. Gene therapy can also be used to deliver trophic factors in a way that avoids the diffusion problems associated with infusion of the drug by catheter. Kordower et al have demonstrated that lentivirus delivery of GDNF by direct injection into the striatum is well tolerated and provides dramatic behavioral and histological benefits to MPTP-treated monkeys.[108] Similar results have been obtained in MPTP monkeys with AAV delivery of nurturin, a trophic factor in the same family as GDNF. Clinical trials testing AAV-nurturin in PD patients are expected to be initiated in the near future.

CONCLUSIONS

There has been a marked resurgence of interest in surgical therapies for PD during the past decade, offering the potential to provide benefits to patients with advanced PD who can no longer be adequately controlled with medical therapy. Ablative procedures have been largely replaced by high-frequency stimulation in order to minimize side-effects, particularly those associated with bilateral procedures. DBS-STN is the most widely employed procedure, although good results have also been reported with DBS-GPi and blinded comparisons have not yet been performed. DBS-VIM is rarely employed even for patients with tremor-dominant PD, as comparable anti-tremor effects can be obtained with DBS-STN and this procedure has the potential to improve other parkinsonian features if they develop later in the course of the illness.

The optimal surgical candidate has PD as diagnosed by the UK brain bank criteria, a good response to levodopa, disability that is largely related to motor complications, and intact cognition. In such patients more than 80% experience a good or excellent response and serious side-effects occur in fewer that 5%. There is no evidence that DBS benefits patients with an atypical or secondary parkinsonism, and surgery is not recommended for these patients.

The anti-parkinsonian effects obtained with surgical therapies are for the most part no greater than can be obtained with levodopa and non-dopaminergic features are not affected. The benefits that are obtained largely reflect a reduction in dyskinesia and an improvement in "off" time. Indeed, it is interesting to consider that the development of a levodopa formulation that provides the benefits of the drug but without motor complications would eliminate the need for the majority of surgery that is performed for PD today. Ablative procedures have largely been abandoned, but may have a place in individual patients who are from remote areas and do not have ready access to follow-up necessary for the postoperative management of DBS patients.

The experimental therapeutics of PD now being tested in the laboratory have captured the imagination of the press and the lay public, offering the promise of transplantation, stem cells, and gene therapies. It is clear, however, that there is much to be done before any of these therapies can be made available as routine treatments for PD, and it is important that expectations be properly managed. We have repeatedly seen that promising results in open-label trials that are subject to placebo effect and physician bias may not be replicated in double-blind placebo-controlled studies. We have also learned that unanticipated side-effects can limit the utility of even the most promising therapy. Perhaps most importantly, it should be appreciated that the major unmet medical need in PD is the management of non-dopaminergic features such as freezing, gait disturbance, postural instability, autonomic disturbances, and dementia. Cell-based or gene therapies that completely restore dopaminergic function may still not deal with these disabling features of PD. The bar needs to be set at a higher standard and we need to seek out therapies that will improve both dopaminergic and non-dopaminergic features of PD. Most surgical procedures are employed late in the course of the illness when PD features can no longer be controlled with medical therapies. It is possible that the dopamine lesion itself contributes to degeneration of non-dopaminergic neurons in the brainstem and cerebral cortex,[32] and that early correction of the dopaminergic deficit would have more widespread benefits. Still, neuroprotective therapies appear to offer the greatest hope for treating both the dopaminergic and non-dopaminergic features of PD, and where surgical approaches will fit in the long-term remains to be determined. It is to be hoped that the development of a neuroprotective therapy that slows or stops disease progression will effectively cure PD and eliminate the need for surgery. For the present, however, surgical approaches warrant a place in the management of PD.

REFERENCES

1. Meyers R. The modification of altering tremors, rigidity and festination by surgery of the basal ganglia. Res Publ Assoc Res Nerv Ment Dis 1942;21:602.
2. Cooper IS. Ligation of the anterior choroidal artery for involuntary movements of parkinsonism. Arch Neurol 1956;75:36–48.
3. Cooper IS, Bravo G. Chemopallidectomy and chemothalamectomy. J Neurosurg 1958;15:244.
4. Lang AP, Lozano AE. Parkinson's disease. New Engl J Med 1998;339;1044–1053.
5. Olanow CW, Watts RL, Koller WC. An algorithm (decision tree) for the management of Parkinson's disease: treatment guidelines. Neurology 2001;56(Suppl. 5):1–88.
6. Albin RL, Young AB, Penney JB. The functional anatomy of basal ganglia disorders. TINS 1989; 12:366–375.
7. DeLong MR. Primate models of movement disorders of basal ganglia origin. TINS 1990;13:281–289.
8. Obeso JA, Rodriguez-Oroz MC, Rodriguez M, Lanciego JL, Artieda J, Gonzalez N, Olanow CW. Pathophysiology of the basal ganglia in PD. Trends Neurosci 2000;23:8–19.
9. Bergman H, Wichmann T, deLong MR. Reversal of experimental parkinsonism by lesions of the subthalamic nuceus. Science 1990;249:1436.
10. Brotchie JM, Mitchell IJ, Sambrook MA, Crossman AR. Alleviation of parkinsonism by antagonist of excitatory amino acid transmission in the medial segment of the globus pallidus in rat and primate. Mov Disord 1991;6:133–138.
11. Fox MW, Ahlskog JE, Kelly PJ. Stereotactic ventrolateralis thalamotomy for medically refractory tremor in post-levodopa era Parkinson's disease patients. J Neurosurg 1991;75:723.
12. Narabayshi H, Yokochi F, Nakajima Y. Levodopa-induced dyskinesia and thalamotomy. J Neurol Neurosurg Psychiatry 1984;47:831.
13. Narabayshi H. Stereotaxic VIM thalamotomy for treatment of tremor. Eur Neurol 1989;29:29.
14. Tasker RR. Thalamotomy. Neurosurg Clin NA 1990;1:841.
15. Laitinen LV, Bergenheim AT, Hariz MI. Leksell's posteroventral pallidotomy in the treatment of Parkinson's disease. J Neurosurg 1992;76:53.
16. Laitinen LV, Bergenheim AT, Hariz MI. Ventroposterolateral pallidotomy can abolish all parkinsonian symptoms. Stereotact Funct Neurosurg 1992;58:14.
17. Bergman H, Wichmann T, Karmon B, DeLong MR. The primate subthalamic nucleus. II: Neuronal activity in the MPTP model of parkinsonism. J Neurophysiol 1994;72:507–519.
18. Crossman AR, Mitchell IJ, Sambrook MA. Regional brain uptake of 2-deoxy glucose in MPTP-induced parkinsonism in the Macaque monkey. Neuropharmacology 1985;24:587–591.
19. Dogali M, Fazzini E, Kolodny E et al. Stereotactic ventral pallidotomy for Parkinson's disease. Neurology 1995;45:753–761.
20. Baron MS, Vitek JL, Bakay RAE et al. Treatment of advanced Parkinson's disease by posterior GPi pallidotomy: 1-year results of a pilot study. Ann Neurol 1996;40:355–366.
21. Lang AE, Lozano AM, Montgomery E, Duff J, Tasker R, Hutchinson W. Posteroventral medial pallidotomy in advanced Parkinson's disease. N Engl J Med 1997;337:1036–1042.
22. Fine J, Duff J, Chen R et al. Long-term follow-up of unilateral pallidotomy in advanced Parkinson's disease. N Engl J Med 2000;342:1708–1714.
23. Obeso JA, Rodriguez-Oroz MC, Rodriguez M, DeLong MR, Olanow CW. Pathophysiology of levodopa-induced dyskinesias in Parkinson's disease: problems with current model. Ann Neurol 2000;47(Suppl. 1):22–32.

24. Samii A, Turnbull IM, Kishore A et al. Reassessment of unilateral pallidotomy in Parkinson's disease: a 2-year follow-up study. Brain 1999;122:417–425.
25. Aziz TZ, Peggs D, Sambrook MA, Crossman AR. Lesion of subthalamic nucleus for the alleviation of MPTP-induced parkinsonism in the primate. Mov Disord 1991;6:288–293.
26. Guridi J, Herrero MT, Luquin MR, Guillen J, Ruberg M, Laguna J, Vila M, Javoy-Agid F, Agid Y, Hirsch E, Obeso JA. Subthalamotomy in parkinsonian monkeys: behavioural and biochemical analysis. Brain 1996;119:1717–1727.
27. Alvarez L, Macias R, Guridi J et al. Dorsal subthalamotomy for Parkinson's disease. Mov Disord 2001;16:72–78.
28. Su PC, Tseng HM, Liu HM, Yen RF, Liou HH. Treatment of advanced Parkinson's disease by subthalamotomy: one-year results. Mov Disord 2003;18:531–538.
29. Alvarez L, Marcias R, Lopez G et al. Bilateral subthalamotomy in Parkinson's disease: initial and long-term response. Brain 2005;128:570–583.
30. Chen CC, Lee ST, Wu T, Chen CJ, Huang CC, Lu CS. Hemiballism after subthalamotomy in patients with Parkinson's disease: report of 2 cases. Mov Disord 2002;17:1367–1371.
31. Tseng HM, Su PC, Liu HM. Persistent hemiballism after subthalamotomy: the size of the lesion matters more than the location. Mov Disord 2003;18:1209–1211.
32. Rodriguez MC, Obeso JA, Olanow CW. Subthalamic nucleus-mediated excitotoxicity in Parkinson's disease; a target for neuroprotection. Ann Neurol 1998;44:175–188.
33. Piallat B, Benazzouz A, Benabid AL. Subthalamic nucleus lesion on rats prevents dopaminergic nigral neuron degeneration after striatal 6-OHDA injection: behavioural and immunohistochemical studies. Eur J Neurosci 1996;8:1408–1414.
34. Benabid Al, Pollak P, Louveau A, Henry S, de Rougemont J. Combined (thalamotomy and stimulation) stereotactic surgery of the VIM thalamic nucleus for bilateral Parkinson's disease. Appl Neurophysiol 1987;50:344.
35. Benazzouz A, Hallett M. Mechanism of action of deep brain stimulation. Neurology 2000;55: 13–16.
36. Benabid AL, Pollak P, Gervason C et al. Long-term suppression of tremor by chronic stimulation of the ventral intermediate thalamic nucleus. Lancet 1991;337:403.
37. Blond S, Caparros-Lefebvre D, Parker F et al. Control of tremor and involuntary movement disorders by chronic stereotactic stimulation of the ventral intermediate thalamic nucleus. J Neurosurg 1992;77:62.
38. Benabid AL, Pollock P, Gao D et al. Chronic electrical stimulation of the ventralis intermedius nucleus of the thalamus as a treatment of movement disorders. J Neurosurg 1996;84:203–214.
39. Koller W, Pahwa R, Busenbark K et al. High-frequency unilateral thalamic stimulation in the treatment of essential and parkinsonian tremor. Ann Neurol 1997;42:292–299.
40. Schuurman PR, Bosch A, Bossuyt PMM, Bonsel GJ, van Someren EJW, de Bie RMA et al. A comparison of continuous thalamic stimulation and thalamotomy for suppression of severe tremor. N Engl J Med 2000;342:461–468.
41. Benazzouz A, Gross C, Feger J. Reversal of rigidity and improvement in motor performance by subthalamic high-frequency stimulation in MPTP-treated monkeys. Eur J Neurosci 1993; 5:382–389.
42. Limousin P, Pollak P, Benazzouz A et al. Effect on parkinsonian signs and symptoms of bilateral subthalamic nucleus stimulation. Lancet 1995;345:91–95.
43. Limousin P, Krack P, Pollak P, Benazzouz A, Ardouin C, Hoffmann D, Benabid AL. Electrical stimulation of the subthalamic nucleus in advanced Parkinson's disease. N Engl J Med 1998; 339:1105–1111.
44. Kumar R, Lozano A, Kim YJ et al: Double blind evaluation of subthalamic nucleus deep brain stimulation in advanced Parkinson's disease. Neurol 1998;51:850–855.
45. Bejjani B, Damier P, Arnulf I et al. Pallidal stimulation for Parkinson's disease. Two targets? Neurology 1997;49:1564–1569.
46. Pahwa R, Wilkinson S, Smith RN et al. High-frequency stimulation of the pallidus for the treatment of Parkinson's disease. Neurology 1997;49:249–253.
47. Siegfried J, Lippitz B. Bilateral chronic stimulation of ventroposterolateral pallidum: new therapeutic approach for alleviating all parkinsonian symptoms. Neurosurgery 1994;35:1126–1129.
48. Volkmann J, Sturm V, Weiss P et al. Bilateral high-frequency stimulation of the internal globus pallidus in advanced Parkinson's disease. Ann Neurol 1998;44: 953–961.
49. The Deep Brain Stimulation for PD study group. Deep brain stimulation of the subthalamic nucleus or globus pallidus pars interna in Parkinson's disease. N Engl J Med 2001;345:956–963.

50. Krack P, Batir A, Van Blercom N, Chabardes S, Fraix V, Ardouin C, Koudsic A, Limousin PD, Benazzouz A, LeBas JF, Benabid AL, Pollak P. Five-year follow-up of bilateral stimulation of the subthalamic nucleus in advanced Parkinson's disease. N Engl J Med 2003;349(20):1925–1934.
51. Rodriguez MC, Obeso JA, Olanow CW. Subthalamic nucleus-mediated excitotoxicity in Parkinson's disease: a target for neuroprotection. Ann Neurol 1998;44:175–188.
52. Piallat B, Benazzouz A, Benabid AL. Subthalamic nucleus lesion on rats prevents dopaminergic nigral neuron degeneration after striatal 6-OHDA injection: behavioural and immunohistochemical studies. Eur J Neurosci 1996;8:1408–414.
53. Wright AK, Atherton JF, Norrie L, Arbuthnott GW. Death of dopaminergic neurones in the rat substantia nigra can be induced by damage to globus pallidus. Eur J Neurosci 2004;20(7):1737–1744.
54. Oh MY, Abosch A, Kim SH, Lang AE, Lozano AM. Long-term hardware-related complications of deep brain stimulation. Neurosurgery 2002;50:1268–1274.
55. Bejjani BP, Damier P, Arnulf I et al. Deep brain stimulation in Parkinson's disease: opposite effects of stimulation in the pallidum. Mov Disord 1998;13:969–970.
56. Krack P, Pollak P, Limousin P, Hoffmann D, Benazzouz A, LeBas JF, Koudsie A, Benabid AL. Opposite effects of pallidal stimulation in Parkinson's disease. Ann Neurol 1998;43:180–192.
57. Gracies JM, Bucobo JC, Danisi F, Weisz D, Brin MF, Olanow CW. Paradoxical impact of unilateral subthalamic stimulation on levodopa-treated parkinsonian symptomatology: one case report. Ann Neurol 1998;44:500–501.
58. Bejjani BP, Damier P, Arnulf I et al. Transient acute depression induced by high-frequency deep-brain stimulation. N Engl J Med 1999;340:1476–1480.
59. Nutt JG, Anderson VC, Peacock JH. DBS and diathermy interaction induces severe CNS damage. Neurology 2001;56:1384–1386.
60. Limousin P, Pollack P, Hoffmann D et al. Abnormal involuntary movements induced by subthalamic nucleus stimulation in Parkinson's disease. Mov Disord 1995;10:672–674.
61. Krack P, Limousin P, Benabid AL, Pollak P. Chronic stimulation of the subthalamic nucleus improves levodopa-induced dyskinesias in Parkinson's disease. Lancet 1997;350:1676.
62. Morrison CE, Borod JC, Brin MF, Raskin SA, Germano IM, Weisz DJ, Olanow CW. A program for neuropsychological investigation of deep brain stimulation (PNIDBS) in movement disorder patients: development, feasibility, and preliminary data. Neuropsychiat Neuropsychol Behav Neurol 2000;13:204–219.
63. Morrison CE, Borod JC, Perrine K, Beric A, Brin MF, Rezai A, Kelly P, Sterio D, Germano I, Weisz D, Olanow CW. Neuropsychological functioning following bilateral subthalamic nucleus stimulation in Parkinson's disease. Arch Clin Neuropsych 2004;19:165–181
64. Saint-Cyr JA, Trépanier LL, Kumar R, Lozano AM, Lang AE. Neuropsychological consequences of chronic bilateral stimulation of the subthalamic nucleus in Parkinson's disease. Brain 2000;123: 2091–2108.
65. Germano IM, Gracies J-M, Weisz DJ, Tse W, Koller WC, Olanow CW. Unilateral stimulation of the subthalamic nucleus in parkinson's disease: a double-blind 12-month study. J Neurosurg 2004; 101:36–42.
66. Olanow CW. The scientific basis for the current treatment of Parkinson's disease. Ann Rev Med 2004;55:41–60.
67. Nandi D, Liu X, Winter JL, Aziz TZ, Stein JF. Deep brain stimulation of the pedunculopontine region in the normal non-human primate. J Clin Neurosci 2002;9:170–174.
68. Drouot X, Oshino S, Jarraya B, Besret L, Kishima H, Remy P, Dauguet J, Lefaucheur JP, Dollé F, Cordé F, Bottlaender M, Peschanski M, Kéravel Y, Hantraye P, Palfi S. Functional recovery in a primate model of Parkinson's disease following motor cortex stimulation. Neuron 2004;44:769–778.
69. Olanow CW, Freeman TB, Kordower JH. Fetal nigral transplantation as a therapy for Parkinson's disease. TINS 1996;19:102–109.
70. Bjorklund A, Stenevi U. Reconstruction of the nigrostriatal dopamine pathway by intracerebral nigral transplants. Brain Res 1979;177:555–560.
71. Perlow MJ, Freed WJ, Hoffer BJ et al. Brain grafts reduce motor abnormalities produced by destruction of nigro-striatal dopamine system. Science 1979;204:643–647.
72. Bankiewicz KS, Plunkett RJ, Jacobawitz DM et al. The effect of fetal mesencephalon implants on primate MPTP-induced parkinsonism. J Neurosurg 1990;72:231–244.
73. Redmond DE, Roth RH, Elsworth JD et al. Fetal neuronal grafts in monkeys given methyl-phenyl-tetrahydro-pyridine. Lancet 1986;i:1125–1127.
74. Madrazo I, Drucker-Colin R, Diaz V et al. Open microsurgical autograft of adrenal medulla to right caudate nucleus in two patients with intractable Parkinson's disease. N Engl J Med 1987; 316:831–834.

75. Lindvall O, Backlund EO, Farde L et al. Transplantation in Parkinson's disease: two cases of adrenal medullary grafts to the putamen. Ann Neurol 1987;22:457–468.
76. Goetz CG, Olanow CW, Koller WC et al. Multicenter study of autologous adrenal medullary transplantation to the corpus striatum in patients with advanced Parkinson's disease. N Engl J Med 1989;320:337–341.
77. Olanow CW, Koller W, Goetz CG et al. Autologous transplantation of adrenal medulla in Parkinson's disease. Arch Neurol 1990;47:1286–1289.
78. Lindvall O, Brundin P, Widner H et al. Grafts of fetal dopamine neurons survive and improve motor function in Parkinson's disease. Science 1990;247:574–577.
79. Lindvall O, Widner H, Rehncrona S et al. Transplantation of fetal dopamine neurons in Parkinson's disease: one-year clinical and neurophysiological observations in two patients with putaminal implants. Ann Neurol 1992;31:155–165.
80. Freed CR, Breeze RE, Rosenberg Nl et al. Survival of implanted fetal dopamine cells and neurologic improvement 12 to 46 months after transplantation for Parkinson's disease. N Engl J Med 1992;327:1549–1555.
81. Spencer DD, Robbins RJ, Naftolin F et al. Unilateral transplantation of human fetal mesencephalic tissue into the caudate nucleus of patients with Parkinson's disease. N Engl J Med 1992;327: 1541–1548.
82. Sawle GV, Bloomfield PM, Bjorklund A et al. Transplantation of fetal dopamine neurons in Parkinson's disease: PET [18F]-6-L-fluorodopa studies in two patients with putaminal implants. Ann Neurol 1992;31:166–173.
83. Remy P, Samson Y, Hantrave P et al. Clinical correlates of [18F] fluorodopa uptake in five grafted parkinsonian patients. Ann Neurol 1995;38: 580–588.
84. Freeman TB, Olanow CW, Hauser RA et al. Bilateral fetal nigral transplantation into the postcommissural putamen in Parkinson's disease. Ann Neurol 1995;38:379–388.
85. Hauser RA, Freeman TB, Snow BJ, Nauert M, Gauger L, Kordower JH, Olanow CW. Long-term evaluation of bilateral fetal nigral transplantation in Parkinson's disease. Arch Neurol 1999;56:179–187.
86. Kordower JH, Freeman TB, Snow BJ, Vingerhoets FJG, Mufson EJ, Sanberg PR, Hauser RA, Smith DA, Nauert M, Perl DP, Olanow CW. Post mortem evidence of dopamine graft survival and striatal reinnervation in a Parkinson's disease patient displaying improved motor fucntion following fetal nigral transplantation. N Eng J Med 1995;332:1118–1124.
87. Kordower JH, Rosenstein JM, Collier TM, Burke MA, Chen E-Y, Li JM, Martel L, Levey AE, Mufson EJ, Freeman TB, Olanow CW. Functional fetal nigral grafts in a patient with Parkinson's disease: chemoanatomic, quantatative, ultrastructural, and metabolic studies. J Comp Neurol 1996; 370: 203–230
88. Freed CR, Greene PE, Breeze RE et al. Transplantation of embryonic dopamine neurons for severe Parkinson's disease. N Engl J Med 2001;344:710–719.
89. Greene PE, Fahn S, Tsai WY et al. Severe spontaneous dyskinesias: a disabling complication of embryonic dopaminergic tissue implants in a subset of transplanted patients with advanced Parkinson's disease. Mov Disord 1999;14:904.
90. Olanow CW, Goetz CG, Kordower JH, Stoessl J, Sossi V, Brin MF, Shannon KM, Perl DP, Godbold J, Freeman TB. A double-blind controlled trial of bilateral fetal nigral transplantation in Parkinson's disease. Ann Neurol 2003;54:403–414.
91. Dhawan V, Nakamura T, Margouleff C, Freed CR, Breeze RE, Fahn S, Greene PE, Tsai WY, Kao R, Eidelberg D. Double-blind controlled trial of human embryonic dopaminergic tissue transplants in advanced Parkinson's disease: fluorodopa PET imaging. Neurology 1999;52:405.
92. Hagell P, Piccini P, Bjorklund A et al. Dyskinesias following neural transplantation in Parkinson's disease. Nat Neurosci 2002;5:627–628.
93. Brundin P, Pogarell O, Hagell P et al. Bilateral caudate and putamen grafts of embryonic mesencephalic tissue treated with lazaroids in Parkinson's disease. Brain 2000;123:1380–1390.
94. Mendez I, Dagher A, Hong M et al. Simultaneous intrastriatal and intranigral fetal dopaminergic grafts in patients with Parkinson disease: a pilot study. Report of three cases. J Neurosurg 2002;96:589–596.
95. Deacon T, Schumacher J, Dinsmore J et al. Histological evidence of fetal pig neural cell survival after transplantation into a patient with parkinson's disease. Nature Med 1997;3:350–353.
96. Bakay RA, Raiser CD, Stover NP et al. Implantation of spheramine in advanced Parkinson's disease (PD). Front Biosci 2004;9:592–602.
97. Langston JW. The promise of stem cells in Parkinson disease. J Clin Invest 2005;115:23–25.

98. Bjorklund LM, Sanchez-Pernaute R, Chung S et al. Embryonic stem cells develop into functional dopaminergic neurons after transplantation in a Parkinson rat model. Proc Natl Acad Sci USA 2002;99:2344–2349.
99. Snyder BJ, Olanow CW. Stem cell treatment for Parkinson's disease: an update for 2005. Curr Opin Neurol (in press).
100. Kim JH, Auerbach JM, Rodriguez-Gomez JA et al. Dopamine neurons derived from embryonic stem cells function in an animal model of Parkinson's disease. Nature 2002;4:50–56.
101. Takagi Y, Takahashi J, Saiki H et al. Dopaminergic neurons generated from monkey embryonic stem cells function in a Parkinson primate model. J Clin Invest 2005;115:102–109.
102. Lin L-F, Doherty DH, Lile JD et al. A glial cell-line-derived neurotrophic factor for midbrain dopaminergic neurons. Science 1993;260:1130–1132.
103. Gash D, M Zhang, Z Ovadia A et al. Functional recovery in parkinsonian monkeys treated with GDNF. Nature 1996;380:252–255.
104. Gash DM, Zhang Z, Cass WA. Morphological and functional effects of intranigrally administered GDNF in normal rhesus monkeys. J Comp Neurol 1995;363:345–358.
105. Nutt JG, Burchiel KJ, Comella CL et al. Randomized, double-blind trial of glial cell line-derived neurotrophic factor (GDNF) in PD. Neurology 2003;60:69–73.
106. Gill SS, Patel NK, Hotton GR et al. Direct brain infusion of glial cell line-derived neurotrophic factor in Parkinson disease. Nat Med 2003;9:589–595.
107. Morrison PF, Laske DW, Bobo H, Oldfield EH, Dedrick RL. High-flow microinfusion: tissue penetration and pharmacodynamics. Am J Physiol 1994;266:292–305.
108. Kordower JH, Emborg ME, Bloch J et al. Neurodegeneration prevented by lentiviral vector delivery of GDNF in primate models of Parkinson's disease Science 2000;290:767–773.

SECTION 5

NON-MOTOR ASPECTS OF PARKINSON'S DISEASE

11

Depression, Psychosis, and Cognitive Dysfunction in Parkinson's Disease

Karen A. Sawabini, Jorge L. Juncos, and Ray L. Watts

INTRODUCTION

Historically much emphasis has been placed on the treatment and management of the motor symptoms of Parkinson's disease (PD). Non-motor symptoms such as depression, cognitive dysfunction, and psychosis have only recently been recognized as important treatment issues. In fact, several recent surveys assessing quality of life in Parkinson's disease revealed depression and other psychiatric symptoms to have a greater impact on quality of life than motor symptoms.[1] These non-motor phenomena may have catastrophic effects on the quality of life of the patient as well as a negative effect on caregivers. Suboptimal management of non-motor symptoms may lead to frequent, recurrent hospitalizations and ultimately earlier institutionalization of patients. In fact, Goetz et al. found that drug-induced hallucinations and delusions were a significant risk factor for nursing home placement.[2] This chapter examines appropriate treatment strategies for the management of several of the neurobehavioral non-motor complications of Parkinson's disease.

DEPRESSION

Epidemiology, Etiology, and Clinical Features

The estimated prevalence of depression in patients with Parkinson's disease varies from 25% to 40%.[3–5] It can occur at any stage of the disease and may even predate motor symptoms.[6] In fact, depression may actually be part of the spectrum of PD itself. Approximately 50% of depressed patients with PD do not meet full criteria for major depressive disorder but do meet criteria for dysthymia.[3] Dysthymia is more common in females and has an insidious onset. Either of these may affect quality of life negatively. Patients with long-term stress are at particular risk, as are those with a previous history of depression. Gender, age of onset of PD, and degree of functional disability may also be risk factors, although evidence is conflicting.[7–9]

The etiology of depression in PD remains unclear. Deficits of the neurotransmitter serotonin do occur. Depressed PD patients have lower CSF 5-hydroxyindoacetic acid levels than non-depressed PD patients.[10,11] The role of dopamine and norepinephrine loss in the development of depression has not been fully elucidated. It is most likely that depression is mediated by noradrenergic, serotonergic, and dopaminergic neuronal loss. This view is supported by postmortem evidence of loss of the aforementioned neurotransmitters.

The physician and caregiver should remain vigilant for symptoms of depression–including fatigue, apathy, psychomotor retardation, poor motivation, sleep disturbance, and anorexia or hyperphagia. Many of these symptoms may be mistaken for the progression of Parkinson's disease itself. Patients may also experience suicidal ideation, although the actual suicide rate is low. In patients with suspected depression, screening with the Beck Depression Inventory and a detailed interview are warranted. "Off state" symptoms, such as anxiety, panic, a feeling of impending doom and dysphoria, may mimic depression in advanced PD patients with motor complications. However, when questioned carefully they exhibit these symptoms only when the antiparkinsonian effect of their medications is "wearing off." In these patients, dopaminergic therapy should be maximized (Figure 11.1). Addition of a dopamine agonist, catechol-O-methyl transferase (COMT) inhibitor, or amantadine may be necessary if the effect of carbidopa/levodopa is wearing off. Dosing intervals of carbidopa/levodopa may need to be shortened for maximum benefit. Patients on controlled or extended-release formulas may benefit from switching to an immediate-release preparation for more reliable gastrointestinal absorption.

Evaluation and Treatment

Patients should be screened for underlying metabolic disturbances, which can often masquerade as depression. Screening for vitamin B_{12} deficiency, hypothyroidism, and anemia is warranted. Testosterone deficiency should be considered in men with depression refractory to conventional treatment.[12] Screening with the St Louis Testosterone Deficiency Questionnaire is a quick and useful tool that can be performed easily in the outpatient setting.[13] A free testosterone level, preferentially drawn in the morning, is recommended. Testosterone replacement may be given either transdermally (5 mg/day) or intramuscularly (50–400 mg every 2–4 weeks). Prostate-specific antigen (PSA) levels should be measured before treatment is initiated and monitored carefully while on testosterone replacement therapy.

Even though the risk of suicide is low, if depression is interfering with the patient's quality of life, antidepressant therapy should be instituted. Although there are no controlled clinical trials regarding the use of serotonin reuptake inhibitors (SSRIs) in patients with PD, short-acting SSRIs are preferentially

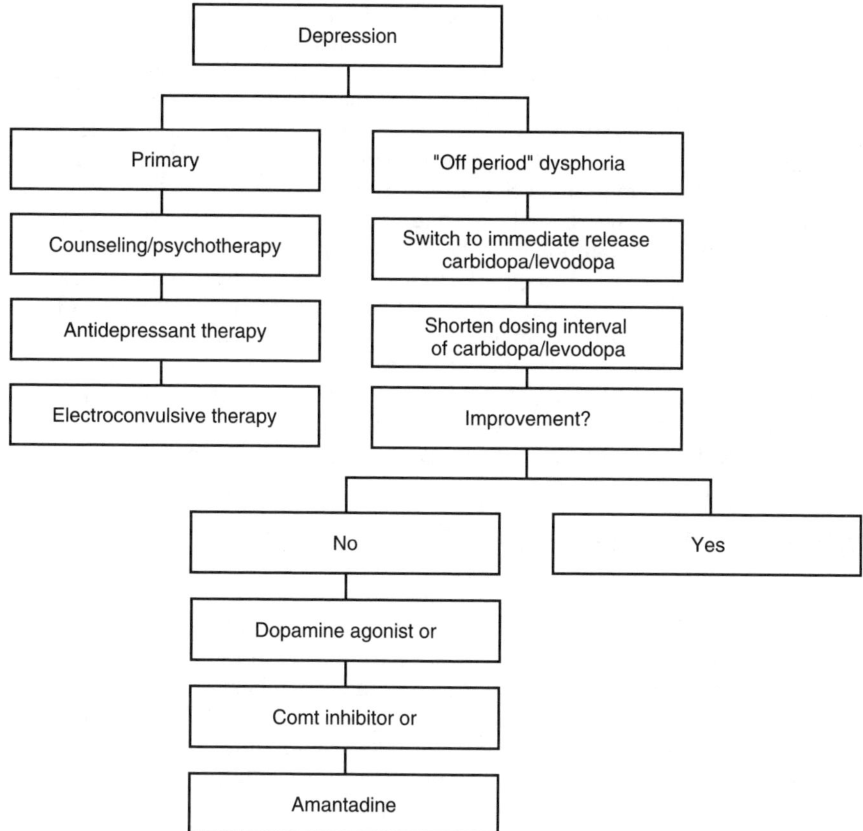

FIGURE 11.1 Approach to treatment of depression in PD patients.

used in clinical practice. Escitalopram, citalopram, paroxetine, and sertraline are usually well tolerated in a majority of patients. Serotonin syndrome has been described rarely in patients concomitantly taking selegiline, a monoamine oxidase (MAO-B) inhibitor, and an SSRI. MAO-B inhibitors may impair serotonin metabolism, resulting in excessive stimulation of 5-HT_{1A} receptors. However, the risk of serotonin syndrome is low and thus should not prevent treatment of a depressed individual.

Few clinical trials regarding the use of tricyclic antidepressants in patients with PD have been conducted. Anderson et al.[14] conducted a double-blind crossover study of 22 depressed PD patients who were randomized to either nortriptyline or placebo for a total of 16 weeks. Treatment with nortriptyline resulted in a significantly reduced score on the Anderson Depression Rating Scale. Tricyclic antidepressants may have undesirable anticholinergic side-effects. Clomipramine, amitriptyline, doxepin, imipramine, and protriptyline have the most anticholinergic side-effects. Antidepressants with activating side-effects such as venlafaxine (37.5–150 mg/day) and bupropion (50–20 mg/day) may be of benefit in patients with profound fatigue who lack insomnia.

Dopamine agonists may be effective in the treatment of depression. Corrigan et al.[15] conducted an 8-week double-blind, randomized trial of fluoxetine (20 mg) versus pramipexole (0.375 mg, 1.0 mg, or 5.0 mg) versus placebo. Patients receiving pramipexole, especially at the higher doses, had statistically significant improvement on the Hamilton Psychiatric Rating Scale for Depression, the Montgomery–Ashberg Depression Rating Scale, and the Clinician's Global Impressions-Severity of Illness scale.

General health measures, such as good nutrition, appropriate sleep hygiene, and a regular exercise regimen, may be helpful. Individual or family counseling should be offered. Local PD support groups may also be of benefit.

Unconventional therapies such as transcranial magnetic stimulation (TMS) are being investigated. In a small trial of 10 patients with both Parkinson's disease and depression, prefrontal TMS resulted in a statistically significant decrease in the Hamilton Depression Rating Scale.[16] In patients with severe depression who are refractory to antidepressant medications, a series of electroconvulsive treatments can be lifesaving and should be considered.

DELIRIUM, HALLUCINATIONS, AND PSYCHOSIS

Delirium

An acute or subacute change in level of consciousness or cognition associated with the presence of illusions and/or hallucinations indicates the presence of a delirium. This may initially present with a reduced ability of the patient to sustain or even shift attention. Recent memory is impaired and disruption of sleep/wake cycles is common. Typically delirium develops over a period of hours to days and it may fluctuate throughout the day. Patients may become agitated, irritable, and restless.

Although typically reversible, delirium warrants immediate attention. A good history is key in identifying the cause(s). Any recent changes of medications, including the addition of new agents, should be investigated. Metabolic etiologies–including dehydration, electrolyte imbalance, and hyperthyroidism–should be excluded. Infections, especially of the urinary tract, also should be considered in the work-up even if the person is asymptomatic. Computerized tomography (CT) or magnetic resonance imaging (MRI) of the brain may be beneficial to exclude a structural abnormality such as cerebral infarction or subdural hematoma as the causative factor. Laboratory tests should be performed, including complete blood count, electrolyte levels, blood urea nitrogen, creatinine, liver function tests, erythrocyte sedimentation rate, thyroid stimulating hormone, urinalysis, and possibly urine drug screen. A lumbar puncture may be indicated if meningoencephalitis is suspected (Table 11.1).

If the work-up is normal and it is suspected that the patient's delirium is secondary to medications, immediate changes are mandatory (Table 11.2). Medications with anticholinergic effects should be discontinued first as these are most likely to cause delirium. These include benztropine, trihexiphenidyl, and oxybutinin as well as tricyclic antidepressants. Narcotics and benzodiazepines are also frequent offenders. In the patient who is on multiple antiparkinsonian medications,

TABLE 11.1 Precipitating factors of delirium and/or psychosis in PD

Dehydration
Electrolyte imbalance
Thyroid disease (hypothyroidism or hyperthyroidism)
Infection (especially of the urinary tract or tracheobronchial tracts/lungs)
Recent change in antiparkinsonian or other CNS active medications

those with the most potential to induce delirium and the least effect on motor symptoms should be excluded first. This includes amantadine and selegiline. If there is no improvement, COMT inhibitors or dopamine agonists should be reduced or excluded next. In patients who are solely on carbidopa/levodopa therapy, bedtime or nocturnal doses should be reduced or excluded. Sustained-release formulations should be avoided as their absorption may vary and lead to fluctuations of delirium. An abrupt cessation of all dopaminergic medications should not occur so as to lessen the risk of neuroleptic malignant syndrome.[17,18] Patients on carbidopa/levodopa alone who cannot reduce their dose due to the degree of motor symptoms should be started on a selective antipsychotic agent (see below).

Hallucinations

Hallucinations in the patient with Parkinson's disease most commonly are secondary to dopaminergic therapies. It is estimated that 20% of patients with PD will develop hallucinations at some point in the course of their disease.[19] Frequently it is the family member or caregiver who brings them to the physician's attention. Risk factors include cognitive dysfunction, older age, and history of depression, as well as sleep disorders. It is quite common for the patient with PD to relate a history of sleep disruption prior to the onset of hallucinations. Moreover, hallucinations are more common at night and they are almost exclusively visual. People, typically strangers, are a common theme, although patients sometimes complain of seeing deceased relatives as well. Patients typically describe these strangers as watchful but not menacing. Rarely do these "strangers" attempt communication. Animals, including rodents and dogs, as well as insects, are other common hallucinations. Tactile hallucinations can

TABLE 11.2 Management of hallucinations and psychosis in PD

Correct/treat metabolic imbalances or infection
Eliminate sedatives, hypnotics, and narcotic analgesics
Eliminate anticholinergic agents
Eliminate amantadine
Reduce doses/Eliminate COMT inhibitors
Reduce doses/Eliminate dopamine agonists
Discontinue bedtime or nocturnal doses of carbidopa/levodopa
Discontinue controlled-release carbidopa/levodopa and use immediate-release formulation
If no improvement, begin low-dose quetiapine before bedtime and titrate accordingly (see text)

occur also (e.g. insects crawling on the skin), but they are much less common. Often these hallucinations are "benign" – the patient retains insight and does not progress to exhibit frank psychosis. The presence of auditory hallucinations is seen primarily in patients with prior history of major depression or evolving dementia with paranoid psychosis. Illusions, in which a patient misperceives a sensory stimulus, may predate or coexist with visual hallucinations.

Hallucinations may occur at any time in the course of the disease, but hallucinations early in the course of the disease or in response to minimal dopaminergic stimulation may be indicative of diffuse Lewy body disease or Lewy body dementia (LBD) (see below). The etiology of visual hallucinations in patients with PD has been postulated to be due to hypersensitivity of mesolimbic as well as mesocortical D3 receptors. However, Makoff et al. found no difference between D2 and D3 polymorphisms in non-hallucinating and hallucinating patients with PD.[20]

Psychosis

Psychosis can occur in up to 30% of patients with Parkinson's disease.[21] It usually presents with hallucinations and/or illusions, as well as delusions, and patients are often agitated and aggressive. They may become paranoid and suspicious of others, especially family members, accusing them of stealing or betraying them in some manner. Sleep disruption is common, especially at night (Table 11.3). Psychosis can be induced by even a small change in medication including anticholinergics, selegiline, dopamine agonists, and levodopa, especially in susceptible patients. Psychosis is typically dose-dependent and it may therefore respond to lowering of medications.

The biochemical basis of psychosis in the PD patient has not been fully elucidated. It is thought to be mediated by the loss of dopaminergic neurons in the nigrocortical and nigromesolimbic projections.[22] Serotonin may play a role as well in the development of visual hallucinations present in psychosis. Djaldetti et al. postulate that visual hallucinations may be due to release or displacement of serotonin from corticolimbic nerve terminals.[23] Left temporal lobe dysfunction may play a role in the development of visual hallucinations as well. Cerebral hypoperfusion of the left temporal lobe was found in patients who were experiencing hallucinations versus non-hallucinatory patients.[24]

Treatment

Use of an antipsychotic agent is warranted in patients with psychosis or in those patients who have retained insight but are bothered by their hallucinations.

TABLE 11.3 Signs of impending or active psychosis in PD

Visual hallucinations and/or illusions (usually "benign" initially)
Sleep disruption (especially nocturnal)
Agitation, restlessness, aggressive behavior
Delirium
Delusions, especially paranoid

Most of the older antipsychotic agents can result in D2 receptor blockade, which can worsen motor symptoms of PD patients. The newer "atypical" agents are more selective for limbic and cortical dopamine receptors as well as 5-HT_{2A} receptors, and they have a lower incidence of extrapyramidal side-effects (Table 11.4). Clozapine and quetiapine have been found to dissociate from D2 receptors in the striatum at a faster rate than other antipsychotic agents.

Quetiapine is currently the first-choice antipsychotic agent for PD patients.[25] It has minimal extrapyramidal side-effects. It is generally well tolerated and has minimal risk of serious toxicity. It is particularly beneficial in patients with sleep disruption due to its sedative effect. A typical starting dose is 12.5 mg before bedtime with a gradual titration every few days up to 50–100 mg daily if needed. Higher doses may be required in patients with a history of current or pre-existing affective disorder, especially if bipolar. Higher doses should be used cautiously, and built up slowly, particularly in elderly patients or those with dementia. Risperidone and olanzapine, both atypical antipsychotics, are generally not well tolerated due to extrapyramidal side-effects.

Clozapine is a D1/D5 antagonist which also has a high affinity for 5-HT_2, H1, and α_1-adrenergic receptors. It is considered the first atypical antipsychotic agent and was approved in 1994 by the US Food and Drug Administration (FDA). Clozapine dosing is similar to quetiapine, usually starting with 12.5 mg at bedtime and gradually titrating upward to 50–75 mg/day in non-demented patients. Serial monitoring of white blood cell counts is required each week as there is a 1% risk of agranulocytosis. It is an effective antipsychotic agent, but due to the risk of agranulocytosis it is reserved for patients who fail treatment with other antipsychotic medications (i.e. quetiapine). At high dosages it has anticholinergic effects, so cognitive function, including short-term memory, should be monitored closely. Ziprasidone is a more recently developed atypical antipsychotic agent. Daily dosage is in the range of 40–160 mg. It can cause prolongation of the QT interval, so periodic electrocardiograms are recommended for patients at risk. The purported risk of extrapyramidal side-effects is low; however, anecdotal evidence suggests it can cause worsening of motor symptoms in PD patients.

Acetylcholinesterase inhibitors may prove beneficial for hallucinations and delusions in PD patients. Fabbrini et al.[26] conducted an open study of 8 patients with Parkinson's disease who had visual hallucinations and/or delusions. Patients received 5 mg of donepezil at bedtime for 2 months. A statistically significant reduction in visual hallucinations and paranoid delusions was observed on the Parkinson's Disease Psychosis Rating Scale. Patients who are on a trial of an acetylcholinesterase inhibitor should be closely monitored for worsening of their motor symptoms.

COGNITIVE DYSFUNCTION AND DEMENTIA

Cognitive Dysfunction

Bradyphrenia is a common finding in patients with Parkinson's disease. It is defined as "cognitive slowing," but it actually indicates a more pervasive

TABLE 11.4 "Atypical" selective antipsychotic agents for hallucinations/psychosis in PD

Class	*Generic name*	*Trade name*	*Dosage range (mg)*	*EPS risk*	*Anticholinergic side-effects*	*Comments/Side effects*
Dibenzodiazepine	Clozapine	Clozaril	12.5–100 daily	Rare	Yes: high risk at higher doses	Risk of agranulocytosis Requires weekly WBC
Thienbenzodiazepine[a]	Olanzapine	Zyprexa	5–10 daily	Low	Yes: low risk	Weight gain, elevated prolactin levels
Dibenzothiazepine	Quetiapine	Seroquel	12.5–100 daily	Rare	Yes: low risk	Weight gain, elevated LFT
Benzisoxazole[a]	Risperidone	Risperdal	0.5–1.0 b.i.d.	Low	Yes: low risk	Nausea, insomnia
Benzisothiazolylpiperazine[b]	Ziprasidone	Geodon	20–80 b.i.d.	Low	Yes: low risk	Risk of prolonged QT interval

[a]Not recommended. [b]New, little experience.

EPS, extrapyramidal symptoms; WBC, white blood cell count; LFT, liver function tests; b.i.d., twice daily.

cognitive dysfunction affecting attention span and word fluency. Visuospatial deficits occur as well and appear to be related to the presence of cognitive impairment.[27] Impaired color discrimination and contrast sensitivity have also been found in patients with PD. Typically these impairments progress over time.[28] Higher cortical executive functions such as the initiation and planning of complex motor activities may also be impaired. The Wisconsin Card Sorting Test and Trail Making Test to assess set-shifting, and the Stroop Test for set maintenance, reveal impairment in PD patients.[29,30]

The etiology of cognitive dysfunction has not been clearly defined. It is most likely that the basal ganglia are involved. Cognitive information processing does occur in the basal ganglia but the intricacies of this are not completely understood. Disruption of thalamic projections to the dorsolateral, anterior cingulate, and orbitofrontal are likely to mediate some aspects of cognitive dysfunction in PD patients. This hypothesis of frontal and prefrontal dysfunction would also explain the development of apathy, which is indicative of frontal lobe dysfunction, in non-demented patients. Apathy presents as a loss of interest, concern, and motivation. It is commonly associated with depression but may also occur in non-depresssed PD patients as well.

Dementia

Dementia occurs in up to one-third of patients with Parkinson's disease.[31] It is a source of much concern to family and caregivers. Risk factors include advanced age, degree of motor disability, and depression. Historically, dementia associated with PD has been described as "subcortical" due to the absence of aphasia. Bradyphrenia, psychomotor slowing, and mild memory impairment complete the constellation of "subcortical dementia." Typically dementia does not occur early in the course of Parkinson's disease. Early-onset dementia warrants careful examination of the diagnosis of PD and if it occurs early it more likely represents Lewy body dementia, Alzheimer's disease, or Creutzfeld–Jacob disease (if the course is very rapid). Standardized dementia rating scales such as the Mattis Dementia Rating Scale are useful tools for assessing cognitive abilities including executive function and attention.[32] Medications, especially anticholinergic agents, may cause memory impairment and cognitive dysfunction, especially in elderly patients. Blood work including thyroid function tests, rapid plasminogen reactant, vitamin B_{12} level, and an antinuclear antibody titer should be performed to exclude potentially treatable causes. Neuroimaging (CT or MRI of the brain) may be helpful in excluding underlying structural abnormalities, such as subacute or chronic subdural hematoma, and is indicated if any lateralizing signs are present or if there is a history of falling or head trauma. Frontal release signs such as grasp, suck, snout, palmomental and root reflexes, as well as Myerson's sign, are indicative of loss of frontal lobe inhibition but may not be present early in the course of dementia.

The pathophysiologic etiology of dementia in Parkinson's disease has not been fully elucidated. In principle, however, it is associated with an evolution of the pathological changes (synucleinopathy) spreading outside of the nigrostriatal dopaminergic motor pathways to affect brain regions that are involved in memory and cognitive processes. Neuronal cell loss in the cholinergic circuits, including the nucleus basalis of Meynert and anterior cingulate gyrus, have been demonstrated in patients with both dementia and Parkinson's disease.[33]

Lewy Body Dementia

Lewy body dementia is characterized by progressive cognitive decline accompanied by parkinsonian features. After Alzheimer's disease, it is the second most frequently occurring neurodegenerative dementia.[34] Typically, postural tremor is more common than the classical rest tremor of Parkinson's disease, but both may occur. Other motor symptoms are often present, including generalized bradykinesia, hypomimia, and cogwheel rigidity. The pathologic basis of LBD is widespread involvement of cortical and subcortical cognitive regions by the synucleinopathy process. In fact, so-called "diffuse Lewy body disease" is best visualized in cortical and subcortical regions microscopically using immunocytochemical stains against alpha-synuclein. Psychiatric disturbances including apathy, visual hallucinations, delusions and fluctuating cognition are pathognomonic. Cognitive disturbances include memory disorder and impaired visuospatial function. The degree of cognitive dysfunction in these patients tends to be mild in the earlier stages with Mini-Mental Status Exam scores in the low to mid-20s range.[35]

Rapid-eye-movement (REM) sleep behavior disorder, in which an individual acts out his or her dreams with vocalizations as well as motor phenomena, is common. If the degree of REM sleep behavior disorder is troublesome, a low dose of clonazepam (0.5–1.0 mg) at bedtime may be helpful but can be associated with worsening encephalopathy in many of these patients.

LBD presents a treatment dilemma as patients typically do poorly with antipsychotic agents. Early in the course, however, low-dose quetiapine or clozapine can block hallucinations and psychosis well enough to allow modest doses of carbidopa/levodopa to help improve motor function to some extent. However, as a whole, patients with Lewy body dementia are not as dopa-responsive as patients with idiopathic PD. Psychiatric symptoms including hallucinations and delusions, as well as cognitive performance on attentional tasks, were improved in a randomized double-blind, placebo-controlled study in which patients with Lewy body dementia were placed on up to 12 mg of rivastigmine daily.[36] Rivastigmine is generally well tolerated but it should be started at a low dosage (e.g. 1.5 mg once or twice daily) and built up very gradually over 6–12 weeks to a full dosage of 6 mg twice daily if tolerated (see Treatment, below). Patients should be closely monitored for worsening of their motor symptoms. Due to the limitations of antipsychotic and dopaminergic agents in this patient population, a trial of an acteylcholinesterase inhibitor should be attempted.

Alzheimer's Disease and Parkinsonism

Alzheimer's disease (AD) is the most prevalent type of neurodegenerative dementia. It was classically described as a "cortical" dementia resulting in apraxia and agnosia in affected individuals; however, subcortical pathology does occur, predominately in the nucleus basalis of Meynert.[37] Unlike LBD, visuospatial skills, verbal fluency, and attention tend to be relatively spared until late in the course. However, extrapyramidal parkinsonian signs may accompany or even predate significant cognitive dysfunction in the patients who are later confirmed to have dementia and pathological changes consistent with Alzheimer's disease.[38] Extrapyramidal signs in these patients most often include symmetric, rather than asymmetric, rigidity, generalized bradykinesia, and hypomimia.[39] Rest tremor is uncommon.

The motor signs do not always respond to dopaminergic therapy, but a careful trial of antiparkinsonian medication is warranted in patients whose motor symptoms are disabling.[40,41] Low-dose carbidopa/levodopa is the treatment of choice. Amantadine and anticholinergic agents should be avoided due to the risk of further impairment of memory and cognition. If no improvement in motor signs is noted, or if improvement is minimal at best, dopaminergic therapy should be discontinued as it can precipitate hallucinations and psychosis. Older, nonselective antipsychotic agents may worsen extrapyramidal signs in these patients and should be avoided. Atypical antipsychotic agents such as quetiapine (12.5–200 mg) may be of benefit if treatment is required. However, starting with a low dose in the evening (e.g. 12.5 mg before bedtime) and very gradual titration of the dosage upward is the best approach to avoid a sudden worsening of encephalopathy.

Treatment

An attempt should be made to improve the memory disorder and cognitive decline in patients with dementia, so treatment with an acetylcholinesterase inhibitor should be instituted. Several double-blind, randomized trials involving donepezil and tacrine resulted in improved cognitive function in patients with dementia and Parkinson's disease.[42,43] Tacrine was the first acetylcholinesterase inhibitor approved by the US Food and Drug Administration (FDA). It was a mildly effective agent, but due to required close monitoring of liver function and dosing four times a day, it lost favor. Donepezil was the second FDA-approved acetylcholinesterase inhibitor. It is generally well tolerated and requires a single daily dose of 5 mg initially. After 4–6 weeks patients should be placed on 10 mg daily for maximum benefit. Galantamine and rivastigmine are newer agents. Both are generally well tolerated except for the gastrointestinal side-effects which can occur with any of the acetylcholinesterase inhibitors. Galantamine should be initiated at 4 mg twice daily for 4 weeks, then increased if tolerated to 8 mg twice daily for another 4 weeks and increased again to 12 mg twice daily. Rivastigmine inhibits both acetylcholinesterase and butylcholinesterase. The recommended starting dose of rivastigmine is 1.5 mg twice daily. This should be maintained for 2–4 weeks at which time the dose can be increased to 3 mg twice daily. In 2- to 4-week increments the dose may be increased further to 4.5 mg twice daily and up to a maximum of 6 mg twice daily. Patients should be monitored for worsening of their motor symptoms while on these agents, but the incidence of this is probably low.

Often patients and family members are interested in non-traditional therapies. Lay press reports regarding Gingko biloba have touted it as beneficial in patients with cognitive dysfunction. Several randomized, double-blind studies of Ginkgo biloba extract Egb 761 revealed improvement in the scores of several standardized tests including the ADAS-Cog (cognitive subscale of the Alzheimer's Disease Assessment Scale).[44,45] Patients taking Gingko biloba should be cautioned of the risk of bleeding as it is a platelet inhibitor.

CONCLUSIONS

Appropriate management of non-motor manifestations of Parkinson's disease such as depression, psychosis and cognitive dysfunction may be key in reducing disability in PD patients. However, these phenomena can present a difficult challenge for the treating physician. Antidepressants, atypical antipsychotic agents, and acetylcholinesterase inhibitors are the mainstays of treatment. Investigation of potential neuroprotective agents is an area of need and holds promise for the future.

Acknowledgments

This work was supported in part by NIH/NIA P50 AG16582-06 (UAB Alzheimer's Disease Research Center), the Lanier Family Foundation, the Mary Louise Brown Foundation, the Frances Hollis Brain Foundation, and the Emory University and University of Alabama at Birmingham Parkinson's Disease Research Funds.

REFERENCES

1. Global Parkinson's Disease Survey. Mov Disord 2002;17:60–67.
2. Goetz CG, Stebbins GT. Risk factors for nursing home placement in advanced Parkinson's disease. Neurology 1993;43:2227–2229.
3. Cummings JL. Depression and Parkinson's disease a review. Am J Psychiatry 1992;149:443–454.
4. Doonreief G, Mirabello E et al. An estimate of the incidence of depression in idiopathic Parkinson's disease. Arch Neurol 1992;49:305–307.
5. Yamamoto M. Depression in Parkinson's disease: its prevalence, diagnosis, and neurochemical background. J Neurol 2001;248(3):5–11.
6. Allain H, Schuck S, Mauuit N. Depression in Parkinson's disease. Br Med J 2000;320:1287–1288.
7. Schrag A, Jahanshahi M et al. What contributes to depression in Parkinson's disease? Psychol Med 2001;31(1):65–73.
8. Giladi N, Treves TA et al. Risk factors for dementia, depression and psychosis in longstanding Parkinson's disease. J Neural Trans 2000;107(1):59–71.
9. Leentjens AF, Lousberg R et al. Markers for depression in Parkinson's disease. Acta Psychiatr Scand 2002;106:196–201.
10. Sano M, Stern Y, Cote L et al. Depression in Parkinson's disease: a comparison with disabled control subjects. J Geriatr Psychiatry 1990;2:3–9.
11. Mayeux R, Stern Y, Sano M et al. The relationship of serotonin to depression in Parkinson's disease. Mov Disord 1988;3:237–244.
12. Okun M et al. Beneficial effects of testosterone replacement for the non-motor symptoms of Parkinson's disease. Arch Neurol 2002;59:1750–1753.
13. Morley JE, Charlton E et al. Validation of a screening questionnaire for androgen deficiency in aging males. Metabolism 2000;49:1239–1242.
14. Anderson J et al. Antidepressive treatment in Parkinson's disease: a controlled trial of the effect of nortriptyline in patients with Parkinson's disease treated with L-dopa. Acta Neurol Scand 1980;62:210–219.

15. Corrigan MH, Denahan AQ et al. Comparison of pramipexole, fluoxetine, and placebo in patients with depression. Depress Anxiety 2000;11(2):58–65.
16. Dragasevic N, Potebic A et al. Therapeutic efficacy of bilateral prefrontal slow repetitive transcranial magnetic stimulation in depressed patients with Parkinson's disease: an open study. Mov Disord 2002;17:528–532.
17. Ikebe S, Harada T et al. Prevention and treatment of malignant syndrome in Parkinson's disease: a consensus statement of the malignant syndrome research group. Parkinsonism Rel Disord 2003;9(suppl. 1):s47–49.
18. Hahimoto T, Tokuda T et al. Withdrawal of levodopa and other risk factors for malignant syndrome in Parkinson's disease. Parkinsonism Rel Disord 2003;9(suppl. 1):s25–30.
19. Sanchez-Ramos JR, Ortoll R et al. Visual hallucinations associated with Parkinson's disease. Arch Neurol 1996;53:1265–1268.
20. Makoff AJ, Greaham JM et al. Association study of dopamine receptor gene polymorphisms with drug-induced hallucinations in patients with idiopathic Parkinson's disease. Pharmacogenetics 2000;10:43–48.
21. Naimark D, Jackson E et al. Psychotic symptoms in Parkinson's disease with dementia. J Am Geriatr Soc 1996;44(3):252–253.
22. Agid Y, Javoy-Agid F et al. Biochemistry of neurotransmitters of Parkinson's disease. In: Marden CD, Fahn S (eds), Movement Disorders. London: Butterworth, 1987, pp. 166–230.
23. Djaldetti R, Melamed E. Neurobehavioral abnormalities in Parkinson's disease. In: Watts R, Koller W (eds), Movement Disorders: Neurologic Principles and Practice, 2nd edn. New York: McGraw-Hill, 2004.
24. Okada K, Suyama N et al. Medication induced hallucination and cerebral blood flow in Parkinson's disease. J Neurol 1999;246:365–368.
25. Friedman J, Factor S. Atypical antipsychotics in the treatment of drug-induced psychosis in Parkinson's disease. Mov Disord 2000;15:201–211.
26. Fabbrini G, Barbant P et al. Donepezil in the treatment of hallucination and delusions in Parkinson's disease. Neurol Sci 2002;23(1):41–43.
27. Levin BE, Llabre MM et al. Visuospatial impairment in Parkinson's disease. Neurology 1991;3:365–369.
28. Diederich N, Raman R et al. Progressive worsening of spatial and chromatic processing deficits in Parkinson's disease. Arch Neurol 2002;59:1249–1252.
29. Tamura I, Kikuchi S et al. Deficits of working memory during mental calculation in patients with Parkinson's disease. J Neurol Sci 2003;209(1/2):19–23.
30. Kanazawa A, Mizuno Y et al. Executive function in Parkinson's disease. Rinsho Shinkeigaku 2001;41(4/5):167–172.
31. Brown RG, Marsden CD. How common is dementia in Parkinson's disease. Lancet 1984;ii(8414):1262–1265.
32. Mattis S. Dementia Rating Scale. Odessa, FL: Psychological Assessment Resources Inc., 1988.
33. Zweig RM, Cardillo JE et al. The locus ceruleus and dementia in Parkinson's disease. Neurology 1993;43:986–991.
34. Barker WW, Luis CA et al. Relative frequencies of Alzheimer disease, Lewy body, vascular and frontotemporal dementia and hippocampal sclerosis in the state of Florida Brain Bank. Alzheimer Dis Assoc Disord 2002;16(4):203–212.
35. Salmon DP et al. Neuropsychological deficits associated with diffuse Lewy body disease. Brain Cog 1996;31:141–165.
36. McKeith I et al. Efficacy of rivastigmine in dementia with Lewy bodies: a randomised, double-blind, placebo-controlled international study. Lancet 2000;356(247):2031–2036.
37. Whitehouse P, Struble R et al. Alzheimer's disease: evidence of selective loss of cholinergic neurons in the basal forebrain. Science 1982;215:1237–1239.
38. Ditter SM, Mirra SS. Neuropathologic and clinical features of Parkinson's disease in Alzheimer's disease patients. Neurology 1987;37:754–760.
39. Lopez OL, Wisnieski JT et al. Extrapyramidal signs in patients with probable Alzheimer's disease. Arch Neurol 1997;54:969–975.
40. Mitchell S. Extrapyramidal features in Alzheimer's disease. Age Ageing 1999;28:401–409.
41. Rajput AH, Rozdilsky B et al. Levodopa efficacy and pathological basis of Parkinson syndrome. Clin Neuropharmacol 1990;13:553–558.
42. Werber EA, Rabey JM. The beneficial effect of cholinesterase inhibitors on patients suffering from Parkinson's disease and dementia. J Neural Trans 2001;108:1319–1325.

43. Aarsland D, Laake K et al. Donepezil for cognitive impairment in Parkinson's disease: a randomised controlled study. J Neurol Neurosurg Psychiatry 2002;72:708–712.
44. Le Bars PL, Velasco FM et al. Influence of the severity of cognitive impairment on the effect of Ginkgo biloba extract Egb 761 in Alzheimer's disease. Neuropsychobiology 2002;45(1):19–26.
45. Mix JA, Crews WD. A double-blind placebo-controlled, randomized trial of Ginkgo biloba extract Egb 761 in a sample of cognitively intact older adults: neuropsychological findings. Hum Psychopharmacol 2002;17(6):267–277.

12

Gastrointestinal, Urological, and Sleep Problems in Parkinson's Disease

Fabrizio Stocchi

INTRODUCTION

In his classic 1817 monograph, Sir James Parkinson described gastrointestinal dysfunction in patients with shaking palsy:[1]

> *". . . food is with difficulty retained in the mouth until masticated; and then as difficultly swallowed . . . the saliva fails of being directed to the back part of the fauces, and hence is continually draining from the mouth . . . the bowels which all along had been torpid, now in most cases, demand stimulating medicines of very considerable power: the expulsion of the faeces from the rectum sometimes requiring mechanical aid."*

Since then, many authors have described systemic symptoms in patients with Parkinson's disease (PD) and other parkinsonisms.[2–4] These are not only very distressing for the patients but interfere with the treatment of their disease. The majority of parkinsonian patients depend for their mobility and activities of daily living on the level of levodopa in their blood. Levodopa (L-dihydroxyphenilalanine) is a large neutral amino acid (LNAA) and is absorbed only from the small bowel–mostly in the duodenum, but there is some absorption in the jejunum and ileum–which contains LNAA transporters. This drug has a short half-life, so any factor that limits or delays levodopa absorption results in a reappearance of parkinsonian symptoms. In addition, PD affects swallowing, esophageal motility, colonic, and bladder function.

NEUROPHYSIOLOGY OF GASTROINTESTINAL FUNCTION

Control of gastrointestinal (GI) function is complex and involves components of the central, autonomic, and enteric nervous systems. Cortical localization for a number of aspects of GI function–including hunger, vomiting, swallowing, salivation, and defecation–have been identified.[5–7] Subcortical centers, including the basal ganglia, are presumed to play some role in modulating GI function, but exactly where and how is not clear. Except for the oropharyngeal and proximal esophageal musculature and the external anal sphincter, which are under somatic control, the gut is controlled by the central nervous system (CNS) via the autonomic nervous system and circulating hormones.

It has been proposed that swallowing is regulated by central pattern generators, which reside in the medial reticular formation of the rostral medulla and the reticulum adjacent to the nucleus tractus solitarius and project to the nucleus ambiguus and dorsal motor nucleus of the vagus (DMV).[7,8] These generators contain the neural programs that direct the sequential movements of the multitude of oral, pharyngeal, and esophageal muscles that produce normal swallowing. In PD, the nucleus ambiguus is spared, but the pedunculopontine tegmental nucleus and the DMV are not.[9] Therefore, it seems likely that dysphagia in PD is primarily due to defective coordination of the oral, pharyngeal, and esophageal musculature, produced by the combination of dysfunction in the medullary central pattern generators and increased inhibitory outflow from the pallidum to the pedunculopontine tegmental nucleus.[7] Within the esophageal myenteric plexus, however, Lewy bodies have been identified, raising the possibility that at least some portion of parkinsonian dysphagia might be the result of direct damage to the enteric nervous system.[10]

Stomach and intestinal function are more directly controlled by the autonomic and enteric nervous systems. The bulk of parasympathetic inervation of the GI tract is derived from the DMV, which supplies the stomach, small intestine, and proximal colon. Parasympathetic supply to the mid and distal colon travels via sacral nerves. Sympathetic supply to the entire GI tract derives from cells of the intermediolateral column of the spinal cord at T5 to L3 levels. Information is passed by both parasympathetic and sympathetic sources to the enteric nervous system, where cholinergic neurons in the myenteric plexus can either stimulate contraction of smooth muscle cells in the gut wall or excite surface epithelial cells to absorb or secrete fluid and electrolytes.[10] In general terms, parasympathetic signals stimulate GI function, while sympathetic signals inhibit its mobility. In PD, the involvement of the DMV is well documented, but involvement of other centers, such as the median raphe nucleus of the pons, has also been described.[11–13] Available data suggest that neurons in the DMV containing substance P are damaged by PD.[14] While these changes in parasympathetic autonomic supply to the gut could certainly account for the impairment of GI function in PD, abnormalities in the enteric nervous system within the gut itself have also been identified, including both Lewy body formation and actual dopaminergic neuronal loss.[15–17]

SWALLOWING ABNORMALITIES AND ESOPHAGEAL ALTERATIONS

Dysphagia and a variety of swallowing abnormalities are well-recognized complications of PD. Logemann et al.[18] reported abnormal lingual control of swallowing. Blonsky et al.[19] described lingual festination in which the elevated tongue prevented passage of the bolus into the pharynx. Logemann et al.[20] discussed a delayed swallowing reflex and noted aspiration. Bushmann et al.[21] reported a repetitive and involuntary reflux from the vallecula and piriform sinuses into the oral cavity. They also observed that some patients have great difficulty swallowing pills, with retention in the vallecula for long periods. Dopaminergic drugs improve swallowing in some patients, whereas anticholinergics may inhibit the process.[21]

The main esophageal alterations in patients with parkinsonism are non-peristaltic swallowing, belching, segmental spasms, esophageal dilatation, and gastro-esophageal reflux.[22,23] Belching can be related to "on"/"off" fluctuations[24] and may disappear when the patient is "on" (mobile state). Bramble et al.[25] suggested that cholinergic rather than dopaminergic mechanisms are more important in the control of esophageal motility in patients with parkinsonism, and showed that intravenous administration of atropine sulfate produced marked disruption of coordination in response to swallowing in patients with PD compared with control subjects. Therefore, anticholinergic drugs may worsen coordination in response to swallowing.

Patients with swallowing and/or esophageal problems may benefit from the use of a liquid formulation of levodopa (melevodopa, Dispersible Madopar)[26] or from the subcutaneous injection of the dopamine receptor agonist apomorphine.[27] Anticholinergic drugs should be withdrawn.

Some patients suffer from achalasia which can be treated with botulinum toxin injection into the cardia.[28]

DROOLING SALIVA (SIALORRHEA)

The presence of excessive saliva in the mouth, with consequent drooling, was initially noted by James Parkinson[1] and has been considered a cardinal sign of PD for many years. Surveys record the presence of excess saliva or drooling in 70–78% of PD patients, compared to 6% of control subjects.[3,4] It has become clear that the overabundance of saliva is not the result of excessive saliva formation, but rather the consequence of inefficient and infrequent swallowing. In fact, saliva production in PD is typically diminished, rather than increased.[29–31] Moreover, drooling saliva is not usually present in treated non-fluctuating parkinsonian patients but it appears in advanced patients during their "off" periods. In fact, antiparkinsonian therapy that improves swallowing prevents the drooling of saliva.

Although excessive saliva and drooling are not dangerous or life-threatening, they are a source of considerable embarrassment to patients. This has led to a variety of treatment approaches to this problem. Potent anticholinergic drugs, such as trihexyphenidyl and benztropine, are frequently prescribed in an attempt to "dry up" the excess saliva. Unfortunately, these drugs can also produce very troublesome systemic and CNS toxic effects and further impair deglutition. Recently it has been suggested that sublingual administration of a drop of 1% atropine ophthalmic solution twice daily can control excess saliva in affected patients without the systemic toxicity associated with oral ingestion,[32] but formal studies of this approach are still lacking.

Intraparotid injections of botulinum toxin A (BTX-A) have also been employed in attempts to eradicate excessive saliva in PD patients. Different studies have shown that intraparotid BTX-A injection significantly reduces saliva production and improves drooling saliva.[33–35] Although no significant adverse effects were reported in these studies, caution regarding potential complications of this technique–such as excessively dry mouth, dysphagia due to pharyngeal muscle weakness, and even facial nerve and artery damage from the injection–has been advised by other investigators.[36] Moreover, the treatment cannot be very successful if submandibular glands are not injected. The ultrasound-guided technique eliminates most of the possible side-effects, providing a method to inject the four glands safely. Recently, botulinum toxin B was used in some patients who had not improved with BTX-A, with excellent results.[37,38]

Other approaches to drooling saliva include surgery (tympanic neurectomy[39]), speech and language therapy,[40] and the use of chewing gum. The results are not always positive, and unpleasant side-effects may occur after surgery.

THE STOMACH

Gastroparesis, or delayed gastric emptying, can occur in Parkinson's disease[41,42] and other parkinsonisms and can produce a variety of symptoms, such as early satiety, abnormal discomfort with bloating, nausea, vomiting, weight loss, and even malnutrition.

Levodopa is not absorbed from the stomach, so that delayed gastric emptying may delay and blunt the achievement of peak plasma levodopa levels, adversely affecting the clinical response to the dose.[43] Levodopa taken after meals may be poorly absorbed because of the delayed gastric emptying due to the bulk, tonicity, and composition of the food.[44,45] Lipids and carbohydrates as well as some drugs such as dopamine agonists anticholinergics may delay gastric emptying as well. Excessive gastric acidity also delays gastric emptying, but too much neutralization of stomach contents may lead to incomplete dissolution of the levodopa tablets and thus incomplete absorption.[46] Gastric emptying may be also delayed by PD itself or by constipation because of the colon–gastric reflex.

It has been demonstrated that in parkinsonian patients a levodopa tablet may remain in the stomach for very long time. The enzyme dopa-decarboxylase is present in the gastric mucosa and can convert levodopa trapped in the stomach into dopamine, making it unavailable for CNS delivery and utilization.[47] Furthermore, the dopamine formed in the stomach may stimulate gastric dopamine receptors, which promote stomach relaxation and inhibit gastric motility, with the potential consequence of worsening the gastroparesis.[48,49]

Many authors have reported that direct infusion of liquid levodopa into the duodenum ensures a more reliable and predictable response to the drug.[50] Moreover, levodopa plasma levels after intraduodenal infusion are much more stable then after intragastric infusion.[51] These studies emphasize the role of the stomach in the pathophysiology of motor fluctuations in parkinsonian patients.

Since levodopa is absorbed only from the small bowel, the competition in the stomach between levodopa and other dietary LNAAs (e.g. valine, leucine, and isoleucine) is not common, although it may occur.

Liquid levodopa may improve patients with motor fluctuations, ensuring a better absorption. Subcutaneous infusion of dopamine agonists (apomorphine and lisuride)[53] is very effective in controlling motor fluctuations by bypassing the gastrointestinal tract.

Parkinsonian patients should be advised to eat small meals and avoid protein during the day and to take the drugs when fasting. Domperidone sometimes may help gastric emptying.

SMALL BOWEL

The literature contains references both to symptoms and radiological signs suggestive of small intestine motor dysfunction in Parkinson's disease, but the frequency and the functional significance of some of these findings remain uncertain.

Weight loss is a frequent finding in elderly patients with PD,[54,55] although the reasons have not been fully explained. An increase in energy expenditure has been shown in two studies,[55,56] whilst other possible contributing factors include dietary deficiency, or malabsorption due to small bowel bacterial overgrowth. Dietary deficiency is unlikely to be the cause.[57] Davies et al.[58] showed a reduced absorption of mannitol with an increase in the lactulose/mannitol ratio, suggesting a reduction in the absorptive surface area of the small intestine in parkinsonian patients. The authors explained these results by means of a specific alteration in the enterocyte brush border membrane. The same authors did not find any evidence of small bowel bacterial contamination, whereas other studies have suggested small bowel bacterial overgrowth being implicated in malabsorption, even when the small bowel is anatomically normal.[59,60]

Davies and associates[58] also found a significantly prolonged orocecal transit time in PD patients compared to healthy elderly subjects, and this was not related to disease severity or duration. This phenomenon may be due to disordered gastrointestinal autonomic function. Lewy bodies have been found in the sympathetic vertebral chain and in the ganglionic coeliacum of PD patients.[16,61] Thus autonomic or enteric nervous system dysfunction may be responsible for the increased orocecal transit time.

WEIGHT LOSS

Although commonly perceived by both patients and physicians to be a frequent feature of PD, unintended weight loss has actually received surprisingly little direct study. Different studies reported weight loss in the majority of PD patients observed,[62] and the weight loss was significantly higher than in control subjects.[63] PD patients were four times as likely to have reported a weight loss of greater than 4 kg than were controls. Other investigators have noted gender differences in weight loss among PD patients, with a larger percentage of women experiencing weight loss than men (8.5% vs 4.3%).[64]

The reason for progressive, unintended weight loss in PD is not yet clear, although various hypotheses have been advanced. Weight loss in any situation must be accounted for by one of two mechanisms: reduced energy intake or increased energy expenditure (or a combination of the two). Reduced energy intake could be the consequence of either decreased food intake or impaired food absorption. Individuals with PD often display impairment of olfaction[65] with consequent reduction in sense of taste. However, when dietary intake in PD patients has been assessed, no significant differences, compared to control subjects, have been uncovered,[62,66] even though approximately two-thirds of persons with PD do describe some eating difficulties.[62] The possibility that dysphagia might lead to reduced caloric intake and weight loss has also been suggested by some investigators,[67] but discounted by others.[68] Malabsorption is not generally considered to be a component of PD, but Davies and colleagues demonstrated decreased mannitol absorption in persons with PD and suggested that decreased non-mediated uptake across the enterocyte brush border membrane might be at least one factor contributing to weight loss in PD.[58]

The issue of increased energy expenditure in PD has been the subject of some controversy and disagreement. Energy expenditure can be divided into two components: energy expended at rest, accounting for 60–80% of energy expenditure, and physical activity expenditure, which takes up the remaining 20–40%.[66] While some investigators have reported increased resting energy expenditure in both treated and untreated PD patients,[69,70] others have demonstrated a 15% reduction in total energy expenditure, due to a reduction in the physical activity component.[66] It has also been suggested that levodopa-induced dyskinesia might be one cause of increased resting energy expenditure and, indeed, moderate or severe dyskinesia has been noted to be the strongest correlate of undernutrition in PD.[71] Toth and colleagues, however, note that it would take severe dyskinesia to counterbalance the 430 kcal reduction in total energy expenditure they noted in PD patients.[66]

Other mechanisms have also been postulated for unintended weight loss in PD. Evidente et al.[72] measured leptin in PD patients and found no significant difference between individuals who had lost weight compared with weight-stable patients. Contrary to expectations, levels actually showed a trend toward being lower in patients who had lost weight. These investigators suggested, however, that some interaction between levodopa and leptin could still be playing a role in parkinsonian weight loss. It has also been proposed that weight loss in PD may be due to increased lipolytic activity induced by high levels of circulating insulin.[72,73]

An interesting insight to the unresolved issue of unintended weight loss in PD has been the recent recognition that PD patients often gain weight following stereotactic surgery for treatment of motor PD symptoms. Weight gain occurs following both pallidal and subthalamic procedures and is more pronounced following bilateral surgery.[74] While some investigators suggest the weight gain is the result of reduced energy expenditure because of reduced dyskinesia, others have noted no correlation with changes in dyskinesia, food intake, dysphagia, levodopa dose, or PD duration.[74] Indeed, other therapeutic strategies which reduce the severity of dyskinesias, such as continuous subcutaneous infusion of dopamine agonists, induce weight gain.[75] Thus, at the present time the basis for unintended weight loss in PD remains largely unexplained. While increased energy expenditure due to the presence of dyskinesia may be a contributing factor in some, it certainly does not provide an explanation for all. Other factors, as yet unstudied, such as alterations in neuropeptides, might conceivably be involved

LARGE BOWEL

As far as large bowel is concerned, symptoms and signs are more clear and their frequency is high in the PD population.[15,76] Constipation is by far the most frequent symptom complained of by patients. In one survey, 50% of patients had a defecation frequency of less than once daily, compared with 12% in age-matched control subjects.[77] In a recent study at the author's institution, using a questionnaire, 76.5% of the PD patients reported a bowel frequency of less than three evacuations per week; 94% had hard stools and straining for difficult defecation, and 88% had continuous use of laxatives or enemas or both. In our series, 24% of the patients referred to fecal incontinence, 6 for liquid stools and one for solid feces. Seventy-six percent of the patients reported that the onset, orthe worsening, of the bowel dysfunctions followed the onset of neurological symptoms.

Constipation is defined as a decreased frequency of bowel movements to <3 bowel movements per week.[78] The stools may be hard and pellet-like or large and difficult to pass. Constipation may be caused by one or several mechanisms: (1) functional obstruction due to increased segmenting contractions; (2) poor colonic contractions (colonic inertia or pseudo-obstruction), or (3) functional outlet obstruction.[79] Specific symptoms may suggest the underlying etiology of the constipation. All patients usually have abdominal pain, although those with increased segmental contractions are more likely to have lower abdominal cramps associated with irritable bowel syndrome. In contrast, patients with nausea and vomiting are more likely to have an absence of colonic postprandial colonic contractions.[80] Straining at stool and incomplete evacuation may suggest an outlet obstruction.

However, especially in PD, constipation is the result of several mechanisms. For stool expulsion to occur, fecal material must first be propelled through the colon by colonic muscle contractions and then expelled through the coordinated actions of the rectum, anal sphincters, and pelvic floor muscles, as well as the musculature of the abdominal wall and diaphragm.[81] In parkinsonism, constipation is due to colon inertia or to outlet-type dysfunction or both.[82–84] In colon inertia the problem seems to be in the colonic musculature which induces slow transit of feces through the colon.[84,85]

Many authors have reported that the mean colon transit time (MCT) is considerably prolonged in PD patients.[86–89] Thus, slow colon transit is clearly a component of disturbed bowel function in PD patients. Although the role of dopamine in colonic motility has not been defined, constipation may be related to direct involvement of the colonic myenteric plexus by the PD process. Singaram et al.[90] compared colonic tissue from 11 patients with advanced PD, 17 with adenocarcinoma (normal tissue was studied), and 5 who underwent colectomy for severe constipation. Immunohistochemistry was used to stain myenteric and submucosal neurons for dopamine, tyrosine hydroxylase, and vasoactive intestinal polypeptide (VIP). Each class of neurons was quantified as a percentage of the total neuronal population stained for the marker protein gene product 9.5. Nine of the eleven PD patients had substantially fewer dopaminergic myenteric neurons than the other subjects. There was very little difference between the groups in numbers of tyrosine hydroxylase and VIP neurons. High-performance liquid chromatography showed lower levels of dopamine in the muscularis externa (but not mucosa) in four PD patients than in four controls, but levels of dopamine metabolites were similar in two groups. The authors also confirmed the findings of others authors[16,91] who showed that in the gut most Lewy bodies were in VIP-immunoreactive neurons, whereas in the sympathetic ganglia all Lewy body-containing neurons were immunoreactive for tyrosine hydroxylase. These finding suggest that slow colonic transit may be related to a direct involvement of the colonic myenteric plexus by the PD process.

The outlet-type dysfunction is mainly due to the inability of the patients to relax the pelvic floor and therefore to straighten the anorectal angle.[82,92]

Normal defecation occurs at a socially convenient time after rectal distention by fecal material is perceived. Tonic-resting activity in the striated sphincter musculature is inhibited and relaxation of the puborectalis (PR) muscle sling permits straightening of the rectoanal angle, allowing access of rectal contents to the anal canal. Simultaneously, relaxation occurs in the external anal sphincter (EAS) muscle. During defecation straining, there is cocontraction of glottic, diaphragmatic, and abdominal wall muscles, and rectal evacuation is achieved by a combination of raised intra-abdominal pressure and relaxation of the anal sphincter muscles, often aided by colonic pressure waves. Previous descriptions of activity during simulated defecation straining have confirmed that, in normal subjects, there is inhibition of the EAS and PR muscles.[93] In subjects with normal sphincter muscle relaxation, activity in the adjacent gluteal muscles does not change when recorded under the laboratory conditions of this study.[92] Mathers et al.[81] showed that the selective pattern of muscle contraction and inhibition that accompanies defecation straining is disturbed in some parkinsonian patients suffering from constipation. Paradoxical activation of the PR and EAS muscles occurred and some patients also showed a tendency to recruit gluteal muscles during simulated defecation straining.

Sometimes paradoxical anal sphincter muscle contraction resembling anismus-type pelvic outlet obstruction may occur too.[92]

Anorectal manometry has revealed several abnormalities in parkinsonian patients which included low basal and impaired squeeze pressures, prominent phasic fluctuations during squeeze, and a hypercontractile response to recto-sphinteric reflex.[88]

At the author's institution we studied the anorectal function in 17 parkinsonian patients. The mean duration of their disease was 10.5 years (SD = 5 yrs) and the Hoehn–Yahr stage ranged from 2 to 5.[94] Four hours after receiving an enema, patients underwent anorectal manometry with a multilumen catheter (outer diameter 4 mm) with distal side openings spaced 5 mm apart. Three lumens were continuously perfused (0.5 mL/min) with bubble-free distilled water by means of a low-compliance pneumohydraulic capillary-infusion system and were connected through P23 Db Statham external transducers to a multichannel polygraph. A latex balloon was attached to the tip of the catheter, 5 cm from the nearest recording side-hole. When suspended in air and inflated with 50 mL of air, the balloon was 6.5 cm long and 4 cm wide. Intra-balloon pressures were recorded and transmitted to the polygraph via a fourth lumen. With the subject lying on the left side, the manometric probe was introduced through the anus so that all recording holes were positioned within the rectal ampulla. The manometric catheter was then withdrawn through the anal canal with a station pullthrough technique. The probe was then reintroduced into the rectum and withdrawn to be positioned in the anal canal, with the recording sensors at 10, 15, and 20 mm from the anal verge. The operator kept the manometric probe firmly in place throughout the study period. The protocol included three tasks: act of squeezing; progressive intermittent distention of the intrarectal balloon; and straining on two separate occasions.

Resting anal pressure was 49 ± 19 mmHg and maximal contraction pressure was 99 ± 40 mmHg lasting for 15.6 ± 6.8 seconds, all remaining under the normal values. Three patients were unable to contract the anus. Resting and squeezing anal pressures showed an inverse direct relationship with disease duration. Maximal anal contraction pressure was higher in patients with a lower degree of disability (Hoehn–Yahr stages 2/3) than in the more severe patients (stages 4/5). A significant relationship between anal pressure and age of the patients and disease duration was found. The threshold of the inhibitory anal reflex and rectal compliance was within the normal range, and the mean threshold of rectal sensitivity (70 ± 58 mL of air) was in the upper range of the normal value. Manometric recordings during straining showed a lack of anal inhibition in 11 patients (65%).

Altered voluntary anal contraction and paradoxical anal contraction during straining have been repeatedly reported in PD patients.[88] In our study we found also an insufficient relaxation of the anal canal during straining. A possible explanation is a manometric expression of the abdominopelvic dysynergia, recorded with electromyography in other studies,[95] manifesting as an insufficient decrease in anal pressure accompanied by a paradoxical contraction.

The manometric finding of a paradoxical contraction or insufficient inhibition of the anal canal during straining could reflect the generalized extrapyramidal motor disorder, and hence be unrelated to degeneration of the sacral nuclei. Its frequent occurrence in patients with idiopathic constipation,[96] and in children with functional megarectum,[97] indicates that the abnormality is strictly related not to the specific neurological alterations of idiopathic PD but rather to a focal dystonic condition[92] of the abdominopelvic muscles compounded by Parkinson's disease.

The finding of a low resting anal tone has not been consistently reported in PD patients. The investigation described above confirms that, although resting anal pressure may be within normal range in PD, some patients have marked hypotonia. Because the resting anal pressure is essentially due to the contractile activity of the internal anal sphincter–a function mainly regulated by the orthosympatic nervous system–this abnormality may reflect a degenerative lesion of the spinal cord intermediolateral columns or autonomic ganglia, or both.[61]

Alternative explanations for the reduced anal pressure in resting conditions and during voluntary contraction can be found in the possible presence of anatomical changes in the internal and external anal sphincters consequent to age-related degeneration or continuous straining efforts, or both–which, in the attempt to overcome the difficulty to defecate, may lead to traction neuropathy involving the distal fibers of the pudendal nerves.

Irrespective of its pathophysiologic mechanism, the reduced anal tone during resting conditions and voluntary contraction could explain the relatively high frequency of episodes of fecal incontinence for liquid stools reported by PD patients, especially after laxative intake. The inefficient voluntary anal contraction found in PD patients may be due to their inability to recruit properly the muscle fibers of the external anal sphincter.

While many therapies have been advocated for the treatment of constipation in PD, few have been subjected to clinical trial. Ashraf et al.[98] reported that psyllium increased stool frequency and weight but did not alter colonic transit or anorectal function in PD patients with confirmed constipation. Astarloa et al.[99] reported that a diet rich in insoluble fiber produced a significant improvement in constipation, as indicated by an increase in stool frequency and an improvement in stool consistency. A fascinating observation in this study was a parallel improvement in extrapyramidal function, which in turn appeared to be related to an increase in the bioavailability of orally administered levodopa. The authors suggested that this increase in levodopa absorption and resultant improvement in clinical status were related to an augmentation in GI motility and thereby drug delivery. Suppression of defecation can result in delayed gastric emptying, perhaps through a cologastic reflex.[100,101] This could be the explanation of the beneficial effect of treatments improving constipation on extrapyramidal symptoms.

The difficulty in relaxing the pelvic floor and paradoxical puborectalis contraction generally respond dramatically to dopaminergic drugs.[81] Paradoxical electromyographic activity in anal sphincter muscles tends to persist even in the "on" phase. However, a definite improvement in pelvic outlet obstruction has been demonstrated with proctography after apomorphine administration.[81] This evidence extends the concept of an "off"-period pelvic floor dystonia in PD, advanced by Mathers and colleagues.[92] Therefore, patients should try to pass feces when "on" or take a quick-acting drug (apomorphine[53]) before starting defecation. Unfortunately some patients still experience difficulty defecating when motor disability has otherwise been reversed by dopaminergic drugs. In these patients the injection of botulinum toxin in the puburectalis muscle and/or in the external anal sphincter may be useful. Botulinum toxin injection may be used also in those patients with painful anismus-type dystonia.

Laxatives are useful in patients with normal pelvic floor relaxation. On the other hand, continuing to prescribe laxatives to patients who cannot achieve effective defecation due to pelvic floor dystonia will only produce adverse effects from the laxatives and further increase the patients' frustration.

Megacolon and even sigmoid volvulus may be a complication of the impaired colonic motor function in PD. Although uncommon, these complications may be life-threatening, and volvulus should certainly be considered in any PD patient who presents with an acute abdomen.

BLADDER DYSFUNCTION

There is a general perception that bladder control can be a major problem in patients with Parkinson's disease.[102–104] The prevalence of urinary disturbances in studies of PD patients diagnosed according to modern criteria was about 27%.[105,106] In these studies the severity of urological symptoms correlated with disease duration and severity.

The cause and nature of bladder symptoms in patients with genuine PD may be difficult to establish, and treatment is often unsatisfactory. Patients complain of urgency and frequency which may be severe, and urge incontinence particularly if poor mobility compounds their bladder disorder.[105,107] Many male patients with PD will be in the age group in whom bladder outflow obstruction due to benign prostatic hyperplasia (BPH) is a common coexistent disorder.[108] Those with outflow obstruction complain of voiding symptoms such as a hesitancy and a poor flow and furthermore may also have urgency since obstruction itself can cause detrusor overactivity. It is likely that a number of the earlier studies on "Parkinson's disease" and the bladder included patients with multiple-system atrophy (MSA), and the reputation that patients with PD have a poor outcome following prostatic sugery may be due to the inadvertent inclusion of some men with MSA in the surveys.[108] Urological intervention is not contraindicated in men with PD, but it is reasonable to try these patients on anticholinergic medication first if urinary frequency symptoms are prominent. If conservative measures fail, then a voiding cystometrogram to demonstrate obstructed voiding should be performed before transurethral resection of prostate is considered.

Female patients with urinary complaints seem to be similarly affected and approximately 70% complain of urgency with or without urge incontinence.[109]

If no urological cause for bladder symptoms is demonstrated, a neurological cause can be considered. There are several possible neurogenic causes of bladder symptoms in PD. Urodynamic studies of several series of patients have found that the most common abnormality is detrusor hyperreflexia, the incidence varying from 45% to 93%.[110,111] In a large study conducted with urodynamic evaluation in PD and MSA patients, it was shown that hyperreflexia with vesicosphincteric synergy was a more frequent finding in PD patients who had more severe motor disorders and longer disease duration.[106] In multiple system atrophy, hyperreflexia was already present even in patients with less advanced disease.

The hypothesis most widely held as to the cause of detrusor hyperreflexia in PD is that, in health, the basal ganglia have an inhibitory effect on the micturition reflex, and with cell loss in the substantia nigra this is lost. Experimental evidence of an inhibitory role for the basal ganglia comes from animal MPTP (1-methyl-4-phenyl-1,2,3,6-tetrahydropyridine) models.[112] It is likely that the degeneration of dopaminergic neurons in the substantia nigra and subsequent loss of striatal dopamine concentration may lead to detrusor hyperactivity, by an inability to activate the tonic inhibition executed by D1 receptors. Indeed selective D1 agonist SKF 38393 depressed detrusor overactivity in experimental animals.[112]

Clinical studies which have looked at the effect of levodopa or apomorphine on bladder behavior in patients with PD have produced conflicting results. In patients showing "on"/"off" phenomena, cystometry done in both states showed a lessening of hyperreflexia with levodopa in some patients and a worsening in others.[113] A similar unpredictable effect was found on detrusor hyperreflexia when subcutaneous apomorphine was given in one study, although in another all those with detrusor hyperreflexia improved.[114]

Some authors have suggested that an impaired relaxation or "bradykinesia" of the urethral sphincter can result in voiding dysfunction due to bladder outflow obstruction, while an earlier study suggested the effect of levodopa was to increase bladder neck obstruction. A study in which subcutaneous apomorphine was given to patients with PD and urinary symptoms showed that apomorphine reduced bladder outflow resistance and improved voiding in all 10 patients. It was proposed that this intervention be used to demonstrate the reversibility of outflow obstruction in men with PD before prostatic surgery is undertaken – an excellent suggestion but unfortunately rarely done.[106,109,110]

Addressing a correct diagnosis in PD patients suffering from bladder disturbances is very important to avoid inappropriate urologic surgery. Cystometry or even videourethrography is mandatory in men with PD in whom prostatic surgery is being considered. Cystometry can be useful to demonstrate detrusor overactivity; being a rare finding in the early stage of PD, this can be a pointer to consider another diagnosis. However, in cases of detrusor overactivity an anticholinergic therapy can be considered.

Treatment can be considered also on the basis of symptoms alone. It is, however, important to measure the post-micturition residual volume since incomplete emptying and a raised residual contributes significantly to neurogenic bladder dysfunction. This can be easily done with an ultrasound scan.

Treatment of a neurogenic bladder is generally successful,[115] especially in the early stage. The drugs of choice are oxybutinin and tolderodine. These anticholinergics usually improve urgency and frequency as they reduce the parasympathetic effect on the bladder. Treatment with an anticholinergic can be initiated when the micturition residual volume is under 100 mL. When the volume is over 100 mL, drug therapy can be started but the volume has to be monitored. In patients with micturition residual volume, a daily administration of vitamin C (1 g) reduces the risk of infection by increasing urine acidity.

Side-effects of oxybutinin and tolderodine are related to their anticholinergic proprieties. Tolderodine should have less propensity than oxybutinin to cross the blood–brain barrier, being less lipophilic. However, a recent double-blind controlled trial with extended-release oxybutinin and tolderodine has shown a similar reduction in total incontinence episodes and comparable adverse events involving the central nervous system.[116]

SLEEP DISORDERS

Problems at night are common in Parkinson's disease and, because of their debilitating effect on performance during the daytime, merit special attention.

In 1999, sudden and irresistible sleep attacks with subsequent automobile accidents were reported in nine PD patients on ropinirole and pramipexole therapy.[117] This report had the merit of drawing attention to sleep problems in parkinsonism. However, in 1817, James Parkinson wrote "tremor may occur during sleep," and Gowers, in 1901, underlined the persistence of tremor during sleep.[118]

Nowadays it is clear that tremor and rigidity are alleviated during sleep, but other sleep disorders are common in patients suffering from PD.[119] Their prevalence is difficult to ascertain due to the heterogeneity of patients and to the different criteria used to categorize sleep disorders, but it seems to vary from 98% to 74–81%.[120,121] At the author's institution we conducted a questionnaire survey on 200 PD patients and 100 normal controls; 78.5% of patients and 47% of the controls complained of sleep disorders.[122]

The role of gender is not clear. No sex differences for difficulty in initiating sleep have been reported, while female patients experience more disturbed sleep maintenance and excessive dreaming.[121]

Difficult sleep maintenance (light and fragmented sleep), and difficulties in initiating sleep, are often the earliest and most frequent symptoms observed in PD patients. In more advanced stages, insomnia, excessive daytime sleepiness, nightmares, and restlessness syndrome (possibly associated with periodic leg movements) can also be observed. In fluctuating patients, nocturnal akinesia, dystonia, painful cramps, and parasomnias may aggravate nocturnal problems.

Insomnia

Initial insomnia, sleep maintenance insomnia, and sleep fragmentation are the three disorders reported.

In a recent survey, insomnia was present in about 40% of the patients,[122] and in another study it was reported in 59% of patients compared to 35% of controls.[121] Insomnia was mainly due to difficulties in sleep maintenance (21.5%). The percentage of patients who complained of frequent awakenings and early-morning awakening was twice that of controls. In the study by Kumar and associates, 49% of PD patients suffered from nighttime awakenings.[123]

The prevalence of initial insomnia is similar in PD patients and elderly controls. In normal elderly population it is often due to anxiety and depression, whereas severity of diseases, restless legs syndrome, and akathisia seem to be the most common causes in PD patients.[123,124]

Insomnia can be idiopathic, due to nocturnal parkinsonian symptoms (difficulty in turning over in bed, painful leg cramps, vivid dreams/nightmares, pain, stiffness, jerks), or to an initial cognitive decline. Moreover it may be caused by neuropsychiatric/behavioral problems (anxiety or agitated depression) or be induced by medications.[124–127] Benzodiazepine antidepressants (tricyclics, MAOIs), antipsychotics, and anticholinergics may cause alteration of sleep architecture.[128–131]

Whereas tremor and rigidity are alleviated during sleep, from a neurophysiological point of view in PD patients there is an increase in muscle activity, such as repetitive muscle contractions (RMCs) that appear during non-REM sleep. RMCs, the equivalent of tremor during wakefulness, are subclinical and are inhibited by REM sleep. It is therefore possible that repetitive muscle contractions prevent progression to deep slow-wave sleep, resulting in light and fragmented sleep throughout the night. Also, sleep breathing disorders, predominantly obstructive, seem to be common in PD. Degenerative changes in the CNS affecting centers for sleep regulation may contribute to these problems.

Sleep fragmentation can be made worse by a need to pass urine frequently during the night. Nocturia is a very common problem in PD patients, being reported by Lees et al. in 70% of their patients,[125] and by 43.5% of the patients in another study.[122] Nocturia is a consequence of an abnormal bladder sensitivity. Hyperreflexia with vesicosphincteric synergy is present in up to two-thirds of parkinsonian patients,[106] as a consequence of which the bladder of these patients can hold only about 250 mL of urine. Bladder overactivity worsens during drug-free periods such as during the night. Patients should avoid drinking liquids just before retiring to bed.

Daytime Sleepiness and Excessive Daytime Sleepiness

Daytime sleepiness (DS) and excessive daytime sleepiness (EDS) are widely reported to be common in patients with Parkinson's disease.[132–135] Mild DS consists of increased sleepiness with a tendency to fall asleep a few times. EDS represents a more severe increased somnolence during normal waking hours, with longer and more frequent sleep episodes. Factors interfering with nocturnal sleep such as awakenings, loud snoring, depression, limitation of daily activity, and drug consumption may contribute to EDS.

The circadian rhythm of sleep is biphasic in the normal elderly population and they have more pronounced afternoon drowsiness. Surveys have shown that between 0.5% and 5% complained of EDS,[136] and in a large study of an elderly population (4578 people) about 20% of the subjects reported to be "usually sleepy in the daytime."[137]

An association has been postulated between EDS and the neurobiology of PD,[125] while other authors do not agree with this and suggest that EDS is a consequence of dopaminergic therapy[119,138] or of the biologic aging process. However, in most of the studies where PD patients were compared with age-matched controls, EDS was significantly more prevalent in the PD patients; in one study only was no significant difference reported between PD patients and controls. Indeed, an increased Epworth Sleepiness score was found in parkinsonian patients compared with normal controls in most other relevant studies.

Frucht et al.[117] reported eight cases of "sleep attacks" in parkinsonian patients while they were driving a car. The authors cited the dopamine agonists the people were taking (pramipexole and ropinirole) as the cause of the accidents. Sleep attacks have since been described also with pergolide, bromocriptine, and levodopa. However, the term "sleep attack" should not be used because it is not recognized in sleep disturbance classifications. "Sudden-onset somnolence" or "irresistible somnolence" would be more appropriate to define these events.[139]

Hobson et al.[134] reported on a large study which had the objective of determining the frequency of, and predictors for, sudden-onset somnolence and, particularly, episodes of falling asleep while driving among patients with PD.[133] The authors conducted a prospective survey in 18 clinics directed by members of the Canadian Movement Disorders Group. Six-hundred and thirty-eight consecutive highly functional PD patients without dementia were enrolled, of whom 420 were currently drivers. The patients were evaluated using the Epworth Sleepiness Scale, and a scale designed for this study to address falling asleep in unusual circumstances (Inappropriate Sleep Composite Score). EDS was present overall in 327 (51%) of the patients and in 213 (51%) of the PD drivers. Patients taking a variety of different dopamine agonists had no differences in their Epworth Sleepiness scores, in the composite score, or in the risk of falling asleep while driving. Sixteen patients (3.8%) had experienced at least one episode of sudden onset of sleep while driving (after the diagnosis of PD); in 3 (0.7%), it occurred without warning. The two risk factors associated with falling asleep at the wheel were the Epworth Sleepiness score and the composite score. A standard Epworth Sleepiness score of 7 or higher predicted 75% of episodes of sleep behind the wheel.

The main conclusion of this large study was that excessive daytime sleepiness is common *even in patients with PD who are independent and do not have dementia*, and sudden-onset sleep without warning is infrequent.

Arnulf et al.[140] performed nighttime polysomnography and daytime multiple sleep latency tests in 54 consecutive levodopa-treated PD patients referred for sleepiness, 27 of whom were also receiving dopamine agonists. A narcolepsy-like phenotype was found in 39% of the patients. Severity of sleepiness was weakly correlated with Epworth score and daily levodopa dose but not with DA-agonist treatment, age, disease duration, motor disability, total sleep time, periodic leg movements, apnea/hypopnea, or arousal indices. The authors concluded that in PD patients preselected for sleepiness, severity of sleepiness was not dependent on nocturnal sleep abnormalities, motor and cognitive impairment, or antiparkinsonian treatment. The results suggest that sleepiness and the sudden onset of sleep does not result from pharmacotherapy but is related to the pathology of PD.

Roth et al.[141] performed a study to determine whether PD patients taking dopamine agonists and reporting unintended sleep episodes (SEs) exhibited physiologically defined daytime sleepiness, and might thus be differentiated from those taking DAs but not reporting such sleep episodes. Twenty-four patients with abnormal Epworth Sleepiness scores greater than 10 who were taking DAs were enrolled into one of two groups: those with SEs (n = 16) and those without (n = 8). The patients underwent three consecutive days of testing that included two nights of polysomnography followed by the Multiple Sleep Latency Test (MSLT). Overall frequency of pathological sleepiness (MSLT > 5 minutes) was 42% (10/24). Mean levels of sleepiness, frequencies of pathological sleepiness, and naps with stage 2 or REM-sleep were similar between the two groups. Sleep tendency was similar in patients prescribed pergolide, ropinirole, or pramipexole combined with levodopa. Polysomnography testing revealed no significant differences between the groups in total sleep time, sleep efficiency, sleep architecture, or presence of restless legs syndrome or periodic leg movements. There was no relationship between degree of nocturnal sleep disturbance and level of daytime sleepiness. The authors concluded that unintended sleep episodes in PD patients occur against a background of excessive daytime sleepiness and are unrelated to nocturnal sleep or the use of a specific dopamine agonist.

Paus et al.[142] performed a survey (structured telephone interviews) of 2952 PD patients to study the putative association of dopamine agonists with sleep attacks. In 177 patients, sudden, unexpected, and irresistible sleep episodes while engaged in some activity were identified. Ninety-one of these patients denied the occurrence of appropriate warning signs. A total of 133 patients (75%) had an Epworth Sleepiness score above 10, with 65 (37%) having a score above 15. Thirty-one patients (18%) had a score ≤10 and yet experienced sleep attacks without warning signs. Thus, although a significant proportion of patients at risk for sleep attacks might be identified using the Epworth Sleepiness Scale, roughly 1% of the PD patient population seems to be at risk for sleep attacks without appropriate warning signs and without accompanying daytime sleepiness.

In this study, sleep attacks occurred with all dopamine agonists marketed in Germany (alpha-dihydroergocryptine, bromocriptine, cabergoline, lisuride, pergolide, pramipexole, ropinirole), and no significant difference between ergot and non-ergot drugs was evident. Levodopa monotherapy carried the lowest risk for sleep attacks (2.9%; 95% confidence interval [CI]: 1.7–4.0%), followed by dopamine agonist monotherapy (5.3%; CI: 1.5–9.2%) and a combination of levodopa and a dopamine agonist (7.3%; CI: 6.1–8.5%). Neither selegeline nor amantadine nor entacapone appeared to influence the occurrence of sleep attacks. The conclusion of this study was that a high Epworth Sleepiness score, intake of dopamine agonists, and duration of PD were the main influencing factors for the occurrence of sleep attacks. The odds ratio for dopamine agonist therapy was 2.9 compared to 1.9 with levodopa therapy and 1.05 for a 1-year-longer disease duration.

Fabbrini et al.[143] compared 25 de-novo PD patients with 50 treated PD patients and 25 healthy control subjects all of whom were matched for age and gender. The authors concluded that de-novo patients did not differ from normal subjects whereas the treated patients had significantly higher Epworth and Pittsburgh sleep quality scores.

Homann et al.[144] reviewed 20 publications between July 1999 and May 2001 in which "sleep attacks" or narcoleptic-like attacks were discussed in PD patients taking dopaminergic drugs. They found that "sleep attacks" occurred with all different dopaminergic agents including levodopa. These attacks may occur without warning and with prodrome drowsiness.

All the studies cited above clearly demonstrate that daytime sleepiness and unintended sleep episodes are common in PD patients. Sleep episodes are more likely to occur against a background of excessive daytime sleepiness and are unrelated to nocturnal sleep or the use of a specific DA. All dopaminergic treatments can induce sleep episodes.

Parasomnias

Another common sleep-associated complaint are parasomnias, undesirable phenomena that occur exclusively during sleep or are exaggerated by sleep. They include vivid dreams, nightmares, night terrors, nocturnal vocalizations, REM-sleep behavior disorder (RBD), nocturnal hallucinosis, sleep-talking, somnambulism, and panic attacks.[145]

Sharf et al.[146] reported a high incidence of levodopa-related parasomnias in PD patients, including vivid dreams, night terrors with nocturnal vocalizations, and nightmares. There was a significant correlation between prevalence and incidence of first episode with the duration of levodopa therapy, but not with the stage of disease, age, disability, concomitant drugs, and family history of psychosis. Parasomnias might further contribute to sleep disturbance, as they can be accompanied by motor disinhibition during REM sleep.

RBD is characterized by vigorous movements during REM sleep, and may also be caused by neuronal degeneration in the central nervous system; however, the site of degeneration remains unclear. Both parkinsonism and RBD become more prevalent with aging, with onset usually occurring in the sixties. Recent findings show that many individuals with RBD eventually develop parkinsonism. Conversely, it is also true that certain patients diagnosed with parkinsonism subsequently develop RBD. Postmortem examination reveals that Lewy bodies, Lewy neurites, and α-synuclein are found in brainstem nuclei in both PD and RBD patients.[147]

Overview of Abnormal Simple and Complex Nocturnal Movements

Abnormal simple and complex nocturnal movements seen in PD patients can be the cause of sleep disruption because of frequent awakenings.[148] Complex movements include fragmentary nocturnal myoclonus, nocturnal akathisia, periodic leg movements of sleep, and restless legs syndrome.

Fragmentary nocturnal myoclonus consists of irregular myoclonic jerks of the extremities, probably related to dopaminergic stimulation.[149] It is most common in subjects affected by levodopa-induced dyskinesias occurring mainly during non-REM sleep.[150]

Periodic leg movements of sleep (PLMS) consists of rhythmic extension of the toe and dorsiflexion of the ankle, with occasional flexion of knee and hip. The condition is often unilateral and, in contrast to myoclonus, has a frequency of one every 20–40 seconds. PLMS is usually reported to occur in the first part of the night and tends to be related to age. PLMS may be associated with a disorder of dopaminergic transmission.[151]

In a polysomnographic study, Wetter et al.[152] assessed periodic leg movement (PLM) patterns in untreated patients with mild to moderate PD. PLM indices during sleep and wakefulness were significantly higher in PD patients than in normal subjects.

Restless legs syndrome (RLS) frequently coexists with PLMS in PD patients. It consists of creeping sensations in the lower limbs and a compulsion to move; it is relieved by movement. Because of dysesthesia, patients with RLS have difficulty falling asleep.[153]

Tan et al.[154] performed a study to investigate the prevalence of RLS amongst a PD outpatient population, using the diagnostic criteria of the International Restless Legs Syndrome Study Group (IRLSSG). Among an unselected population of 125 PD patients, there were 19 patients (15.2%) with motor restlessness. Of these, one patient had RLS-like symptoms very similar to the wearing-off effect of levodopa. None of the patients satisfied the IRLSSG diagnostic criteria of RLS. This was not significantly different from prevalences in the Chinese Asian general population and clinic populations.

Nocturnal akathisia is another cause of sleep disruption. It consists of a sensation of inner restlessness, sometimes accompanied by stereotyped movements due to difficulty in remaining still.[155]

Management of Sleep Problems

There seems to be general agreement that more attention should be paid to sleep problems in PD patients. The Epworth Sleepiness Scale (ESS) is a simple tool that can be used in clinical practice to detect daytime sleepiness.

Chaudhuri et al.[156] have proposed a simple visual sleep scale, a bedside screening instrument to evaluate sleep disturbances in Parkinson's disease. A combination of sub-items may help identify specific aspects of sleep disturbance, which in turn may help target treatment.

When considering the management of a sleep problem in a PD patient, it is important first to establish the nature of the disturbed sleep by means of a detailed history taken from the patient and caregivers. Then it is necessary to identify any concurrent medications, as well as psychological and psychosocial factors contributing to the sleep disorder. Then, two types of strategy are available: non-pharmacological and pharmacological.

Non-pharmacological management

Non-pharmacological management consists of guidance directed at observing good sleep hygiene.[157] Recommend the use of a well-ventilated bedroom with comfortable temperature and an adjustable bed with a firm, non-slippery mattress. Other recommendations are regular exercise, and avoidance of caffeinated drinks, smoking and heavy meals. Having a warm bath two hours before bedtime, and a light bedtime snack, seem to be useful. Relaxation exercises and self-hypnosis, and adequate exposure to morning sunlight to maintain circadian rhythm, may help, as well as reading before lights-out to overcome initial insomnia. A flexible sleep schedule is desirable, such as establishing a regular naptime, taken in the bed, for a predetermined length of time.[158] In patients suffering from nocturia, limit fluid intake after mid-afternoon, and have a device beside the bed in which to urinate.

Pharmacological management

A rationalization of dopaminergic therapy is essential because of the stimulating effect of dopaminergic drugs. High doses should be avoided at bedtime. Selegiline and amantadine should be stopped in patients who have difficulty with sleeping, or should always be taken before noon.

A small dose of slow-release levodopa at bedtime may be helpful in patients with frequent awakenings because of poorly controlled motor symptoms at night. In a double-blind crossover study,[159] the efficacy of a single dose of a controlled-release formulation of levodopa/carbidopa (Sinemet CR 200/50 mg) was compared with that of a placebo in improving sleep-related motor disturbances in a group of 40 fluctuating PD patients. Sinemet CR significantly improved nocturnal akinesia and increased the hours of sleep.

Gabapentin has been reported to improve rigidity, bradykinesia, and tremor in PD patients. It seems to be useful in improving sleep disturbances, and increased sleep phases 3 and 4 in normal subjects.[160]

Among sedatives and hypnotics, benzodiazepines (BZs) are the most commonly used drugs. Side-effects are more frequent in the elderly, and physical dependence and rebound insomnia may occur if they are used continuously.[161]

A short- to medium-acting cyclopirrolone hypnotic, zopiclone, has been shown to be as effective as a BZ in the treatment of chronic insomnia, causing fewer side-effects.[162] Zolpidem, a short-acting amidazopyridine, seems to be useful too, in acute and chronic insomnia, being less involved in disrupting sleep architecture.[163] The efficacy of low doses of the atypical neuroleptic clozapine has been reported, without exacerbation of parkinsonian symptoms.[164] Tricyclic antidepressants (amitriptiline) seems to be similarly useful in treating initial insomnia. Diphenydramine also has an hypnotic effect because of its anticholinergic and antihistaminic proprieties.

For patients with nocturia, a bedtime dose of oxybutinin or tolterodine may improve bladder continence. In the more severe cases, desmopressin nasal spray may be used to reduce the production of urine.

REFERENCES

1. Parkinson J. Essay on the Shaking Palsy. London: Nealy & Jones, 1817.
2. Edwards LL, Quigley EMM, Pfeiffer RF. Gastrointestinal dysfunction in Parkinson's disease: frequency and pathophysiology. Neurology 1992;42:726–732.
3. Edwards LL, Pfeiffer RF, Quigley EMM et al. Gastrointestinal symptoms in Parkinson's disease. Mov Disord 1991;6:151–156.
4. Pfeiffer RF. Gastrointestinal dysfunction in Parkinson's disease. Lancet Neurol 2003;2(2):107–116.
5. Fisher CM. Hunger and the temporal lobe. Neurology 1994;44:1577–1579.
6. Penfield WG, Jasper H. Epilepsy and the Functional Anatomy of the Human Brain. Boston: Little, Brown, 1954.
7. Hunter PC, Crameri J, Austin S, Woodward MC, Hughes AJ. Response of parkinsonian swallowing dysfunction to dopaminergic stimulation. J Neurol Neurosurg Psychiatry 1997;63:579–583.
8. Miller AJ. Neurophysiological basis of swallowing. Dysphagia 1986;1:91–100.
9. Jellinger KA. Pathology of Parkinson's disease: changes other than the nigrostriatal pathway. Mol Chem Neuropathol 1991;14:153–197.
10. Qualman SJ, Haupt HM, Yang P, Hamilton SR. Esophageal Lewy bodies associated with ganglion cell loss in akalasia: similarity to Parkinson's disease. Gastroenterology 1984;87:848–856.
11. Camilleri M, Bharucha AE. Gastrointestinal dysfunction in neurologic disease. Semin Neurol 1996;16:203–216.
12. Gai WP, Blessing WW, Blumbergs PC. Ubiquitin-positive degenerating neurites in the brainstem in Parkinson's disease. Brain 1995;118:1447–1459.
13. Halliday GM, Blumbergs PC, Cotton RG, Blessing WW, Geffen LB. Loss of brainstem serotonin- and substance P-containing neurons in Parkinson's disease. Brain Res 1990;510:104–107.
14. Halliday GM, Li YW, Blumbergs PC et al. Neuropathology of immunohistochemically identified brainstem neurons in Parkinson's disease. Ann Neurol 1990;27:373–385.
15. Kupsky WJ, Grimes MM, Sweeting J, Bertsch R, Cote LJ. Parkinson's disease and megacolon: concentric hyaline inclusions (Lewy bodies) in enteric ganglion cells. Neurology 1987;37:1253–1255.
16. Wakabayashi K, Takahashi H, Ohama E, Ikuta F. Parkinson's disease: an immunohistochemical study of Lewy-body containing neurons in the enteric nervous system. Acta Neuropathol 1990;79:581–583.

17. Singaram C, Ashraf W, Gaumnitz EA et al. Dopaminergic defect of enteric nervous system in Parkinson's disease patients with chronic constipation. Lancet 1995;346:861–864.
18. Logemann JA, Blonsky ER, Boshes B. Lingual control in Parkinson's disease. Trans Am Neurol Assoc 1973;98:276–278.
19. Blonsky ER, Logemann JA, Boshes B et al. Comparison of speech and swallowing function in patients with tremor disorders and in normal geriatric patients: a cinefluorographic study. J Gerontol 1975;30:299–303.
20. Logemann JA, Boshes B, Blonsky ER et al. Speech and swallowing evaluation in the diagnosis of neurologic disease. IVth Am Congress Neurol 1975;18:71–78.
21. Bushmann M, Dobmeyer SM, Leeker L et al. Swallowing abnormalities and their response to treatment in Parkinson's disease. Neurology 1989;39:1309–1314.
22. Calne DB, Shaw DG, Spiers ASD et al. Swallowing in parkinsonism. Br J Radiol 1970;43:456–457.
23. Gibberd FB, Gleeson JA, Gossage AAR et al. Oesophageal dilatation in Parkinson's disease. J Neurol Neurosurg Psychiatry 1974;37:938–940.
24. Kempster PA, Lees AJ, Crichton P et al. Off-period belching due to a reversible disturbance of oesophageal motility in Parkinson's disease and its treatment with apomorphine. Mov Disord 1989;4:47–52.
25. Bramble MG, Cunliffe J, Dellipiani W. Evidence for a change in neurotransmitter affecting oesophageal motility in Parkinson's disease. J Neurol Neurosurg Psychiatry 1978;41:709–712.
26. Steiger MJ, Stocchi F, Bramante L et al. The clinical efficacy of single morning doses of levodopa methil esther, dispersible madopar and Sinemet Plus in Parkinson's disease. Clin Neuropharmacol 1992;15:501–504.
27. Muguet D, Broussolle E, Chazot G. Apomorphine in patients with Parkinson's disease. Biomed Pharmacother 1995;49:197–209.
28. Martinek J, Siroky M, Plottova Z et al. Treatment of patients with akalasia with botulinum toxin: a multicenter prospective cohort study. Dis Esophagus 2003;16(3):204–209.
29. Bagheri H, Damase-Michel C, Lapeyre-Mestre M et al. A study of salivary secretion in Parkinson's disease. Clin Neuropharmacol 1999;22:213–215.
30. Bateson MC, Gibberd FB, Wilson RSE. Salivary symptoms in Parkinson's disease. Arch Neurol 1973;29:274–275.
31. Eadie MJ. Gastric secretion in parkinsonism. Aust Ann Med 1963;12:346–350.
32. Hyson HC, Jog MS, Johnson A. Sublingual atropine for sialorrhea secondary to parkinsonism. Parkinsonism Rel Disord 2001;7(suppl.)[abstract].
33. Bhatia KP, Munchau A, Brown P. Botulinum toxin is a useful treatment in excessive drooling of saliva. J Neurol Neurosurg Psychiatry 1999;67:697.
34. Pal PK, Calne DB, Calne S, Tsui JKC. Botulinum toxin A as a treatment for drooling saliva in PD. Neurology 2000;54:244–247.
35. Friedman A, Potulska A. Quantitative assessment of parkinsonian sialorrhea and results of treatment with botulinum toxin. Parkinsonism Rel Disord 2001;7:329–332.
36. O'Sullivan JD, Bhatia KP, Lees AJ. Botulinum toxin A as a treatment for drooling saliva in PD. Neurology 2000;55:606–607.
37. Stocchi F, Testa A, Vacca L, DePandis MF. XIV International Congress on Parkinson's Disease, Helsinki. Parkinsonism Rel Disord 2001;7(suppl.):s90.
38. Porta M, Ganba M, Bertacchi G, Vaj P. Treatment of sialorrhoea with ultrasound guided butulinum toxin type A injection in patients with neurological disorders. J Neurol Neurosurg Psychiatry. 2001;70:538–540.
39. Mullins WM, Gross CW, Moore JM. Long-term follow-up of tympanic neurectomy for sialorrhea. Laryngoscope 1979;89:1219–1223.
40. Marks L, Turner K, O'Sullivan J, Deighton B, Lees A. Drooling in Parkinson's disease: a novel speech and language therapy intervention. Int J Lang Commun Disord 2001;36(suppl.): s282–287.
41. Hardoff R, Sula M, Tamir A et al. Gastric emptying time and gastric motility in patients with Parkinson's disease. Mov Disord 2001;16:1041–1047.
42. Djaletti R, Baron J, Ziv I et al. Gastric emptying in Parkinson's disease patients with and without response fluctuations. Neurology 1996;46:1051–1054.
43. Baruzzi A, Contin M, Riva R et al. Influence of meal ingestion time on pharmacokinetics of orally administered levodopa in parkinsonian patients. Clin Neuropharmacol 1987;10:527–537.
44. Dubois A. Diet and gastric digestion. Am J Clin Nutr 1985;42:1002–1005.
45. Kelly KA. Motility of the stomach and gastroduodenal junction. In: Johnson LR (ed.), Physiology of the Gastrointestinal Tract. New York: Raven Press, 1981.

46. Leon AS, Spiegel H. The effect of antacid administration on the absorption and metabolism of levodopa. J Clin Pharmacol 12 (1972) 263–267.
47. Evans MA, Broe GA, Triggs EJ et al. Gastric emptying rate and the systemic availability of levodopa in the elderly parkinsonian patient. Neurology 1981;31:1288–1294.
48. Valenzuala JE. Dopamine as a possible neurotransmitter in gastric relaxation. Gastroenterology 1976;71:1019–1022.
49. Berkowitz DM, McCallum RW. Interaction of levodopa and metoclopramide on gastric emptying. Clin Pharmacol Ther 1980;27:414–420.
50. Ruggieri S, Stocchi F, Carta A et al. Jejunal delivery of L-dopa methyl ester. Lancet 1989;ii:45.
51. Kurlan R, Rothfield KP, Woodward WR et al. Erratic gastric emptying of levodopa may cause "random" fluctuations of parkinsonian mobility. Neurology 1988;38:419–421.
52. Wade DN, Mearrik PT, Birkett DJ et al. Active transport of L-dopa in the intestine. Nature 1973;242:463–465.
53. Stocchi F, Ruggieri S, Viselli F et al. Subcutaneous lisuride infusion. In: Lakke JPWF, Delhaas EM, Rutgers AWF (eds), New Trends in Clinical Neurology: Parenteral Drug Therapy in Spasticity and Parkinson's Disease. USA: Parthenon Publishing Group, 1992.
54. Levi S, Cox M, Lugon M et al. Increased energy expenditure in Parkinson's disease. Br Med J 1990;301:1256–1257.
55. Yapa RSS, Playfer JR, Lye M. Anthropometric and nutritional assessment of elderly patients with Parkinson's disease. J Clin Exp Geront 1989;11:155–164.
56. Markus HS, Cox M, Tomkins AM. Raised energy expenditure in Parkinson's disease and its relationship to muscular rigidity. Clin Sci 1992;83:199–204.
57. Davies KN, King D, Davies H. A study of the nutritional status of elderly patients with Parkinson's disease. Age Ageing 1994;23:142–145.
58. Davies KN, King D, Billington D, Barrett JA. Intestinal permeability and orocaecal transit time in elderly patients with Parkinson's disease. Postgrad Med J 1996;72:164–167.
59. McEvoy A, Dutton J, James OFW. Bacterial contamination of the small intestine is an important cause of malabsorption in the elderly. Br Med J 1983;287:789–793.
60. Montgomery RD, Haboubi NY, Mike NH et al. Cause of malabsorption in the elderly. Age Ageing 1986;15:235–240.
61. Den Hartog Jager WA, Bethlem J. The distribution of Lewy bodies in the central and autonomic nervous system in idiopathic paralysis agitans. J Neurol Neurosurg Psychiatry 1960;23:283–290.
62. Abbott RA, Cox M, Markus H, Tomkins A. Diet, body size and micronutrient status in Parkinson's disease. Eur J Clin Nutr 1992;46:879–884.
63. Beyer PL, Palarino MY, Michalek D, Busenbark K, Koller WC. Weight change and body composition in patients with Parkinson's disease. J Am Diet Assoc 1995;95:979–983.
64. Durrieu G, Llau ME, Rascol O et al. Parkinson's disease and weight loss: a study with anthropometric and nutritional assessment. Clin Auton Res 1992;2:153–157.
65. Wszolek ZK, Markopoulou K. Olfactory dysfunction in Parkinson's disease. Clin Neurosci 1998;5:94–101.
66. Toth MJ, Fishman PS, Poehlman ET. Free-living daily energy expenditure in patients with Parkinson's disease. Neurology 1997;48:88–91.
67. Nozaki S, Saito T, Matsumura T, Miyai I, Kang J. Relationship between weight loss and dysphagia in patients with Parkinson's disease. Rinsho Shinkeigaku 1999;39:1010–1014.
68. Jankovic J, Wooten M, Van der Linden C, Jansson B. Low body weight in Parkinson's disease. South Med J 1992;85:351–354.
69. Markus HS, Cox M, Tomkins AM. Raised resting energy expenditure in Parkinson's disease and its relationship to muscle rigidity. Clin Sci (Lond) 1992;83:199–204.
70. Broussolle E, Borson F, Gonzalez de Suso JM et al. Increase of energy expenditure in Parkinson's disease. Rev Neurol (Paris) 1991;147:46–51.
71. Kempster PA, Wahlqvist ML. Dietary factors in the management of Parkinson's disease. Nutr Rev 1994;52:51–58.
72. Evidente VGH, Caviness JN, Adler CH et al. Serum leptin concentrations and satiety in Parkinson's disease patients with and without weight loss. Mov Disord 2001;16:924–927.
73. Vardi J, Oberman Z, Rabey I et al. Weight loss in patients treated long-term with levodopa: metabolic aspects. J Neurol Sci 1976;30:33–40.
74. Ondo WG, Ben-Aire L, Jankovic J et al. Weight gain following unilateral pallidotomy in Parkinson's disease. Acta Neurol Scand 2000;101:79–84.
75. Stocchi F, Ruggieri S, Vacca L, Olanow CW. Prospective randomized trial of lisuride infusion versus oral levodopa in patients with Parkinson's disease. Brain 2002;125:1–9.

76. Lewitan A, Nathanson L, Slade WR. Megacolon and dilatation of the small bowel in Parkinsonism. Gastroenterology 1952;17:367–374.
77. Pallis CA. Parkinsonism: natural history and clinical features. Br Med J 1971;3:683–690.
78. Thompson WG, Dotevall G, Drossman DA et al. Irritable bowel syndrome: guidelines for the diagnosis. Gastroenterol Int 1989;2:92–95.
79. Reynolds JC, Ouyang A, Lee C et al. Chronic severe constipation. Gastroenterology 1987;92:414–420.
80. Bazzocchi G, Ellis J, Villanueva-Meyer J et al. Postprandial colonic transit and motor activity in chronic constipation. Gastroenterology 1990;98:686–693.
81. Mathers SE, Kempster PA, Law PJ et al. Anal sphincter dysfunction in Parkinson's disease. Arch Neurol 1989;46:1061–1064.
82. Lubowski DZ, Swash M, Henry M. Neural mechanisms in disorders of defecation. Baillière's Clin Gastroenterol 1988;2:210–223.
83. Martelli H, Devroede G, Arhan P et al. Mechanisms of idiopathic constipation: outlet obstruction. Gastroenterology 1978;75:623–631.
84. Arhtan P, Devroede G, Jehannin B et al. Segmental colon transit time. Dis Colon Rectum 1981;24:625–629.
85. McLean RG, Smart RC, GastonPerry D et al. Colon transit scintigraphy in health and constipation using oral I-131-cellulose. J Nucl Med 1990;31:985–989.
86. Metcalf AM, Phillips SF, Zinsmeister AR et al. Simplified assessment of segmental colonic transit. Gastroenterology 1987;92:40–47.
87. Jost WH, Schimrigk K. Constipation in Parkinson's disease. Klin Wochenschr 1991;69:906–909.
88. Edwards LL, Quigley EMM, Harned RK et al. Characterization of swallowing and defecation in Parkinson's disease. Am J Gastroenterol 1994;89:15–25.
89. Sakakibara R, Odaka T, Uchiyama T et al. Colonic transit time and rectoanal videomanometry in Parkinson's disease. J Neurol Neurosurg Psychiatry 2003;74:268–272.
90. Singaram C, Ashraf W, Gaumnitz EA et al. Dopaminergic defect of enteric nervous system in Parkinson's disease patients with chronic constipation. Lancet 1995;346:861–864.
91. Wakabayashi K, Takahachi H, Ohama E, Ikuta F. Tyrosine hydroxylase: immune reactive intrinsic neurons in the Auerbah's and Meissner's plexuses of humans. Neurosci Lett 1989; 96:259–263.
92. Mathers SE, Kempster PA, Swash M et al. Constipation and paradoxical puborectalis contraction in anismus and Parkinson's disease: a dystonic phenomenon? J Neurol Neurosurg Psychiatry 1988;51:1503–1507.
93. Floyd WF, Walls EW. Electromyography of the sphincter ani externus in man. J Physiol 1953;122:599–609.
94. Stocchi F, Badiali D, Vacca L et al. Anorectal function in multiple system atrophy and Parkinson's disease. Mov Disord 2000;15:71–76.
95. Ger G-C, Wexner SD, Jorge JMN, Salanga VD. Anorectal manometry in the diagnosis of paradoxical puborectalis syndrome. Dis Colon Rectum 1993;36:816–825.
96. Whitehead WE, Devroede G, Habib FI, Meunier P, Wald A. Functional disorders of the anorectum. Gastroenterol Int 1992;5:92–108.
97. Loening-Baucke VA, Cruikshank BM. Abnormal defecation dynamics in chronic constipated children with encopresis. J Pediatr 1986;108:562–566.
98. Ashraf W, Pfeiffer RP, Park F, Lof J, Quigley EMM. Constipation in Parkinson's disease: objective assessment and response to psyllium. Mov Disord 1997;6:946–951.
99. Astarloa R, Mena MA, Sanchez V, de la Vega L, de Yebenes JG. Clinical and pharmacological effects of a diet rich in insoluble fibres on Parkinson's disease. Clin Neuropharmacol 1992;15:375–380.
100. Kellow JE, Gill RC, Wingate DL. Modulation of human upper gastrointestinal motility by rectal distension. Gut 1987;28:864–868.
101. Tjeerdsma HC, Smout AJPM, Akkermans LMA. Voluntary suppression of defecation delays gastric emptying. Dig Dis Sci 1993;38:832–836.
102. Andersen JT, Hebjorn S, Frimodt-Moller C et al. Disturbances of micturition in Parkinson's disease. Acta Neurol Scand 1976;53:161–170.
103. Pavlakis AJ, Siroky MB, Goldstein IL, Krane RJ. Urologic findings in Parkinson's disease. J Urol 1983;129:80–83.
104. Kirby R, Fowler C, Gosling J, Bannister R. Urethrovesical dysfunction in progressive autonomic failure with multiple system atrophy. J Neurol Neurosurg Psychiatry 1986;49:554–562.

105. Araki I, Kuno S. Assessment of voiding dysfunction in Parkinson's disease by the international prostate symptom score. J Neurol Neurosurg Psychiatry 2000;68:429–433.
106. Stocchi F, Carbone A, Inghilleri M et al. Urodynamic and neurophysiological evaluation in Parkinson's disease and multiple system atrophy. J Neurol Neurosurg Psychiatry 1997;62:507–511.
107. Lemack GE, Dewey RB, Roehrborn CG et al. Questionnaire-based assessment of bladder dysfunction in patients with mild to moderate Parkinson's disease. Urology 2000;56:250–254.
108. Chandiramani VA, Palace J, Fowler CJ. How to recognize patients with parkinsonism who should not have urological surgery. Br J Urol 1997;80:100–104.
109. Dmochowkki RR. Female voiding dysfunction and movement disorders. Int Urogynecol J Pelvic Floor Dysfunct 1999;10:144–151.
110. Araki I, Kitahara M, Oida T, Kuno S. Voiding dysfunction and Parkinson's disease: urodynamic abnormalities and urinary symptoms. J Urol 2000;164:1640–1643.
111. Berger Y, Salinas JN, Blaivas JG. Urodynamic differentiation of Parkinson's disease and Shy–Drager syndrome. Neurourol Urodyn 1990;9:117–121.
112. Yoshimura N, Mizuta E, Kuno S, Sasa M, Yoshida O. The dopamine D1 receptor agonist SKF38393 suppresses detrusor hyperreflexia in the monkey with parkinsonism induced by 1-methyl-4-phenyl-1,2,3,6-tetrahydropyridine (MPTP). Neuropharmacology 1993;32:315–321.
113. Uchiyama T, Sakakibara R, Hattori T, Yamanishi T. Short-term effect of a single levodopa dose on micturition disturbance in Parkinson's disease patients with the wearing-off phenomenon. Mov Disord 2003;18:573–578.
114. Aranda B, Cramer P. Effects of apomorphine and L-dopa on the parkinsonian bladder. Neurol Urodyn 1993;12:203–209.
115. Andersson KE. Treatment of overactive bladder: other drug mechanisms. Urology 2000;55:51–57.
116. Diokno AC, Appell RA, Sand PK et al., for the OPERA Study Group. Prospective, randomized, double-blind study of the efficacy and tolerability of the extended-release formulations of oxybutynin and tolterodine for overactive bladder: results of the OPERA trial. Mayo Clin Proc 2003;78:687–695.
117. Frucht S, Rogers JD, Greene PE, Gordon MF, Fahn S. Falling asleep at the wheel: motor vehicle mishaps in persons taking pramipexole and ropinirole. Neurology 1999;52:1908–1910.
118. Gowers WR. A Manual of Diseases of the Nervous System. Philadelphia: Blakiston, 1901.
119. Nausieda PA, Glantz R, Weber S et al. Psychiatric complications of levodopa therapy in parkinson's disease. Adv Neurol 1984;40:271– 277.
120. Factor SA, Weiner WJ. "Sleep benefit" in Parkinson's disease. Neurology 1998;50:1514–1515.
121. Van Hilten JJ, Weggeman M, Van der Velde EA et al. Excessive daytime sleepiness and fatigue in Parkinson's disease. J Neural Transm 1993;5:235–244.
122. Stocchi F, Vacca L, Torti M et al. Survey on sleep problems in 200 patients with Parkinson's disease. Parkinsonism Rel Disord 2001;7(suppl.):s101.
123. Kumar S, Bhatia M, Behari M. Sleep disorders in Parkinson's disease. Mov Disord 2002;4: 775–781.
124. Factor SA, McAlarney T, Sanchez-Ramos JR, Weiner WJ. Sleep disorders and sleep effect in Parkinson's disease. Mov Disord 1990;5:280–285.
125. Lees AJ, Blackburn NA, Campbell VL. The nighttime problems of Parkinson's disease. Clin Neuropharmacol 1988;11:512–519.
126. Crismond ML. Insomnia. In: Koda Kimble MA, Yung LY (eds), Applied Therapeutics: the Clinical Use of Drugs. Vancouver, WA: Applied Therapeutics, 1992.
127. Lacy C, Armstrong LL, Ingrim N, Lance LL. Drug Information Handbook. Hudson, OH: Lexi-Comp, 1995.
128. Ashton H. The effect of drugs on sleep. In: Cooper R (ed.), Sleep. New York: Chapman & Hall, 1994, pp. 175–211.
129. Sharpley AL, Cowen PJ. Effect of pharmacologic treatments on the sleep of depressed patients. Biol Psychiatry 1995;37:85–98.
130. Kay DC, Blackburn AB, Buckingam JA, Karacan I. Human pharmacology of sleep. In: Williams RL, Karacan I (eds), Pharmacology of Sleep. New York: John Wiley, 1976, p. 83.
131. Gillin JC, Sutton L, Ruoz C et al. Dose-dependent inhibition of REM sleep in normal volunteers by biperidine, a muscarinic antagonist. Biol Psychiatry 1991;31:151–156.
132. Tandberg E, Larsen JP, Karlsen K. Excessive daytime sleepiness and sleep benefit in Parkinson's disease: a community-based study. Mov Disord 1999;14:922–927.

133. Hobson DE, Lang AE, Martin WR et al. Excessive daytime sleepiness and sudden-onset sleep in Parkinson's disease: a survey by the Canadian Movement Disorders Group. JAMA 2002;287:455–463.
134. Brodsky MA, Godbold J, Roth T, Olanow CW. Sleepiness in Parkinson's disease: a controlled study. Mov Disord 2003;18:668–672.
135. Hogl B, Seppi K, Brandauer E et al. Increased daytime sleepiness in Parkinson's disease: a questionnaire survey. Mov Disord 2003;18:319–323.
136. O'Suilleabhain PE, Dewey RB. Contributions of dopaminergic drugs and disease severity to daytime sleepiness in Parkinson's disease. Arch Neurol 2002;59:986–989.
137. Roth T, Rohers TA, Carskadon MA, Dement WC. Daytime sleepiness and alertness. In: Kryger MH, Roth T, Dement WC (eds), Principles and Practise of Sleep Medicine. Philadelphia: WB Saunders, 1994, p. 40.
138. Whitney CW, Enright PL, Newman AB et al. Correlates of daytime sleepiness in 4578 elderly persons: the cardiovascular health study. Sleep 1998;21:27–36.
139. Olanow CW, Schapira AH, Roth T. Waking up to sleep episodes in Parkinson's disease. Mov Disord 2000;15:212–215.
140. Arnulf I, Konofal E, Merino-Andreu M et al. Parkinson's disease and sleepiness: an integral part of PD. Neurology 2002;58:1019–1024.
141. Roth T, Rye DB, Borchert LD et al. Assessment of sleepiness and unintended sleep in Parkinson's disease patients taking dopamine agonists. Sleep Med 2003;4(4):275–280.
142. Paus S, Brecht HM, Koster J et al. Sleep attacks, daytime sleepiness, and dopamine agonists in Parkinson's disease. Mov Disord 2003;18:659–667.
143. Fabbrini G, Barbanti P, Aurilia C et al. Excessive daytime sleepiness in de-novo and treated Parkinson's disease. Mov Disord 2002;5:1026–1030.
144. Homann CN, Wenzel K, Suppan K et al. Sleep attacks in patients taking dopamine agonists: a review. Br Med J 2002;324:1483–1487.
145. Kelly DD. Disorders of sleep and consciousness. In: Kandel ER, Schwartz JH, Jessel TM (eds), Principles of Neuronal Science. Norwalk, CT:Appleton & Lange, 1991, p. 805.
146. Sharf B, Moskovitz C, Lupton MD, Klawans HL. Dream phenomena induced by chronic levodopa therapy. J Neural Transm 1987;43:143–151.
147. Lai YY, Siegel JM. Physiological and anatomical link between Parkinson-like disease and REM sleep behavior disorder. Mol Neurobiol 2003;27(2):137–152.
148. McCarley RW. Dreams and the biology of sleep. In: Kryger MH, Roth T, Dement WC (eds), Principles and Practice of Sleep Medicine. Philadelphia: WB Saunders, 1994, p. 373.
149. Klawans H, Goetz C, Bergen D. L-dopa induced myclonus. Arch Neurol 1975;32:331–334.
150. Nausieda P, Tanner V, Klawans H. Serotonergically active agents in L-dopa-induced psychiatric toxicity reactions. In: Fahn S, Calne DB, Shoulson I (eds), Advances in Neurology: Experimental Therapeutics of Movement Disorders. New York: Raven Press, 1983.
151. Ancoli-Israel S, Kripke D, Klauber M et al. Periodic leg movements in sleep in community-dwelling elderly. Sleep 1991;14:496–500.
152. Wetter TC, Collado-Seidel V, Pollmacher T et al. Sleep and periodic leg movement patterns in drug-free patients with Parkinson's disease and multiple system atrophy. Sleep 2000;23(3):361–367.
153. Montplaisir J, Godbout R, Pelletier G, Warnes H. Restless legs syndrome and periodic limb movements during sleep. In: Kryger MH, Roth T, Dement WC (eds), Principles and Practice of Sleep Medicine. Philadelphia:WB Saunders, 1994, p. 589.
154. Tan EK, Lum SY, Wong MC. Restless legs syndrome in Parkinson's disease. J Neurol Sci 2002;196(1/2):33–36.
155. Linazasoro G, Masso JFM, Suarez JA. Nocturnal akatisia in Parkinson's disease: treatment with clozapine. Mov Disord 1993;8:171–174.
156. Chaudhuri KR, Pal S, DiMarco A et al. The Parkinson's disease sleep scale: a new instrument for assessing sleep and nocturnal disability in Parkinson's disease. J Neurol Neurosurg Psychiatry. 2002;73:629–635.
157. Zarcone VPJ. Sleep hygiene. In: Kryger MH, Roth T, Dement WC (eds), Principles and Practice of Sleep Medicine. Philadelphia: WB Saunders, 1994, p. 542.
158. Pal PK, Calne S, Samii A, Fleming JAE. A review of normal sleep and its disturbances in Parkinson's disease. Parkinsonism Rel Disord 1999;5:1–17.
159. Stocchi F, Barbato L, Nordera G, Berardelli A, Ruggieri S. Sleep disorders in Parkinson's disease. J Neurol 1998;245(suppl. 1):s15–18.

160. Rao ML, Clarenbach P, Vahlensieck M, Kratzschmar S. Gabapentin augments whole blood serotonin in healthy young men. J Neural Transm 1988;73:129–134.
161. Linsen SM, Zitman FG, Breteler MH. Defining benzodiazepine dependence: confusion persists. Eur Psychiatry 1995;10:310–311.
162. Lader M. Zopiclone: is there any dependence and abuse potential? J Neurol 1997;244 (suppl. 1):s19–22.
163. Shaw SH, Curson H, Coquelin JP. A double-blind comparative study of zolpidem and placebo in the treatment of insomnia in elderly psychiatric in-patients. J Int Med Res 1992;20:150–161.
164. Ruggieri S, De Pandis MF, Bonamartini A, Vacca L, Stocchi F. Low dose of clozapine in the treatment of dopaminergic psychosis in Parkinson's disease. Clin Neuropharmacol 1997; 20:204–209.

SECTION 6

NEUROPROTECTION IN PARKINSON'S DISEASE

13

Neuroprotection in Parkinson's Disease

Hideki Mochizuki and Yoshikuni Mizuno

INTRODUCTION

Parkinson's disease (PD) is characterized by neurodegeneration of the pigmented neurons in the brainstem, particularly of the dopaminergic neurons in the substantia nigra pars compacta. The resultant striatal loss of dopamine (DA) is responsible for most of the symptoms of PD.

The prognosis of Parkinson's disease has improved greatly since the introduction of levodopa as treatment. Levodopa is still the gold standard. All the treatment methods currently available are symptomatic. Nigral neurodegeneration progresses slowly despite treatment and may cause long-term problems such as motor fluctuations and drug-induced psychosis. Thus neuroprotective treatment is urgently needed for patients with PD. This chapter reviews the literature on treatment aimed at neuroprotection of the substantia nigra in PD.

LEVODOPA

Levodopa has often been claimed to be neurotoxic to the nigral neurons in experimental conditions. However, recent consensus meetings on levodopa came to the conclusion that there was no evidence to indicate that levodopa enhanced nigral neurodegeneration when it was given to live animals or to humans.[1,2] Levodopa may even be *neuroprotective*, depending on the experimental conditions.

In-vitro studies

Mytilineou et al.[3] treated primary dissociated cultures of rat mesencephalon with levodopa (200 μmol) for 48 hours; they found a decrease in the number of tyrosine hydroxylase-positive neurons (DA neurons) by 69.7% compared to controls.

At the same time, the level of glutathione rose to 125.2% of control values. Thus, exposure of mesencephalic cultures to levodopa induced both damaging and antioxidant effects. In cultures treated with L-buthionine sulfoximine (L-BSO), an inhibitor of glutathione (GSH) synthesis, levodopa prevented cell death by L-BSO.

Mena et al.[4] studied the effect of levodopa on ventral midbrain neuron/cortical astrocyte co-cultures in serum-free, glia-conditioned medium. Levodopa (50 μmol) protected dopaminergic neurons from death and increased the number and branching of neuronal processes. Levodopa increased the level of GSH as well. Inhibition of glutathione peroxidase by L-BSO (3 μmol for 24 h) blocked the neurotrophic action of levodopa. *N*-acetyl-L-cysteine (250 μmol 48 h), which promoted glutathione synthesis, had a neurotrophic effect similar to that of levodopa. These data suggest that the neurotrophic effect of levodopa may be mediated by elevation of GSH content.

Koshimura et al.[5] studied the effects of dopamine and levodopa on the survival of differentiated PC12 cells. Addition of dopamine to the culture medium at 3–30 μmol prevented cell death induced by depletion of serum and nerve growth factor (NGF). Levodopa and NGF at low concentrations also protected PC12 cells from cell death induced by depletion of serum, but high concentrations were neurotoxic. Intracellular Ca^{2+} concentration and mitogen-activated protein (MAP) kinase activity were increased by both dopamine and levodopa. These neuroprotective effects were blunted by a calcium-channel blocker and an inhibitor of MAP kinase. These results raised the possibility that dopamine and levodopa might protect PC12 cells from cell death by activating MAP kinase activity via elevation of intracellular Ca^{2+} concentration.

Han et al.[6] studied the mechanism of GSH elevation by the treatment with levodopa using different cell cultures. They found that auto-oxidizable compounds (α-methyl-dopa, dopamine, apomorphine, catechol, and hydroquinone) behaved similarly to levodopa, whereas structural analogues that were unable to undergo auto-oxidation (3-O-methyl-dopa, tyrosine, 2,4-dihydroxyphenylalanine, and resorcinol) failed to elevate GSH levels. They concluded that up-regulation of GSH was a response to oxidative stress. Cultures pretreated with levodopa or hydroquinone were protected from loss of viability. However, when cultures were pretreated with both levodopa and ascorbate, which prevented the rise in GSH, protection was lost. They concluded that the up-regulation of cellular GSH evoked by auto-oxidizable agents was associated with significant protection of cells.

Thus levodopa appears to be neuroprotective depending on the experimental conditions. Marked improvement in the outcome of patients with Parkinson's disease since the introduction of levodopa may in part be due to neuroprotective effects of levodopa on nigral neurons. But it is not easy to prove this on the patients with PD.

DOPAMINE AGONISTS

Apomorphine

R-apomorphine (APO) is a catechol-derived dopamine D1/D2 receptor agonist.

In-vitro Studies

Gassen et al.[7] showed that 1–10 µmol of apomorphine protected rat PC12 cells from the toxic effects of H_2O_2 (0.6 mmol) and 6-hydroxydopamine (6-OHDA) (150 µmol). These effects were not exhibited by ascorbic acid, desferal, lisuride, or bromocriptine. They suggested that apomorphine might be an ideal drug to study neuroprotection in parkinsonian subjects.

In-vivo Studies

Grunblatt et al.[8] studied in-vivo effects of apomorphine. Pretreatment with 5–10 mg/kg of R-apomorphine administered subcutaneously in C57BL mice protected against 1-methyl-4-phenyl-1,2,3,6-tetrahydropyridine (MPTP; 24 mg/kg i.p.)-induced loss of nigrostriatal dopamine neurons as indicated by striatal dopamine content, tyrosine hydroxylase (TH) content, and TH activity. *In vitro*, R-apomorphine inhibited mice striatal monoamine oxidase (MAO-A and MAO-B) activities with IC_{50} values of 93 µmol and 241 µmol, respectively. The authors suggested that the neuroprotective effect of R-apomorphine against MPTP neurotoxicity was derived from its radical scavenging and MAO inhibitory actions and not from its agonistic activity.

Grunblatt et al.[9] examined the neuroprotective property of R- and S-apomorphine in MPTP models. Both S-APO (0.5–1 mg/kg s.c.) and R-APO (10 mg/kg) pretreatment of C57-BL mice protected against MPTP (24 mg/kg i.p.) induced dopamine depletion and reduction in TH activity. However, only R-APO prevented nigrostriatal neuronal cell degeneration. R-APO prevented the reduction of striatal GSH and the increase in the ratio of GSSG over total glutathione, caused by MPTP treatment. The authors suggested that the antioxidant and iron-chelating properties together with activation of DA receptors might participate in the neuroprotection provided by APO enantiomers.

Bromocriptine

In-vitro Studies

Yoshikawa et al.[10] studied the free-radical scavenging property of bromocriptine. They analyzed superoxide production from a superoxide generating system (hypoxanthine–xanthine oxidase system) by the spin-trapping method using electron spin resonance; bromocriptine scavenged superoxide anions. Bromocriptine also had a strong scavenging effect on the 5,5-dimethyl-1-pyrroline-N-oxide hydroxide signal produced from Fenton's reaction. Furthermore, they also found inhibition of lipid peroxidation in rat brain homogenate by bromocriptine.

Sawada et al.[11] reported neuroprotective properties of bromocriptine on glutamate-induced neuronal death. They used cultured rat mesencephalic neurons: preincubation with bromocriptine (1 and 10 µmol) provided neuroprotection against glutamate-induced (1 mmol) neurotoxicity in mesencephalic neurons (both dopaminergic and non-dopaminergic neurons). Quinpirole (10 µmol), a D2 agonist, showed similar effects as bromocriptine.

Takashima et al.[12] treated cultured rat embryonic ventral mesencephalic neurons with levodopa (100 μmol), which showed selective toxicity to dopaminergic neurons. Bromocriptine (2 μmol) when added to the culture medium protected dopaminergic neurons from levodopa toxicity.

Glutamate transporters play an essential role in keeping the extracellular-glutamate concentration below the neurotoxic level, and their blockade causes neuronal death in both acute and chronic models. Yamashita et al.[13] studied the effect of bromocriptine on glutamate transport using stable cell lines expressing human glutamate transporters (hGluT-1). Bromocriptine (100 μmol/L) enhanced glutamate uptake; this was interpreted that bromocriptine enhanced the removal of extracellular glutamate.

Thus bromocriptine appears to have neuroprotective properties on cultured mesencephalic neurons treated with levodopa or glutamate. These properties may in part be mediated by free-radical scavenging properties of bromocriptine.

In-vivo Studies

Kondo et al.[14] studied effects of bromocriptine on methamphetamine-induced hydroxyl-radical formation. Methamphetamine acts on dopaminergic synaptic vesicles, releasing stored dopamine. Released dopamine is metabolized by monoamine oxidase and by auto-oxidation; hydroxyl radicals are formed in these reactions. They treated rats with methamphetamine. Hydroxyl-radical formation was measured by the salicylate trapping method. Treatment of rats by bromocriptine significantly reduced hydroxyl-radical formation and attenuated methamphetamine-induced striatal dopamine depletion.

Ogawa et al.[15] studied the effect of bromocriptine on striatal dopamine depletion induced by intraventricular injection of 6-OHDA. Pretreatment of mice with bromocriptine (5 mg/kg i.p. for 7 days) completely prevented dopamine decrease. In the same experimental condition, levodopa/carbidopa (75/7.5 mg/kg i.p. for 7 days) showed partial protection.

Liu et al.[16] examined the effects of bromocriptine on ischemia-induced neuronal damage in the CA1 subfield of the Mongolian gerbil. Forebrain ischemia was induced by occlusion of bilateral common carotid arteries for 3 minutes. They observed neuronal damage 7 days after the ischemia in control animals; bromocriptine partially prevented this neuronal damage.

Muralikrishnan and Mohanakumar[17] studied the effects of bromocriptine on hydroxyl-radical formation induced by MPTP in mice. Bromocriptine (10 mg/kg i.p.) completely blocked hydroxyl-radical formation caused by MPTP (30 mg/kg i.p.). They also measured activities of catalase and super-oxide dismutase in substantia nigra on day 7 after MPTP treatment. In the control mice, activities of this enzyme showed 2-fold and 1.5-fold increases, respectively. Bromocriptine significantly attenuated these increases. In addition, bromocriptine blocked MPTP-induced behavioral dysfunction as well as glutathione and dopamine depletion. The authors interpreted these results as indicating the presence of potent neuroprotective action in bromocriptine.

Pergolide

In-vitro Studies

Nishibayashi et al.[18] examined nitric oxide (NO) generation induced by 3-(2-hydroxy-1-methylethyl-2-nitrosohydrazino)-N-methyl-1-propanamine and 2-(4-carboxy-phenyl)-4,4,5,5-tetramethylimidazoline-1-oxyl 3-oxide (carboxy- PTIO) by electron-spin resonance spectrometry. Pergolide attenuated NO generation significantly; bromocriptine showed a similar effect but to a lesser extent. The IC50 was estimated to be approximately 23 µmol for pergolide and 200µmol for bromocriptine.

In-vivo Studies

Felten et al.[19] examined age-related loss of dopaminergic cell bodies in the substantia nigra pars compacta and terminals in the striatum in rats. Chronic pergolide administration (0.5 mg/kg/day for 21 or 23 months) prevented age-related diminution of dopamine fluorescence intensity in the substantia nigra as well as striatum. Pergolide administration also prevented age-related decline in circulating FSH level.

Asanuma et al.[20] studied the effects of pergolide on 6-OHDA-induced dopamine depletion in mice. Intracerebroventricular injection of 6-OHDA (40 µg) induced rapid decrease in the levels of dopamine, DOPAC, and HVA in the striatum to 49%, 29%, and 68% of the controls, respectively, at week 1. Repeated pretreatment with pergolide (0.5 mg/kg, i.p.) for 7 days before administration of 6-OHDA almost completely protected against reduction in striatal dopamine and its metabolites one week after the injection of 6-OHDA. The authors ascribed these effects of pergolide to free-radical scavenging action of pergolide.

Gomez-Vargas et al.[21] examined effects of pergolide on NO generation using a direct detection system by electron-spin resonance. Pergolide dose-dependently scavenged NO. Furthermore, pergolide after repeated administration (0.5 mg/kg/day, i.p. for 7 days) significantly inhibited phospholipid peroxidation of rat brain homogenates.

O'Neill et al.[22] examined the effects of pergolide on ischemia-induced neuronal loss in CA1 region of the hippocampus of Mongolian gerbils. Ischemia was induced by bilateral carotid artery occlusion for 5 minutes. Pergolide 0.5 and 1.0 mg/kg i.p. provided significant ($p < 0.05$ and $p < 0.01$, respectively) neuroprotection against the ischemia-induced neuronal loss. Bromocriptine and lisuride also provided significant ($p < 0.05$) neuroprotection, but only at a high dose (1.0 mg/kg). In contrast, haloperidol, SKF 38393 (a dopamine D1 receptor agonist), and SCH 23390 (a dopamine D1 receptor antagonist) failed to provide neuroprotection.

Human Studies

Zimmerman et al.[23] retrospectively compared the clinical state of 14 patients with PD who took pergolide continuously for 63 ± 17 months (group I) to that of 12 similar patients who started pergolide and then stopped it after 60 ± 5 days (group II). Disability measured during the "on" state did not worsen during the observations period in group I patients, whereas patients in group II showed significant deterioration. The authors interpreted these results as suggesting neuroprotective properties in pergolide.

But symptomatic effects of pergolide likely influenced the "on"-time disability in group I and it is difficult to make any definite conclusion on neuroprotection in a retrospective study. There is no published study that addressed the question as to the potential neuroprotective properties of pergolide in humans.

Cabergoline

Cabergoline, a new ergoline derivative, is a D2-specific dopaminergic agonist that is more potent and longer-acting than other dopamine agonists.

In-vivo Studies

Finotti et al.[24] examined the antioxidant effect of cabergoline in rats. Male Wistar rats were treated with vehicle or with 2.5 mg/kg and 10 mg/kg of cabergoline, 6 or 10 times, at 48-hour intervals. Cabergoline decreased basal lipid peroxide levels in the hippocampus of rats given 10 mg/kg 10 times, and in the striatum of rats given the same dose 6 or 10 times. The authors interpreted these results as indicating the presence of antioxidant properties in cabergoline.

Human Studies

Rinne et al.[25] conducted a multicenter, randomized, double-blind 3- to 5-year trial to assess whether initial therapy with cabergoline alone or in combination with levodopa would prevent or delay the occurrence of long-term motor complications in patients with early PD ($n = 412$; Hoehn–Yahr stages 1 to 3). Patients were randomized to receive either cabergoline (0.25–4 mg once daily) or levodopa (100–600 mg/day) titrated over a maximum period of 24 weeks. The development of motor complications (the endpoint) was significantly less frequent in patients treated with cabergoline than in levodopa recipients (22% vs 34%; $p < 0.02$). The relative risk of developing motor complications during treatment with cabergoline was more than 50% lower than with levodopa. Starting treatment with cabergoline significantly delays the development of motor complications. It is not know whether or not the motor-fluctuation delaying effect of cabergoline is related to a neuroprotective effect on the dopaminergic neurons or to a long-lasting symptomatic effect of cabergoline.

Talipexole

Talipexole (6-allyl-2-amino-5,6,7,8-tetrahydro-4H-thiazolo-[4,5-d]azepine) is a non-ergot compound that is an agonist at α_2-adrenoceptors and at dopamine autoreceptors.

In-vivo Studies

Kondo et al.[26] examined the effects of talipexole on methamphetamine-induced TH decrease in mice. Methamphetamine (5 mg/kg every 2 hours, four times, i.p) induced marked reduction in TH activity in the striatum of C57BL/6N mice 72 hours after the injection. Talipexole (0.25 mg/kg or 1.0 mg/kg, i.p.) prior to the administration of methamphetamine significantly attenuated this decrease (>40% protection). The authors attributed this effect to the hydroxyl-radical scavenging action of talipexole.

Kitamura et al.[27] reported neuroprotective properties of talipexole using Planarians, a flatworm. Planarians treated with MPTP underwent autolysis and individual death in a concentration-dependent manner. Concomitant treatment with talipexole inhibited MPTP-induced autolysis and individual death. Pramipexole showed a similar protective effect. In addition, post-treatment with talipexole at 1 hour after MPTP completely inhibited MPTP-induced individual death.

Pramipexole

Pramipexole is a non-ergot D2/D3 receptor agonist.

In-vitro Studies

Carvey et al.[28] reported that pramipexole reduced levodopa-induced TH cell loss in a dose-dependent and saturable fashion (ED_{50} = 500 pmol); its inactive stereoisomer was significantly less potent and pergolide and bromocriptine had negligible cytoprotective effects. Culture media from mesencephalic cultures incubated with pramipexole for 6 days increased TH cell counts in freshly harvested recipient cultures.

Le et al.[29] studied effects of pramipexole on cytotoxicity induced by dopamine, 6-OHDA, and hydrogen peroxide using a dopaminergic cell line, MES 23.5. Pramipexole was neuroprotective against the cytotoxicity induced by these compounds. The authors ascribed these neuroprotective actions to antioxidant effects of this compound. Selective D2 or D3 antagonists were of no effect using the same experimental system.

Kakimura et al.[30] examined effects of talipexole and pramipexole on the release of cytochrome c and α-synuclein, their aggregations, and activation of caspases. Treatment of human neuroblastoma SH-SY5Y cells with MPTP (1 mmol) induced release of cytochrome c from the organellar fraction to the cytosolic fraction as the initial event, then DNA fragmentation followed, and accumulation of α-synuclein protein in the cytosolic fraction occurred as the last event. Talipexole and pramipexole at low concentrations (0.1–1 mmol) significantly inhibited the accumulation of cytochrome c or α-synuclein in the cytosolic fraction. In addition, the release of cytochrome c by hydrogen peroxide or the aggregation of α-synuclein by cytochrome c plus hydrogen peroxide was inhibited by talipexole and pramipexole at high concentrations (5–10 mmol). In-vitro activation of caspase-9 and -3 induced by cytochrome c and/or dATP (deoxyadenosine 5′-triphosphate) was also inhibited by at high concentrations of these drugs. This is an interesting observation in view of the accumulation of α-synuclein in PD. The same group of investigators also reported inhibition of MPTP-induced apoptotic cell death by talipexole and pramipexole using the same culture system.[31]

Cassarino et al.[32] reported 1-methyl-4-phenylpyridinium ion (MPP^+)-induced oxygen radial production from SH-SY5Y cells and from rat striatum with protection by pramipexole. Pramipexole (100–1000 μmol) also exhibited a concentration-dependent inhibition of opening of the mitochondrial transition pore induced by calcium and phosphate or MPP^+. The opening of the mitochondrial transition pore is an important initial event for the apoptosis cascade.

In-vivo Studies

Hall et al.[33] reported the effects of pramipexole on ischemia-induced cell damage. They produced forebrain ischemia in gerbils by bilateral carotid arterial occlusion for 10 minutes. There was a 40–45% loss of nigrostriatal cell bodies by 28 days after ischemia/reperfusion in vehicle-treated animals. Daily post-ischemic oral dosing of pramipexole (1 mg/kg p.o., twice daily, beginning at 1 hour after insult) decreased the 28-day post-ischemic loss of nigrostriatal dopamine neurons by 36% ($p < 0.01$ vs vehicle-treated). The effect was specific for dopamine neurons. The same team examined pramipexole's effects on methamphetamine-induced (10 mg/kg, i.p. 4 times, each 2 hours apart) nigrostriatal degeneration in male Swiss–Webster mice. In vehicle-treated mice, there was a 40% loss of nigrostriatal neurons by day 5. In contrast, pramipexole dosing (1 mg/kg, p.o., 1 hour after the last methamphetamine dose, plus daily) attenuated the nigrostriatal degeneration from 40% to only 8% ($p < 0.00001$ vs vehicle-treated). The authors ascribed these effects of pramipexole to reduction in dopamine turnover and the resultant decrease in hydroxyl-radical production.

Vu et al.[34] treated rats with pramipexole or saline before and after an intracerebroventricular 6-OHDA injection. Pramipexole treated animals exhibited a 29% and a 27% reduction in striatal dopamine loss and TH-positive cell loss compared with saline-treated animals.

Regarding the neuroprotective mechanism of pramipexole, Takata et al.[35] made an interesting observation in that they found marked increase in bcl-2 immunoreactivity in neuronal dendritic processes in both cerebral cortex and hippocampus after the treatment of rats with talipexole or pramipexole for 4 days.

Zou et al.[36] treated mice with MPTP and found a 38.1% increase in thiobarbituric-acid reactive substance (TBARS) in nigra, a 46.7% decrease of TH-positive nigral dopaminergic neurons, and a 59.4% reduction in striatal dopamine level. Pramipexole treatment significantly inhibited the TBARS production by 76%, and attenuated the nigral dopaminergic neuronal loss and striatal dopamine level by about 50%.

Human studies

Marek et al.[37] reported effects of pramipexole treatment on striatal 2β-carboxymethoxy-3β(4-iodophenyl)tropane (β-CIT) uptake studied by SPECT in patients with Parkinson's disease. The group of patients studied in this report represents a subgroup of patients studied in a large-scale randomized controlled study to compare two treatment methods; i.e. levodopa versus early pramipexole and add-on levodopa as needed.[38] The authors studied 151 early-stage parkinsonian patients treated with levodopa for 4 years and 150 patients treated with pramipexole initially and with additional levodopa as needed for the same period. They analyzed single-photon emission computed tomography (SPECT) using β-CIT labeled with iodine[123] before the treatment and 4 years after the treatment. The reduction in striatal β-CIT uptake during the 4-year period was 28.1% in the levodopa group and 17.1% in the levodopa group. The results were interpreted as suggesting the presence of neuroprotective effect in pramipexole in parkinsonian patients.

Ropinirole

Ropinirole is a non-ergot D2 and D3 receptor agonist.

In-vitro studies

Iida et al.[39] examined in-vitro antioxidant properties of ropinirole. Ropinirole had a low hydroxyl-radical or NO scavenging activity by the electron-spin resonance spectrometric method. Ropinirole had no direct O_2- scavenging activity *in vitro*. A high concentration of ropinirole (25 μmol) suppressed lipid peroxidation (TBARS) in mouse striatal homogenate induced by peroxidant stimulation. But these activities were very weak, suggesting that the antioxidant effect of ropinirole observed *in vitro* might be a minor component of its neuroprotective effect *in vivo*.

In-vivo Studies

Iida et al.[39] treated mice with ropinirole (2 mg/kg, i.p.) for 7 days and analyzed GSH, catalase, and superoxide dismutase (SOD) activities in the striatum. The treatment resulted in increases of these enzyme activities by 130%, 150%, and 120%, respectively. Treatment with ropinirole also resulted in the protection of striatal dopaminergic neurons against 6-OHDA-induced nigral neuronal loss.

Human Studies

Alan et al.[40] studied the potential neuroprotective effect of ropinirole on a parkinsonian nigrostriatal system using PET. This was a 2-year, double-blind, multinational study of 186 de-novo PD patients treated with ropinirole or levodopa. Patients with insufficient therapeutic benefit could supplement medication with open adjunctive levodopa and continue in the study. The primary endpoint was the change in putamen ^{18}F-dopa uptake measured with 3D PET. Ninety-three PD patients were randomized to each treatment; 73% of the ropinirole and 74% of the levodopa patients completed the 2-year study. Central ROI analysis of putamen ^{18}F-dopa uptake showed significantly slower progression with ropinirole (–13% ropinirole vs –20% levodopa; $p = 0.022$). The authors concluded that their data provided clear evidence of significantly slower disease progression in PD patients taking ropinirole compared with levodopa.

MONOAMINE OXIDASE B INHIBITOR

L-Deprenyl (Selegiline)

Selegiline is an inhibitor of monoamine oxidase B (MAO-B). It has been used in the treatment of Parkinson's disease to increase the "on" time in patients with wearing-off phenomena. As free radicals have been claimed to promote nigral neuronal death in PD, it is an interesting question whether or not monoamine oxidase inhibitors can protect nigral neurons. A variety of experimental models suggest that L-deprenyl provides neuroprotection through multiple mechanisms other than the inhibition of MAO-B.

In-vitro Studies

Mytilineou and Cohen[41] studied the effect of L-deprenyl on MPP^+-treated dopaminergic neurons. When the cultures were treated with deprenyl (10 μmol) 24 hours prior to and during exposure to MPP^+, DA neurons were protected from the toxicity of the drug. In the combined deprenyl plus MPP^+ treatment, the levels of DA in the cultures remained at the control range and the [^{3}H]DA uptake was reduced to only 73% of control.

Vizuete et al.[42] reported similar results using slices of rat striatum. They treated rats with L-deprenyl for 3 weeks and then incubated those slices with MPP^+. They measured dopamine and its metabolite concentrations. The effect of MPP^+ in animals treated with L-deprenyl was smaller than in controls, indicating that deprenyl protected against MPP^+. They also analyzed superoxide dismutase (SOD) and catalase activities and carbonyl group content of the proteins. Both activities increased in deprenyl-treated rats, and the amount of carbonyl groups was unchanged. The authors concluded that the protective effect of L-deprenyl was independent of the MAO-B inhibitor and of the induction of SOD and catalase activities.

In-vivo Studies

There are many reports on the protection of the nigral dopaminergic neurons in MPTP-treated animals.[43–45] Neuroprotective effects of deprenyl depend in part on its MAO-B inhibiting action, but other mechanisms are also likely to contribute.

Wu et al.[46] performed stereotaxic infusion of MPP^+ (4.2 nmol) into the substantia nigra; ipsilateral striatal dopamine levels were reduced to 53.4 ± 3.1% of the controls 4 days after the injection. Co-administration of L-deprenyl (4.2 nmol) with MPP^+ significantly attenuated the dopamine loss caused by MPP^+ to 88.0 ± 3.5% of the controls. However, infusion of (+)-deprenyl (4.2 nmol), Ro16-6491 (4.2 nmol), or pargyline (4.2 nmol) along with MPP^+ into substantia nigra did not significantly change the MPP^+-induced dopamine depletion. The authors concluded that L-deprenyl might possess a unique neuroprotective action on nigral neurons against MPP^+ toxicity independent of the MAO-B inhibition.

Tatton et al.[47] used serum and nerve growth factor withdrawal to induce apoptotic death in PC12 cells. L-Deprenyl reduced both cell death and nuclear DNA degradation in a concentration-dependent manner and was effective at concentrations too low to inhibit MAO ($< 10^{-9}$ mol). R-Deprenyl did not increase PC12 cell survival, and, with the exception of pargyline, other MAO-A and MAO-B inhibitors did not alter apoptotic death. The reduction in apoptosis required the induction of new protein synthesis by L-deprenyl. These results indicate an anti-apoptotic property of L-deprenyl.

Wadia et al.[48] studied the effect of L-deprenyl on PC12 cell survival under serum and nerve growth factor withdrawal. They measured mitochondrial membrane potential using epifluorescence and laser confocal microscopy with the mitochondrial potentiometric dyes chloromethyl-tetramethylrosamine methyl ester and 5,59,6,69-tetrachloro-1,19,3,39-tetraethybenzimidazol carbocyanine iodide. L-Deprenyl retained the mitochondrial membrane potential and protected PC12 cells from apoptotic cell death under this culture condition. The authors concluded that this effect might be mediated by increased synthesis of proteins such as bcl-2.

Human Studies

The Parkinson Study Group[49,50] addressed the question whether L-deprenyl would slow down the disease progression of PD (DATATOP study). Levodopa-naive patients were randomly allocated to one of four groups (placebo, L-deprenyl, α-tocopherol, and L-deprenyl + α-tocopherol). The endpoint was set as the time when patients required levodopa treatment. Significantly fewer numbers of patients who received L-deprenyl with or without α-tocopherol reached the endpoint two years from the randomization compared with those patients who did not receive α-tocopherol. But this difference was ascribed to symptomatic effects of L-deprenyl, and neuroprotection by L-deprenyl was not proved in this study.

The same group[51] examined CSF HVA concentrations based on the assumption that if L-deprenyl would offer neuroprotection, the HVA levels should not decrease over time compared with those who received placebo. Measurements of CSF HVA concentrations led them to conclude that (1) duration of MAO inhibition by L-deprenyl was long-lasting; (2) CSF HVA had limited utility as a marker of severity or progression in PD; (3) L-deprenyl did not provide sufficient MAO inhibition to test adequately the oxidative stress hypothesis of the cause of PD; and (4) the study could not prove a protective role of L-deprenyl in slowing the progression of PD.

Miyasaki et al.[52] made a systematic review of the literature performed to identify all human trials of L-deprenyl in de-novo Parkinson's disease between 1966 and 1999 using MEDLINE, EMBASE, and the Cochrane Library. They concluded that L-deprenyl has mild symptomatic benefit with no proven evidence for neuroprotective benefit.

Rasagiline

Rasagiline–R(+)-N-propargyl-1-aminioindan is an irreversible MAO-B inhibitor with potent anti-apoptotic activity. Youdim et al.[53] reported that its S-isomer (TVP1022) and TV 3219, a novel anti-Alzheimer cholinesterase–MAO inhibitor drug derived from rasagiline, also had potent anti-apoptotic and neuroprotective activities. They showed these activities using serum and NGF withdrawal models of partially neuronally differentiated PC12 cells; these compounds prevented the fall in mitochondrial membrane potential, the first step in cell death.

Maruyama et al.[54] studied the neuroprotective mechanism of rasagiline using human dopaminergic neuroblastoma SH-SY5Y cells. Apoptosis was induced by peroxynitrite generated from SIN-1. Rasagiline reduced apoptosis with much more potency than selegiline, and the protection required 20-minute pre-incubation before SIN-1 treatment. The protection by rasagiline was proved to be due to stabilization of mitochondrial membrane potential against the collapse induced by SIN-1, whereas rasagiline did not scavenge peroxynitrite directly.

CGP 3466B

CGP 3466–dibenzo[b,f]oxepin-10-ylmethyl-methyl-prop-2-ynyl-amine) is structurally related to L-deprenyl, but it exhibits virtually no MAO-B or MAO-A inhibiting properties. It is not metabolized to amphetamines.[55]

In-vitro Studies

Kragten et al.[56] reported specific binding of CGP 3466 to glyceraldehyde-3-phosphate dehydrogenase by affinity binding. Apoptosis assays based on the human neuroblastoma cell line PAJU established the importance of this interaction for mediating drug-induced inhibition of programmed cell death.

Waldmeier et al.[57] reported that CGP 3466 or its hydrogen maleate salt, CGP 3466B, at concentrations between 10^{-11} mol and 10^{-7} mol, protected rat embryonic mesencephalic dopaminergic neurons in free-floating or dispersed cell culture from death inflicted by treatment with MPP^+.

In-vivo Studies

Waldmeier et al.[58] reported the effects of CGP 3466 (0.1 mg/kg s.c.) and CGP 3466B (0.014 mg/kg and 0.14 mg/kg p.o.) twice daily for 18 days using mice lesioned with MPTP (2×30 mg/kg, s.c. at a 72-hour interval). These treatments partially prevented the MPTP-induced loss of TH-positive cells in the substantia nigra.

Andringa et al.[59] studied effects of CGP 3466B using 6-OHDA-treated rats. They infused 6-OHDA bilaterally into the substantia nigra pars compacta of rats that had been pretreated with desipramine. Treatment with CGP 3466B (0.0014–1.4 mg/kg s.c.) or its solvent was begun 2 hours after the 6-OHDA injection, and maintained twice daily for 14 days. CGP 3466B prevented all 6-OHDA-induced behavioral and immunocytochemical deficits.

ANTIOXIDANTS

Vitamin E (α-tocopherol)

In-vitro Studies

Hsu et al.[60] studied the effects of vitamin E on α-synuclein over-expressed cell cultures. Alpha-synuclein over-expression in hypothalamic neuronal cell line (GT1-7) resulted in formation of α-synuclein-immunopositive inclusion-like structures and mitochondrial alterations accompanied by increased levels of free radicals. These alterations were ameliorated by pretreatment with antioxidants including vitamin E. Alpha-synuclein over-expression in these cells showed a significant 30% decrease in mitochondrial activity and 60% decrease of gonadotropine-releasing hormone (GnRH) levels compared to non-transfected controls. Treatment with vitamin E restored normal mitochondrial function and normal levels of GnRH in these cells.

In-vivo Studies

Roghani et al.[61] studied the effects of vitamin E using an early model of PD. They made unilateral intrastriatal 6-OHDA (12.5 μg/5 μL) injection in rats. They pretreated these rats with intramuscular D-α-tocopheryl-acid succinate (24 IU/kg, i.m.) 1 hour before and three times per week for 1 month post-surgery. The number of TH-positive cells reduced significantly by 71% in the vitamin E untreated 6-OHDA lesioned group and by 8% in the vitamin E treated 6-OHDA group in comparison with the control group. Apomorphine- and amphetamine-induced rotational behaviors were also reduced by 74% and 68%, respectively, in vitamin E treated rats as compared with the untreated 6-OHDA lesioned rats. The authors concluded that repeated intramuscular administration of vitamin E exerted a rapid protective effect on the nigrostriatal dopaminergic neurons in their model.

Heim et al.[62] examined the effect of α-tocopherol using unilateral striatal 6-OHDA injected rats. Intraperitoneal injection of α-tocopherol for 8 days increased the ability of naive control animals to find the hidden platform positions in the water maze one week later. In intrastriatal sham-operated rats, 8 daily pre-injections of α-tocopherol significantly increased the duration and number of bursts of stereotyped movements for 30 minutes following a subcutaneous injection of apomorphine. In 6-OHDA-lesioned rats, α-tocopherol prevented the increased response to apomorphine, reduced the apomorphine-induced circling at 3 and 13 weeks, and prevented the decrease in spontaneous locomotion at 10 weeks, as well as the perseverative platform crossings which were caused by an impairment in switching behavior-strategies in the navigation task. The authors concluded that α-tocopherol might be an effective drug in the early stages of PD.

But there are three negative studies on the neuroprotective effects of vitamin E in MPTP-treated animals.[63–65] Thus further studies are needed before making a definite conclusion on the neuroprotective properties of vitamin E.

Human Studies

The Parkinson Study Group[49] addressed the question whether α-tocopherol would slow down the disease progression of PD (DATATOP study). They randomly assigned 800 patients to one of four treatments: placebo, active tocopherol and deprenyl placebo, active deprenyl and tocopherol placebo, or both active drugs. The primary endpoint was the onset of disability prompting the clinical decision to begin administering levodopa. They report the results of tocopherol treatment after a mean follow-up of 14 ± 6 months, as well as the follow-up results for deprenyl. There was no beneficial effect of tocopherol or any interaction between tocopherol and deprenyl despite significant ($p < 0.001$) increase in the CSF α-tocopherol level.[66]

Glutathione peroxidase

In-vitro Studies

Colton et al.[67] studied the effects of glutathione peroxidase on the survival of TH-positive cells using primary cultures of embryonic rat mesencephalon in an environment of low oxygen partial pressure. The number of TH-positive neurons increased approximately 2-fold when glutathione peroxidase was added to the culture medium.

Kim-Han et al.[68] investigated the role of glutathione peroxidase in cellular defense against levodopa cytotoxicity. They used a line of PC12 cells overexpressing glutathione peroxidase. The enzymatic activity was 1.5-fold higher in the transfectants. Transfectants were also significantly more resistant to exposure to either levodopa or t-butyl hydroperoxide than mock-transfected cells. The authors suggested that glutathione peroxidase might play an important role in cellular defense against oxidative stress.

In-vivo Studies

Klivenyi et al.[69] examined the susceptibility of mice with a disruption of the glutathione peroxidase gene to the neurotoxic effects of MPTP. Glutathione peroxidase knockout mice showed no evidence of neuropathological or behavioral abnormalities at 2–3 months of age. Administration of MPTP resulted in significantly greater depletions of dopamine, 3,4-dihydroxybenzoic acid, and homovanillic acid in the knockout mice than those seen in wild-type control mice. Striatal 3-nitrotyrosine (3-NT) concentrations after MPTP were significantly increased in the knockout mice as compared with wild-type control mice.

IMMUNOPHILIN LIGANDS

Immunophilins are a family of small protein molecules serving as cytosolic receptors for immunosuppressant drugs. Some of the ligands for these cytosolic receptor proteins have no immunosuppressant activity; instead they may act as cytoprotective agents.[70]

In-vivo Studies

A non-immunosuppressive immunophilin ligand, 3-(3-pyridyl)-1-propyl(2S)-1-(3,3-dimethyl-1,2-dioxopentyl)-2-pyrrolidine-carboxylate (GPI-1046), bound to FK506 binding protein-12, enhances neurite outgrowth from sensory neuronal cultures with picomolar potency with maximal effects comparable to nerve growth factor.[70] Steiner et al.[70] reported that GPI-1046 induced regenerative sprouting from spared nigrostriatal dopaminergic neurons following MPTP toxicity in mice or 6-OHDA toxicity in rats. The rotational abnormality in 6-OHDA-treated rats was alleviated by GPI-1046.

Ross et al.[71] produced extensive unilateral striatal deafferentation by intranigral 6-OHDA in rats. Beginning 60 days after 6-OHDA injection, animals received a 14-day course of treatment with GPI 1046 (10 mg/kg) or its vehicle alone. GPI 1046 treatment did not alter TH fiber density in the contralateral striatum but did produce significantly higher striatal TH fiber density in the ipsilateral caudate-putamen. This striatal re-innervation occurred in the absence of increased nigral sparing, and appeared to reflect the GPI 1046-induced sprouting of residual TH fibers spared by the 6-OHDA lesion.

Zhang et al.[72] investigated the effects of GPI-1046 in 6-OHDA-lesioned rats. In unlesioned rats, tetanic stimulation of the white matter induced long-term potentiation (LTP) of corticostriatal synaptic transmission. Unilateral microinjection of 6-OHDA into the substantia nigra resulted in a loss of corticostriatal LTP and in significant abnormality of motor behavior as assessed by amphetamine-induced ipsilateral rotations. Daily treatment of 6-OHDA-lesioned rats with GPI-1046 (10 mg/kg s.c.) for 1 week reduced amphetamine-induced rotations by 75% and greatly restored the striatal TH immunostaining. In addition, GPI-1046 almost completely restored corticostriatal LTP in 6-OHDA-lesioned animals. The authors suggested that GPI 1046 was a potential therapeutic agent for Parkinson's disease.

But there are two negative studies on the neuroprotective effects of immunophilin ligands.[73,74] Thus further studies are needed before making a conclusion on the neuroprotective properties of immunophilin ligands.

ANTI-INFLAMMATORY AGENTS

Teismann et al.[75] examined the effects of acetylsalicylic acid, a COX-1/COX-2 (cyclooxygenase-1/cyclooxygenase-2) inhibitor, in comparison with meloxicam, a preferential COX-2 inhibitor on MPTP-induced loss of striatal dopamine and nigral TH (+) neurons. They treated male C57BL/6 mice (n = 82) with a single dose of acetylsalicylic acid (10, 50, 100 mg/kg i.p.) or meloxicam (2, 7.5, 50 mg/kg i.p.) immediately prior to administration of MPTP (30 mg/kg s.c.) or saline. In the saline-treated MPTP control group, striatal dopamine levels were reduced to 15.9% of control values. Dopamine depletion was significantly attenuated to values of 37.1% and 38.6% of saline control values by acetylsalicylic acid (50 and 100 mg/kg) and to values of 36% and 40% by meloxicam (7.5 and 50 mg/kg), respectively. The MPTP-induced decrease of TH-immunoreactivity as well as the loss of nigral neurons was nearly completely prevented by acetylsalicylic acid (100 mg/kg) and meloxicam (7.5 and 50 mg/kg). The molecular mechanism of neuroprotection provided by COX-1 and COX-2 inhibitors is unknown.

ADENOSINE A2 RECEPTOR ANTAGONISTS

Adenosine A2 receptor agonist

Adenosine A2 receptors (A2A) are abundant in the caudate-putamen, nucleus accumbens, and olfactory tubercle in several species.[76] In caudate-putamen, adenosine A2A receptors are localized on several neurons and have been shown to modulate the neurotransmission of γ-aminobutyric acid (GABA), acetylcholine, and glutamate.[77–79]

Ikeda et al.[80] examined the effects of an A2A receptor antagonist, (E)-1,3-diethyl-8-(3,4-dimethoxystyryl)-7-methyl-3,7-dihydro-1H-purine-2,6-dione (KW-6002), in 6-OHDA-treated mice. The A2A antagonist (10 mg/kg p.o.) protected 6-OHDA-induced nigral dopaminergic neuronal loss and prevented the functional loss of dopaminergic nerve terminals in the striatum.

Caffeine

The CNS effects of caffeine are mediated by its antagonistic actions at the A1 and A2A subtypes of adenosine receptors.[81]

In-vitro Studies

Xu et al.[82] investigated the effects of caffeine treatment on MPTP-induced dopaminergic toxicity in mice. Acute pretreatment with caffeine attenuated MPTP-induced loss of striatal dopamine and dopamine transporter binding sites. Chronic treatment with caffeine gave identical results in MPTP-treated mice.

Chen et al.[83] studied the adenosine receptor subtypes that would mediate the effects of caffeine. Caffeine, at doses comparable to those of typical human exposure, attenuated MPTP-induced loss of striatal dopamine and dopamine transporter binding sites. The effects of caffeine were mimicked by several A2A antagonists and by genetic inactivation of the A2A receptor, but not by an A1 receptor blocker. The authors concluded that caffeine attenuated MPTP toxicity by A2A receptor blockade.

Casas et al.[84] studied the effects of repeated co-administrations of caffeine and bromocriptine for 9 consecutive days on contralateral turning in unilateral nigrostriatal 6-OHDA denervated rats. They showed that on the first administration, both caffeine and bromocriptine injection plus saline produced a significant increase in contralateral rotational behavior as compared to saline + saline injections. However, with repeated administrations, tolerance was observed to caffeine, but not to bromocriptine. The combination of different doses of bromocriptine (0.1, 0.2, 0.4, and 0.8 mg/kg) with caffeine (40 mg/kg) significantly enhanced the effects of either drug injected with saline on rotational behavior, and no tolerance was observed with repeated treatment. These results demonstrate that when caffeine is administered repeatedly in combination with bromocriptine, tolerance to its psychostimulant effects would not develop. The authors concluded that caffeine could be used as an adjunctive therapeutic agent with dopamine agonists for the treatment of Parkinson's disease.

Human Studies

In a case–control study, Hellenbrand et al.[85] compared the past dietary habits of 342 PD patients recruited from nine German clinics with those of 342 controls from the same neighborhood or region. They also found that patients consumed less beer (odds ratio [OR]: 0.26; 95% confidence interval [CI]: 0.14–0.49) and spirits (OR: 0.56; CI: 0.36–0.86), but not wine, and they consumed less coffee (OR: 0.27; CI: 0.14–0.52, highest versus lowest quartile), but not tea, than controls. This may relate to a possible interaction between dopaminergic activity and the intake of ethanol or caffeine. Significantly more patients than controls reported ever consuming raw meat (OR: 1.78; CI: 1.21–2.63). These results suggest that the intake of certain foods may be associated with the development of PD.

To explore the association of coffee and dietary caffeine intake with risk of PD, Ross et al. [86] analyzed 8004 Japanese–American men (aged 45–68 years) enrolled in the prospective longitudinal Honolulu Heart Program between 1965 and 1968 by amount of coffee intake (measured at study enrollment and 6-year follow-up) and by total dietary caffeine intake (measured at enrollment). Their findings indicated that higher coffee and caffeine intake was associated with a significantly lower incidence of PD. This effect appeared to be independent of smoking. The data suggested that the mechanism was related to caffeine intake and not to other nutrients contained in coffee.

Ascherio et al.[87] examined the relationship between coffee and caffeine consumption and the risk of this disease among participants in two cohorts. Among men, after adjustment for age and smoking, the relative risk of PD was 0.42 (CI: 0.23–0.78; p for trend < 0.001) for men in the top one-fifth of caffeine intake compared to those in the bottom one-fifth. An inverse association was also observed with consumption of coffee (p for trend $= 0.004$), caffeine from non-coffee sources (p for trend < 0.001), and tea (p for trend $= 0.02$) but not decaffeinated coffee. Among women, the relationship between caffeine or coffee intake and risk of PD was U-shaped, with the lowest risk observed at moderate intakes (1–3 cups of coffee/day, or the third quintile of caffeine consumption). The authors concluded that moderate doses of caffeine might have a protective effect on the risk of PD.

Checkoway et al.[88] studied associations of PD with smoking, caffeine intake, and alcohol consumption in a case–control study conducted in western Washington State in 1992–2000. Clinical subjects consisted of 210 PD patients and 247 controls matched for gender and age. No associations were detected for coffee consumption or total caffeine intake or for alcohol consumption. However, reduced risks were observed for consumption of two cups/day or more of tea (OR: 0.4; CI: 0.2–0.9) and two or more cola drinks/day (OR: 0.6; CI: 0.3–1.4). The associations for tea and cola drinks were not confounded by smoking or coffee consumption.

A possible neuroprotective effect of caffeine is an interesting subject that warrants further studies.

GLUTAMATE RECEPTOR ANTAGONISTS

Amantadine

In-vitro Studies

Weller et al.[89] studied the effects of amantadine and memantine on NMDA receptor-mediated glutamate toxicity in cultured cerebellar, cortical, and mesencephalic neurons. Both drugs protected cerebellar and cortical neurons against glutamate toxicity. Glutamate toxicity (200 μmol) of dopaminergic neurons in mesencephalic cultures was only mildly attenuated by memantine. These findings suggested that amantadine would act by inhibiting NMDA receptor-mediated excitatory neurotransmission.

In-vivo Studies

Wenk et al.[90] compared the side-effects and neuroprotective potency of amantadine, memantine, and (+)-MK-801. They injected NMDA directly into the nucleus basalis magnocellularis of rats. Each test compound significantly attenuated the loss of nucleus basalis magnocellularis cholinergic cells. ED_{50} was 0.077, 2.81, and 43.5 mg/kg for (+)-MK-801, memantine, and amantadine, respectively, giving a relative potency ratio of 1:36:565. The side-effects included ataxia, myorelaxation, and stereotypy, and the ED_{50} for neuroprotective ability was highest for memantine and the lowest for (+)-MK-801. The authors concluded that NMDA receptor antagonists, memantine and amantadine, had a neuroprotective potency in particular at low doses before side-effects appeared.

NEUROTROPHIC FACTORS

Glial Cell Line-derived Neurotrophic Factor (GDNF)

GDNF is a glycosylated, disulfide-bonded homodimer that is a distantly related member of the transforming growth factor-beta superfamily. In embryonic midbrain cultures, recombinant human GDNF promoted the survival and morphological differentiation of dopaminergic neurons and increased their high-affinity dopamine uptake.[91]

More than 100 papers have been published on the neuroprotective effects of GDNF. Only papers pertinent to PD will be discussed here.

In-vitro Studies

Hou et al.[92] studied the effects of GDNF on growth of mesencephalic dopaminergic neurons following exposure to MPP^+. GDNF supported the growth of normally developing dopaminergic neurons and stimulated their survival and recovery after the damage induced by MPP^+.

In-vivo Studies

Beck et al.[93] performed axotomy within the medial forebrain bundle; half the TH-expressing neurons in the substantia nigra were destroyed. This loss was largely prevented by repeated injections of GDNF adjacent to the substantia nigra.

Tomac et al.[94] studied effects of GDNH in MPTP-treated mice. GDNF injected over the substantia nigra or in striatum before MPTP potently protected the dopamine system, as shown by numbers of mesencephalic dopamine nerve cell bodies, dopamine nerve terminal densities, and dopamine levels. When GDNF was given after MPTP, dopamine levels and fiber densities were significantly restored. In both experiments, motor behavior was increased above normal levels.

Arenas et al.[95] grafted genetically engineered fibroblasts expressing high levels of GDNF into locus coeruleus. This procedure prevented more than 80% of the 6-OHDA-induced degeneration of noradrenergic neurons in the locus coeruleus *in vivo*. Moreover, GDNF induced a fasciculated sprouting and increased by 2.5-fold both TH levels and the soma size of lesioned locus coeruleus neurons.

Tseng et al.[96] performed a unilateral medial forebrain bundle (MFB) axotomy in rats. Then they injected low amounts of GDNF that was continuously released from polymer-encapsulated genetically engineered cells grafted close to the substantia nigra. This procedure protected the nigral dopaminergic neurons from an axotomy-induced lesion and significantly improved pharmacological rotational behavior by a mechanism other than dopaminergic striatal reinnervation; loss of TH immunoreactivity in the nigral neurons was prevented and the amphetamine-induced rotational asymmetry was also ameliorated.

Choi-Lundberg et al.[97] injected a replication-defective adenoviral vector encoding human GDNF near the substantia nigra of rats. This procedure protected dopamine neurons from the progressive degeneration induced by 6-OHDA. Bilang-Bleuel et al.[98] reported similar results in MPTP-treated mice.

Mandel et al.[99] made midbrain injection in rats of recombinant adeno-associated virus encoding rat GDNF, which also protected nigral neurons in a progressive 6-OHDA-induced degeneration model.

Kirik et al.[100] used an rAAV-GDNF vector to express GDNF long-term (6 months) in either the nigral dopamine neurons themselves, in the striatal target cells, or in both of these structures. The rats receiving rAAV-GDNF in the striatum displayed behavioral recovery, accompanied by significant reinnervation of the lesioned striatum, which developed gradually over the first 4–5 months after the 6-OHDA lesion (a total of 28 µg).

Wang et al.[101] investigated whether adeno-associated viral (AAV) vector-mediated delivery of a GDNF gene in a delayed manner could prevent progressive degeneration of dopaminergic neurons, while preserving a functional nigrostriatal pathway. Four weeks after a unilateral intrastriatal injection of 6-OHDA, rats received injection of AAV vectors expressing GDNF tagged with FLAG peptide (AAV-GDNFflag) or β-galactosidase (AAV-LacZ) into the lesioned striatum. Consistent with anatomical and biochemical changes, significant behavioral recovery was observed 4–20 weeks following AAV-GDNFflag injection. The authors concluded that a delayed delivery of GDNF gene using AAV vector was efficacious even 4 weeks after the onset of progressive degeneration in a rat model of PD.

Gash et al.[102] extended the rodent studies to rhesus monkeys. They injected GDNF intracerebrally in monkey MPTP models. The recipients of GDNF displayed significant improvements in three of the cardinal symptoms of parkinsonism–bradykinesia, rigidity, and postural instability. GDNF administered every 4 weeks maintained functional recovery. On the lesioned side of GDNF-treated animals, dopamine levels in the midbrain and globus pallidus were twice as high, and nigral dopamine neurons were, on average, 20% larger, with an increased fiber density.

GDNF delivery using a lentiviral vector system also could prevent nigrostriatal degeneration and induce regeneration in primate models of PD.[103]

Human Studies

Kordower et al.[104] reported clinicopathologic findings of a patient who had received intraventricular GDNF treatment. The patient was a 65-year-old man with Parkinson's disease; he received monthly intracerebroventricular injections of GDNF. His parkinsonism continued to worsen following this treatment. Side-effects included nausea, loss of appetite, tingling, L'hermitte's sign, intermittent hallucinations, depression, and inappropriate sexual conduct. There was no evidence of significant regeneration of nigrostriatal neurons or intraparenchymal diffusion of the intracerebroventricular GDNF to relevant brain regions.

Brain-derived Neurotrophic Factor (BDNF)

In-vitro Studies

Hyman et al.[105] studied the effects of BDNF on the survival of dopaminergic neurons of the developing substantia nigra. BDNF (50 ng/mL) enhanced the survival of dopaminergic neurons in serum-free mesencephalic cultures. BDNF (50 ng/mL) also protected cultured nigral dopaminergic neurons from the neurotoxic effects of MPP^+. The authors concluded that BDNF might be a trophic factor for mesencephalic dopaminergic neurons.

Beck et al.[106] also reported that pretreatment of cultured dopaminergic neurons with BDNF reduced their susceptibility to MPP^+ toxicity. In cultures grown in the presence of BDNF (100 ng/mL medium) before MPP^+ treatment, such toxic decrease of dopaminergic parameters was prevented.

Spina et al.[107] studied the effects of BDNF on mesencephalic and SH-SY5Y cell cultures. Exposure of mesencephalic cells to either 6-OHDA or MPP^+ resulted in a loss of 70–80% of dopaminergic neurons. In BDNF-treated cultures, loss of TH-positive cells after exposure to either toxin was reduced to only 30%. BDNF also protected SH-SY5Y cells. Treatment of SH-SY5Y cells with 10 μmol of 6-OHDA for 24 hours caused a 5-fold increase in the levels of oxidized glutathione (GSSG). Pretreatment with BDNF for 24 hours completely prevented the rise in GSSG. BDNF increased the activity of glutathione reductase by 100%.

In-vivo Studies

Frim et al.[108] engineered immortalized rat fibroblasts to secrete human BDNF and implanted these cells near the substantia nigra 7 days before striatal MPP^+ infusion. They found that BDNF-secreting fibroblasts markedly increased nigral dopaminergic neuronal survival compared to control fibroblast implants.

Tsukahara et al.[109] studied the effects of intrathecal infusion of BDNF in MPTP-induced parkinsonian (a total of 1 mg/kg) in monkeys. Nine Japanese monkeys were divided randomly into three groups, an untreated control ($n = 3$), a BDNF group ($n = 3$), and a non-BDNF group ($n = 3$). Animals in the BDNF group received continuous intrathecal infusion of 10 mL of cell culture medium containing 10 μg of BDNF protein. The BDNF-treated animals remained asymptomatic during the first week and showed mild parkinsonism during the second week, whereas the non-BDNF group showed typical parkinsonian syndrome during the first week, with deterioration in the second week. Histological damage in the substantia nigra correlated well with the clinical features.

Levivier et al.[110] reported that intrastriatal grafts of fibroblasts genetically engineered to produce BDNF partially prevented the loss of nerve terminals and completely prevented the loss of cell bodies of the nigrostriatal dopaminergic pathway that had been induced by the intrastriatal injection of 6-OHDA.

ANTI-APOPTOTIC AGENTS

Apoptosis is an important mechanism of physiological and pathological cell death, and is known to occur in various neurological disorders including Parkinson's disease.

Inhibitor of Apoptosis Proteins (IAPs)

IAPs were originally identified in mutant baculovirus lacking p35 based on their ability to rescue cells from apoptosis.[111]

In-vitro Studies

Simon et al.[112] studied one of the members of IAP, X-chromosome-linked IAP (XIAP). XIAP specifically inhibited caspase-3, -7, and -9. Adenoviral gene transfer of XIAP promoted survival of potassium-deprived cerebellar granule neurons.

In-vivo Studies

Eberhardt et al.[113] reported that adenoviral gene transfer of XIAP prevented cell death of dopaminergic substantia pars compacta neurons in a mouse MPTP model.

Virus vector mediating the pan-caspase inhibitor baculovirus p35, and a specific class of caspase inhibitory proteins such as cytokine response modifier A (CrmA) and XIAP, were also effective *in vivo*, especially under pathological conditions.[114]

Bcl-2 and Bcl-xL

The human oncoprotein bcl-2 was the first identified member of a large family of proapoptotic (Bax, Bad, bcl-xs) and anti-apoptotic (bcl-2, bcl-xL) molecules, active in neuronal and non-neuronal cells that form homodimers and heterodimers with each other. The bcl-2 inhibited neuronal apoptosis induced by a variety of noxious stimuli and preserved the functional integrity of injured cells.[115,116] Bcl-xL, one of three isoforms of bcl-x, protects cells from the damaging effect of reactive oxygen species (e.g. lipid peroxidation) which has been shown to induce apoptotic cell death.

In-vitro Studies

Offen et al.[117] examined the potential protective effect of bcl-2 in PC12 cells that had been transfected with the protooncogene. Bcl-2-producing cells showed a marked resistance to dopamine toxicity. The percentage of nuclear condensation and DNA fragmentation visualized by the end-labeling method following dopamine treatment was significantly lower in bcl-2-expressing cells. Furthermore, the presence of bcl-2 protected cells from thiol imbalance and prevented thiol loss following exposure to dopamine. The authors concluded that the protective effects of bcl-2 against dopamine toxicity might be explained, in part, by its action as an antioxidant and by its interference with the production of toxic agents.

In-vivo Studies

Azzouz et al.[118] investigated the potential of recombinant AAV (rAAV) to transfer neuroprotective molecules in an animal model of ALS. They demonstrated that injection of an rAAV encoding the anti-apoptotic protein bcl-2 into the lumbar spinal cord in SOD1G93A mice resulted in sustained bcl-2 expression in motoneurons and significantly increased the number of surviving motor neurons at the end-stage of the disease. Herpes simplex virus vector-mediated expression of bcl-2 was also applied to prevent 6-OHDA-induced degeneration of neurons.[119]

Blömer et al.[120] also reported that intracellular delivery of lentiviral vectors expressing bcl-xL prevented apoptotic death of axotomized cholinergic neurons. Thus, virus vector mediated bcl-2 or bcl-x expression *in vivo* can prevent neuronal death in certain pathological conditions.

Dominant Negative Inhibitors of Caspases

In the mitochondrial pathway of apoptosis, the formation of Apaf-1/caspase-9 complex is accomplished by the heteromeric CARD/CARD (Caspase

Recruitment Domain) interaction. In addition, homophilic CARD/CARD interactions are also found in an array of other proteins involved in apoptotic regulation, including the majority of the initiator pro-caspases, adapter proteins, and cellular apoptosis inhibitors. The recombinant wild-type CARD domain inhibited proteolytic cleavage of pro-caspase-9.[121] Thus over-expression of Apaf-1 CARD can act as a dominant negative inhibitor.

For inhibiting the mitochondrial apoptotic cascade *in vivo*, at the authors' institution we generated an rAAV vector that contained the CARD of Apaf-1 to block the Apaf-1/caspase-9 pathway of cell death via dominant negative interference with the formation of a functional Apaf-1–caspase 9 complex.[122] We injected the wild-type CARD of Apaf-1 as a dominant negative inhibitor of Apaf-1 (rAAV-Apaf-1-DN-FLAG-EGFP) using AAV virus vector into the striatum of C57 black mouse, and then treated with MPTP. Two weeks after the virus injection, mice received four intraperitoneal injections of MPTP (30 mg/kg) in saline at 24-hour intervals. The number of dopaminergic neurons in the rAAV-Apaf-1-DN-EGFP-injected side was significantly greater than the number of neurons on the non-injection side by immunohistochemical analysis. These data indicate that Apaf-1-dominant negative delivery using an AAV vector system can prevent nigrostriatal degeneration in MPTP mice, suggesting that it might be a valuable therapeutic strategy for PD.

OTHER POSSIBLE NEUROPROTECTORS

Estrogen

Estrogen is a gonadal hormone that exerts diverse non-reproductive actions on multiple organs and in multiple physiological systems. Amongst these, estrogen has profound effects on plasticity and cell survival of the adult brain.

In-vitro Studies

Sawada et al.[123] studied neuroprotective effects of estradiol against oxidative stress using primary neuronal culture of the rat ventral mesencephalon. Oxidative stress induced by glutamate, superoxide anions, and hydrogen peroxide caused significant neuronal death. 17α-estradiol provided neuroprotection against glutamate-induced toxicity in dopaminergic neurons, as well as the 17β isoform. The authors concluded that 17α-estradiol might be a potential therapeutic agent for Parkinson's disease.

Singer et al.[124] examined the effects of mitogen-activated protein kinase (MAPK) inhibitor, PD98059, on neuroprotection provided by NGF and estrogen in primary cortical neurons after glutamate excitotoxicity. MAPK signaling pathways were activated by growth factors such as NGF. Inhibition of MAPK signaling with PD98059 blocked both NGF and estrogen neuroprotection in these neurons. These results suggest that cytoplasmic actions of the estrogen receptor may activate the MAPK pathway and this may be a part of neuroprotective mechanisms provided by estrogen.

Sawada et al.[125] demonstrated that ligand-activated estrogen receptor β suppressed dopaminergic neuronal death in an in-vitro MPP^+ model. They treated with MPP^+ (1–100 μmol) and found up-regulation of c-Jun amino-terminal kinase (JNK) and dopaminergic neuronal death, the latter being blocked by curcumin, an inhibitor of the c-Jun/AP-1 cascade. 17α- and 17β-estradiol both protected dopaminergic neurons from MPP^+-induced neuronal death and this was blocked by a pure antagonist of the estrogen receptor, ICI 182,780, but not by an inhibitor of estrogen receptor dimerization, YP537. The authors concluded that the neuroprotection provided by 17α-estradiol was via inhibitory transcriptional regulation at the activator protein-1 (AP-1) site mediated by estrogen receptor β.

In-vivo Studies

Callier et al.[126] studied neuroprotection provided by estrogens using a mouse MPTP model. The MPTP-induced decrease of striatal dopamine transporter binding was prevented by 17β-estradiol (2 μg/day), progesterone (2 μg/day), or raloxifene (5 mg/kg/day) but not by 17α-estradiol (2 μg/day) or raloxifene (1 mg/kg/day).

Dubal et al.[127] reported that physiological levels of estradiol exerted profound protective effects on the cerebral cortex in ischemia induced by permanent middle cerebral artery occlusion. Estradiol prevented the injury-induced down-regulation of bcl-2 expression. This effect was specific to bcl-2. They also found that estrogen receptors were differentially modulated in injury, with estrogen receptor β expression paralleling bcl-2 expression. The authors concluded that estradiol modulated the expression of bcl-2 in ischemic injury.

Green Tea Polyphenol

In-vitro Studies

Levites et al.[128] studied the effects of (-)-epigallocatechin-3-gallate (EGCG). Pretreatment with EGCG (0.1–10 mol) attenuated SH-SY5Y cell death induced by 24-hour exposure to 6-OHDA. EGCG restored the reduced protein kinase C (PKC) and extracellular signal-regulated kinases (ERK1/2) activities, caused by 6-OHDA toxicity. Since EGCG increased phosphorylated PKC, the authors suggested that PKC isoenzymes were involved in the neuroprotective action of EGCG against 6-OHDA.

In-vivo Studies

Levites et al.[129] reported prevention of MPTP-induced dopaminergic toxicity by pretreatment of mice with either green tea extract (0.5 and 1 mg/kg) or EGCG (2 and 10 mg/kg). In addition, the neurotoxin caused an elevation in striatal antioxidant enzymes superoxide dismutase (240%) and catalase (165%) activities, both effects being prevented by EGCG. EGCG itself also increased the activities of both enzymes in the brain. The authors concluded that the brain penetrating property of polyphenols, as well as their antioxidant and iron-chelating properties, might make such compounds an important class of drugs for neurodegenerative disorders.

Nicotine

Nicotine is a natural alkaloid that has considerable stimulatory effects on the central nervous system (CNS). Its effects on the CNS are mediated by the activation of neuronal heteromeric acetylcholine-gated ion channel receptors (also termed nicotinic acetylcholine receptors, nAChR).

In-vitro Studies

Ferger et al.[130] examined the effects of nicotine on hydroxyl free-radical formation *in vitro*. Nicotine and α-phenyl-N-tert-butyl nitrone (PBN) were examined in a cell-free in-vitro Fenton system (Fe^{3+}/EDTA + H_2O_2) for their radical scavenging properties using the salicylate trapping method. Salicylic acid (0.5 mmol) was incubated in the presence and absence of nicotine or PBN and the main products of the reaction of hydroxyl radicals with salicylic acid, namely 2,3- and 2,5-dihydroxybenzoic acid, were immediately determined using HPLC. Nicotine and PBN were both able to significantly reduce hydroxyl-radical levels at concentrations of 1, 2.5, and 5 mmol.

In-vivo Studies

Ferger et al.[130] also studied in-vivo effects of nicotine using a mouse MPTP model. Nicotine (0.1 or 0.4 mg/kg s.c.) was administered twice daily for a period of 14 days. On day 8, a single injection of MPTP (30 mg/kg s.c.) was given. High-dosage nicotine treatment significantly increased the MPTP-induced loss of bodyweight and resulted in a significantly decreased striatal dopamine content and an increased dopamine turnover in comparison with the MPTP-treated controls at day 15. The lower dosage of nicotine did not significantly alleviate the MPTP-induced effects. Thus nicotine was not neuroprotective *in vivo*.

Maggio et al.[131] reported on the neuroprotective effects of (–)nicotine in two animal models of parkinsonism: the diethyldithiocarbamate (DDC)-induced enhancement of MPTP toxicity in mice, and the methamphetamine-induced neurotoxicity in rats and mice. In parallel experiments, they found that (–)nicotine induced the basic fibroblast growth factor (FGF-2) and the brain-derived neurotrophic factor (BDNF) in rat striatum. They concluded that the increase in neurotrophic factors was a possible mechanism by which (–)nicotine protected experimental parkinsonisms. Moreover, they suggested that nAChR agonists could be of potential benefit in the progression of PD.

Costa et al.[132] also reported that nicotine prevented striatal dopamine loss produced by 6-OHDA in the substantia nigra. Subcutaneous nicotine (1 mg/kg) administered 4 hours before and 20, 44, and 68 hours after 6 μg of 6-OHDA prevented significantly the striatal dopamine loss. Chlorisondamine, a long-lasting nicotinic acetylcholine receptor antagonist, prevented the nicotinic protective effects on dopamine concentrations. The authors concluded that putative neuroprotective effects of nicotine *in vivo* depended on an acute intermittent administration schedule and on the extent of the brain lesion.

Human Studies

Gorell et al.[133] analyzed smoking consumption in 144 patients with PD and 464 control subjects, who were frequency matched for sex, race, and age (±5 years), in a population-based case–control study of men and women ≥50 years old. With never-smokers as the reference category, there was an inverse association between current light smokers (>0 to 30 pack-years) and parkinsonian patients, and stronger inverse association of PD with current heavy smokers (>30 pack-years). They concluded that smoking was biologically protective.

Fowler et al.[134] reported 40% decrease in the brain level of monoamine oxidase B in smokers relative to non-smokers or former smokers. MAO-B inhibition is associated with enhanced activity of dopamine, as well as with decreased production of hydrogen peroxide. They proposed that reduction of MAO-B activity might synergize with nicotine to produce the diverse behavioral and epidemiological effects of smoking.

On the other hand, Haack et al.[135] failed to find an association between smoking histories and Parkinson's disease. Furthermore, Behmand et al.[136] studied the effect of chronic nicotine on MPTP neurotoxicity in two strains of mice and found that nicotine increased rather than decreased MPTP toxicity.

CONCLUSION

In summary, many drugs and chemical compounds were studied for neuroprotective properties in experimental parkinsonian cell lines and animal models. Most of the compounds so far reported showed neuroprotective properties against nigral cell death induced by various toxic compounds such as 6-OHDA and MPTP. But very few human studies have been conducted. The results of human studies are not very convincing for proving or excluding neuroprotective properties. In humans, the methods to prove neuroprotective effects for any given compound may not be sensitive enough even if a compound does have a neuroprotective actions against nigral neuronal death. But it is encouraging to say that many compounds showed neuroprotective effects in in-vitro and in-vivo models of PD. Further human studies are warranted.

REFERENCES

1. Agid Y, Ahlskog E, Albanese A et al. Levodopa in the treatment of Parkinson's disease: a consensus meeting. Mov Disord 1999;14:911–913.
2. Agid Y, Olanow CW, Mizuno Y. Levodopa: why the controversy? Lancet 2002;360:575.
3. Mytilineou C, Han SK, Cohen G. Toxic and protective effects of L-dopa on mesencephalic cell cultures. J Neurochem 1993;61:1470–1478.
4. Mena MA, Davila V, Sulzer D. Neurotrophic effects of L-dopa in postnatal midbrain dopamine neuron/cortical astrocyte cocultures. J Neurochem 1997;69:1398–1408.

5. Koshimura K, Tanaka J, Murakami Y, Kato Y. Effects of dopamine and L-dopa on survival of PC12 cells. J Neurosci Res 2000;62:112–119.
6. Han SK, Mytilineou C, Cohen G. L-dopa up-regulates glutathione and protects mesencephalic cultures against oxidative stress. J Neurochem 1996;66:501–510.
7. Gassen M, Gross A, Youdim MB. Apomorphine enantiomers protect cultured pheochromocytoma (PC12) cells from oxidative stress induced by H_2O_2 and 6-hydroxydopamine. Mov Disord 1998; 13:242–248.
8. Grunblatt E, Mandel S, Berkuzki T, Youdim MB. Apomorphine protects against MPTP-induced neurotoxicity in mice. Mov Disord 1999;14:612–618.
9. Grunblatt E, Mandel S, Maor G, Youdim MB. Effects of R- and S-apomorphine on MPTP-induced nigro-striatal dopamine neuronal loss. J Neurochem 2001;77:146–156.
10. Yoshikawa T, Minamiyama Y, Naito Y, Kondo M. Antioxidant properties of bromocriptine, a dopamine agonist. J Neurochem 1994;62:1034–1038.
11. Sawada H, Ibi M, Kihara T et al. Dopamine D2-type agonists protect mesencephalic neurons from glutamate neurotoxicity: mechanisms of neuroprotective treatment against oxidative stress. Ann Neurol 1998;44:110–119.
12. Takashima H, Tsujihata M, Kishikawa M, Freed WJ. Bromocriptine protects dopaminergic neurons from levodopa-induced toxicity by stimulating D(2) receptors: 1. Exp Neurol 1999;159:98–104.
13. Yamashita H, Kawakami H, Zhang Y, Tanaka K, Nakamura S. Neuroprotective mechanism of bromocriptine. Lancet 1995;346:1305.
14. Kondo T, Ito T, Sugita Y. Bromocriptine scavenges methamphetamine-induced hydroxyl radicals and attenuates dopamine depletion in mouse striatum. Ann N Y Acad Sci 1994;738:222–229.
15. Ogawa N, Tanaka K, Asanuma M et al. Bromocriptine protects mice against 6-hydroxydopamine and scavenges hydroxyl free radicals *in vitro*. Brain Res 1994;657:207–213.
16. Liu XH, Kato H, Chen T, Kato K, Itoyama Y. Bromocriptine protects against delayed neuronal death of hippocampal neurons following cerebral ischemia in the gerbil. J Neurol Sci 1995;129:9–14.
17. Muralikrishnan D, Mohanakumar KP. Neuroprotection by bromocriptine against 1-methyl-4-phenyl-1,2,3,6-tetrahydropyridine-induced neurotoxicity in mice. FASEB J 1998;12:905–912.
18. Nishibayashi S, Asanuma M, Kohno M et al. Scavenging effects of dopamine agonists on nitric oxide radicals. J Neurochem 1996;67:2208–2211.
19. Felten DL, Felten SY, Fuller RW et al. Chronic dietary pergolide preserves nigrostriatal neuronal integrity in aged-Fischer-344 rats. Neurobiol Aging 1992;13:339–351.
20. Asanuma M, Ogawa N, Nishibayashi S et al. Protective effects of pergolide on dopamine levels in the 6-hydroxydopamine-lesioned mouse brain. Arch Int Pharmacodyn Ther 1995;329:221–230.
21. Gomez-Vargas M, Nishibayashi-Asanuma S, Asanuma M et al. Pergolide scavenges both hydroxyl and nitric oxide free radicals *in vitro* and inhibits lipid peroxidation in different regions of the rat brain. Brain Res 1998;790(1/2):202–208.
22. O'Neill MJ, Hicks CA, Ward MA et al. Dopamine D2 receptor agonists protect against ischaemia-induced hippocampal neurodegeneration in global cerebral ischaemia. Eur J Pharmacol 1998; 352(1):37–46.
23. Zimmerman T, Sage JI. Comparison of combination pergolide and levodopa to levodopa alone after 63 months of treatment. Clin Neuropharmacol 1991;14:165–169.
24. Finotti N, Castagna L, Moretti A, Marzatico F. Reduction of lipid peroxidation in different rat brain areas after cabergoline treatment. Pharmacol Res 2000;42:287–291.
25. Rinne UK, Bracco F, Chouza C et al. Early treatment of Parkinson's disease with cabergoline delays the onset of motor complications: results of a double-blind levodopa controlled trial. The PKDS009 Study Group. Drugs 1998;55(suppl. 1):s23–30.
26. Kondo T, Shimada H, Hatori K, Sugita Y, Mizuno Y. Talipexole protects dopaminergic neurons from methamphetamine toxicity in C57BL/6N mouse. Neurosci Lett 1998;247(2/3):143–146.
27. Kitamura Y, Kakimura J, Taniguchi T. Protective effect of talipexole on MPTP-treated planarian, a unique parkinsonian worm model. Jpn J Pharmacol 1998;78(1):23–29.
28. Carvey PM, Pieri S, Ling ZD. Attenuation of levodopa-induced toxicity in mesencephalic cultures by pramipexole. J Neural Transm 1997;104(2/3):209–228.
29. Le WD, Jankovic J, Xie W, Appel SH. Antioxidant property of pramipexole independent of dopamine receptor activation in neuroprotection. J Neural Transm 2000;107:1165–1173.
30. Kakimura J, Kitamura Y, Takata K et al. Release and aggregation of cytochrome c and alpha-synuclein are inhibited by the antiparkinsonian drugs, talipexole and pramipexole. Eur J Pharmacol 2001;417(1/2):59–67.

31. Kitamura Y, Kosaka T, Kakimura JI et al. Protective effects of the antiparkinsonian drugs talipexole and pramipexole against 1-methyl-4-phenylpyridinium-induced apoptotic death in human neuroblastoma SH-SY5Y. Mol Pharmacol 1998;54:1046–1054.
32. Cassarino DS, Fall CP, Smith TS, Bennett JP. Pramipexole reduces reactive oxygen species production *in vivo* and *in vitro* and inhibits the mitochondrial permeability transition produced by the parkinsonian neurotoxin methylpyridinium ion. J Neurochem 1998;71:295–301.
33. Hall ED, Andrus PK, Oostveen JA et al. Neuroprotective effects of the dopamine D2/D3 agonist pramipexole against postischemic or methamphetamine-induced degeneration of nigrostriatal neurons. Brain Res 1996;742(1/2):80–88.
34. Vu TQ, Ling ZD, Ma SY et al. Pramipexole attenuates the dopaminergic cell loss induced by intraventricular 6-hydroxydopamine. J Neural Transm 2000;107:159–176.
35. Takata K, Kitamura Y, Kakimura J, Kohno Y, Taniguchi T. Increase of bcl-2 protein in neuronal dendritic processes of cerebral cortex and hippocampus by the antiparkinsonian drugs, talipexole and pramipexole. Brain Res 2000;872(1/2):236–241.
36. Zou L, Xu J, Jankovic J et al. Pramipexole inhibits lipid peroxidation and reduces injury in the substantia nigra induced by the dopaminergic neurotoxin 1-methyl-4-phenyl-1,2,3,6-tetrahydropyridine in C57BL/6 mice. Neurosci Lett 2000;281(2/3):167–170.
37. Marek K, Seibyl J, Shoulson I et al., for the Parkinson Study Group. Dopamine transporter brain imaging to assess the effects of pramipexole vs levodopa on Parkinson disease progression. JAMA 2002;287:1653–1661.
38. Parkinson Study Group. Pramipexole vs levodopa as initial treatment for Parkinson's disease: a randomized controlled trial. JAMA 2000;284:1931–1938.
39. Iida M, Miyazaki I, Tanaka K et al. Dopamine D2 receptor-mediated antioxidant and neuroprotective effects of ropinirole, a dopamine agonist. Brain Res 1999;838(1/2):51–59.
40. Whone AL, Remy P, Davis MR et al. The REAL–PET Study: Slower progression in early Parkinson's disease treated with ropinirole compared with L-dopa. Neurology 2002;58 (suppl. 7):82–83 [abstract].
41. Mytilineou C, Cohen G. Deprenyl protects dopamine neurons from the neurotoxic effect of 1-methyl-4-phenylpyridinium ion. J Neurochem 1985;45:1951–1953.
42. Vizuete ML, Steffen V, Ayala A, Cano J, Machado A. Protective effect of deprenyl against 1-methyl-4-phenylpyridinium neurotoxicity in rat striatum. Neurosci Lett 1993;152(1/2):113–116.
43. Tatton WG, Greenwood CE. Rescue of dying neurons: a new action for deprenyl in MPTP parkinsonism. J Neurosci Res 1991;30:666–672.
44. Chiueh CC, Huang SJ, Murphy DL. Enhanced hydroxyl radical generation by 2′-methyl analog of MPTP: suppression by clorgyline and deprenyl. Synapse 1992;11:346–348.
45. Wu RM, Chiueh CC, Pert A, Murphy DL. Apparent antioxidant effect of l-deprenyl on hydroxyl radical formation and nigral injury elicited by MPP^+ *in vivo*. Eur J Pharmacol 1993;243(3):241–247.
46. Wu RM, Chen RC, Chiueh CC. Effect of MAO-B inhibitors on MPP^+ toxicity *in vivo*. Ann N Y Acad Sci 2000;899:255–261.
47. Tatton WG, Ju WY, Holland DP, Tai C, Kwan M. (–)-Deprenyl reduces PC12 cell apoptosis by inducing new protein synthesis. J Neurochem 1994;63:1572–1575.
48. Wadia JS, Chalmers-Redman RM, Ju WJ et al. Mitochondrial membrane potential and nuclear changes in apoptosis caused by serum and nerve growth factor withdrawal: time course and modification by (–)-deprenyl. J Neurosci 1998;18:932–947.
49. Parkinson Study Group. Effect of deprenyl on the progression of disability in early Parkinson's disease. N Engl J Med 1989;321:1364–1371.
50. Parkinson Study Group. Effect of tocopherol and deprenyl on the progression of disability in early Parkinson's disease. N Engl J Med 1993;328:176–183.
51. Parkinson Study Group. Cerebrospinal fluid homovanillic acid in the DATATOP study on Parkinson's disease. Arch Neurol 1995;52:237–245.
52. Miyasaki JM, Martin W, Suchowersky O, Weiner WJ, Lang AE. Practice parameter: initiation of treatment for Parkinson's disease. An evidence-based review. Report of the Quality Standards Subcommittee of the American Academy of Neurology. Neurology 2002;58:11–17.
53. Youdim MB, Wadia A, Tatton W, Weinstock M. The anti-Parkinson drug rasagiline and its cholinesterase inhibitor derivatives exert neuroprotection unrelated to MAO inhibition in cell culture and *in vivo*. Ann N Y Acad Sci 2001;939:450–458.
54. Maruyama W, Takahashi T, Youdim M, Naoi M. The anti-parkinson drug, rasagiline, prevents apoptotic DNA damage induced by peroxynitrite in human dopaminergic neuroblastoma SH-SY5Y cells. J Neural Transm 2002;109:467–481.

55. Simonian NA, Coyle JT. Oxidative stress in neurodegenerative diseases. Annu Rev Pharmacol Toxicol 1996;36:83–106.
56. Kragten E, Lalande I, Zimmermann K et al. Glyceraldehyde-3-phosphate dehydrogenase, the putative target of the antiapoptotic compounds CGP 3466 and R-(-)-deprenyl. J Biol Chem 1998; 273:5821–5828.
57. Waldmeier PC, Spooren WP, Hengerer B. CGP 3466 protects dopaminergic neurons in lesion models of Parkinson's disease. Naunyn Schmiedebergs Arch Pharmacol 2000;362:526–537.
58. Waldmeier PC, Boulton AA, Cools AR, Kato AC, Tatton WG. Neurorescuing effects of the GAPDH ligand CGP 3466B. J Neural Transm 2000;60(suppl.):s197–214.
59. Andringa G, van Oosten RV, Unger W et al. Systemic administration of the propargylamine CGP 3466B prevents behavioural and morphological deficits in rats with 6-hydroxydopamine-induced lesions in the substantia nigra. Eur J Neurosci 2000;12:3033–3043.
60. Hsu LJ, Sagara Y, Arroyo A et al. Alpha-synuclein promotes mitochondrial deficit and oxidative stress. Am J Pathol 2000;157:401–410.
61. Roghani M, Behzadi G. Neuroprotective effect of vitamin E on the early model of Parkinson's disease in rat: behavioral and histochemical evidence. Brain Res 2001;892:211–217.
62. Heim C, Kolasiewicz W, Kurz T, Sontag KH. Behavioral alterations after unilateral 6-hydroxydopamine lesions of the striatum: effect of alpha-tocopherol. Pol J Pharmacol 2001;53(5):435–448.
63. Martinovits G, Melamed E, Cohen O, Rosenthal J, Uzzan A. Systemic administration of antioxidants does not protect mice against the dopaminergic neurotoxicity of 1-methyl-4-phenyl-1,2,5,6-tetrahydropyridine (MPTP). Neurosci Lett 1986;69(2):192–197.
64. Perry TL, Yong VW, Hansen S et al. Alpha-tocopherol and beta-carotene do not protect marmosets against the dopaminergic neurotoxicity of N-methyl-4-phenyl-1,2,3,6-tetrahydropyridine. J Neurol Sci 1987;81(2/3):321–331.
65. Gong L, Daigneault EA, Acuff RV, Kostrzewa RM. Vitamin E supplements fail to protect mice from acute MPTP neurotoxicity. Neuroreport 1991;2:544–546.
66. Vatassery GT, Fahn S, Kuskowski MA. Alpha tocopherol in CSF of subjects taking high-dose vitamin E in the DATATOP study. Parkinson Study Group. Neurology 1998;50:1900–1902.
67. Colton CA, Pagan F, Snell J et al. Protection from oxidation enhances the survival of cultured mesencephalic neurons. Exp Neurol 1995;132:54–61.
68. Kim-Han JS, Sun AY. Protection of PC12 cells glutathione peroxidase in L-dopa-induced cytotoxicity. Free Radic Biol Med 1998;25(4/5):512–518.
69. Klivenyi P, Andreassen OA, Ferrante RJ et al. Mice deficient in cellular glutathione peroxidase show increased vulnerability to malonate, 3-nitropropionic acid, and 1-methyl-4-phenyl-1,2,5,6-tetrahydropyridine. J Neurosci 2000;20:1–7.
70. Steiner JP, Hamilton GS, Ross DT et al. Neurotrophic immunophilin ligands stimulate structural and functional recovery in neurodegenerative animal models. Proc Natl Acad Sci USA 1997;94: 2019–2024.
71. Ross DT, Guo H, Howorth P et al. The small molecule FKBP ligand GPI 1046 induces partial striatal re-innervation after intranigral 6-hydroxydopamine lesion in rats. Neurosci Lett 2001;297(2):113–116.
72. Zhang C, Steiner JP, Hamilton GS, Hicks TP, Poulter MO. Regeneration of dopaminergic function in 6-hydroxydopamine-lesioned rats by neuroimmunophilin ligand treatment. J Neurosci 2001;21(15):RC156.
73. Bocquet A, Lorent G, Fuks B et al. Failure of GPI compounds to display neurotrophic activity *in vitro* and *in vivo*. Eur J Pharmacol 2001;415(2/3):173–180.
74. Emborg ME, Shin P, Roitberg B et al. Systemic administration of the immunophilin ligand GPI 1046 in MPTP-treated monkeys. Exp Neurol 2001;168:171–182.
75. Teismann P, Ferger B. Inhibition of the cyclooxygenase isoenzymes COX-1 and COX-2 provide neuroprotection in the MPTP-mouse model of Parkinson's disease. Synapse 2001;39:167–174.
76. Svenningsson P, Le Moine C, Fisone G, Fredholm BB. Distribution, biochemistry and function of striatal adenosine A2A receptors. Prog Neurobiol 1999;59:355–396.
77. Kurokawa M, Koga K, Kase H, Nakamura J, Kuwana Y. Adenosine A2a receptor-mediated modulation of striatal acetylcholine release *in vivo*. J Neurochem 1996;66:1882–1888.
78. Mori A, Shindou T, Ichimura M, Nonaka H, Kase H. The role of adenosine A2a receptors in regulating GABAergic synaptic transmission in striatal medium spiny neurons. J Neurosci 1996;16: 605–611.
79. Ochi M, Koga K, Kurokawa M et al. Systemic administration of adenosine A2A receptor antagonist reverses increased GABA release in the globus pallidus of unilateral 6-hydroxydopamine-lesioned rats: a microdialysis study. Neuroscience 2000;100:53–62.

80. Ikeda K, Kurokawa M, Aoyama S, Kuwana Y. Neuroprotection by adenosine A2A receptor blockade in experimental models of Parkinson's disease. J Neurochem 2002;80:262–270.
81. Fredholm BB, Battig K, Holmen J, Nehlg A, Zvartau EE. Actions of the caffeine with the brain with special reference to factors that contribute to its widespread use. Pharmacol Rev 1999; 51:83–133.
82. Xu K, Xu YH, Chen JF, Schwarzschild MA. Caffeine's neuroprotection against 1-methyl-4-phenyl-1,2,3,6-tetrahydropyridine toxicity shows no tolerance to chronic caffeine administration in mice. Neurosci Lett 2002;322(1):13–16.
83. Chen JF, Xu K, Petzer JP et al. Neuroprotection by caffeine and A(2A) adenosine receptor inactivation in a model of Parkinson's disease. J Neurosci 2001;21(10):RC143.
84. Casas M, Prat G, Robledo P et al. Repeated co-administration of caffeine and bromocriptine prevents tolerance to the effects of caffeine in the turning behavior animal model. Eur Neuropsychopharmacol 1999;9:515–521.
85. Hellenbrand W, Seidler A, Boeing H et al. Diet and Parkinson's disease. I: A possible role for the past intake of specific foods and food groups. Results from a self-administered food-frequency questionnaire in a case–control study. Neurology 1996;47:636–643.
86. Ross GW, Abbott RD, Petrovitch H et al. Association of coffee and caffeine intake with the risk of Parkinson's disease. JAMA 2000;283:2674–2679.
87. Ascherio A, Zhang SM, Hernan MA et al. Prospective study of caffeine consumption and risk of Parkinson's disease in men and women. Ann Neurol 2001;50:56–63.
88. Checkoway H, Powers K, Smith-Weller T et al. Parkinson's disease risks associated with cigarette smoking, alcohol consumption, and caffeine intake. Am J Epidemiol 2002;155:732–738.
89. Weller M, Finiels-Marlier F, Paul SM. NMDA receptor-mediated glutamate toxicity of cultured cerebellar, cortical and mesencephalic neurons: neuroprotective properties of amantadine and memantine. Brain Res 1993;613:143–148.
90. Wenk GL, Danysz W, Mobley SL. MK-801, memantine and amantadine show neuroprotective activity in the nucleus basalis magnocellularis. Eur J Pharmacol 1995;293(3):267–270.
91. Lin LF, Doherty DH, Lile JD, Bektesh S, Collins F. GDNF: a glial cell line-derived neurotrophic factor for midbrain dopaminergic neurons. Science 1993;260:1130–1132.
92. Hou JG, Lin LF, Mytilineou C. Glial cell line-derived neurotrophic factor exerts neurotrophic effects on dopaminergic neurons *in vitro* and promotes their survival and regrowth after damage by 1-methyl-4-phenylpyridinium. J Neurochem 1996;66:74–82.
93. Beck KD, Valverde J, Alexi T et al. Mesencephalic dopaminergic neurons protected by GDNF from axotomy-induced degeneration in the adult brain. Nature 1995;373:339–341.
94. Tomac A, Lindqvist E, Lin LF et al. Protection and repair of the nigrostriatal dopaminergic system by GDNF *in vivo*. Nature 1995;373:335–339.
95. Arenas E, Trupp M, Akerud P, Ibanez CF. GDNF prevents degeneration and promotes the phenotype of brain noradrenergic neurons *in vivo*. Neuron 1995;15:1465–1473.
96. Tseng JL, Baetge EE, Zurn AD, Aebischer P. GDNF reduces drug-induced rotational behavior after medial forebrain bundle transection by a mechanism not involving striatal dopamine. J Neurosci 1997;17:325–333.
97. Choi-Lundberg DL, Lin Q, Chang YN et al. Dopaminergic neurons protected from degeneration by GDNF gene therapy. Science 1997;275:838–841.
98. Bilang-Bleuel A, Revah F, Colin P et al. Intrastriatal injection of an adenoviral vector expressing glial-cell-line-derived neurotrophic factor prevents dopaminergic neuron degeneration and behavioral impairment in a rat model of Parkinson disease. Proc Natl Acad Sci USA 1997;94:8818–8823.
99. Mandel RJ, Spratt SK, Snyder RO, Leff SE. Midbrain injection of recombinant adeno-associated virus encoding rat glial cell line-derived neurotrophic factor protects nigral neurons in a progressive 6-hydroxydopamine-induced degeneration model of Parkinson's disease in rats. Proc Natl Acad Sci USA 1997;94:14083–14088.
100. Kirik D, Rosenblad C, Bjorklund A, Mandel RJ. Long-term rAAV-mediated gene transfer of GDNF in the rat Parkinson's model: intrastriatal but not intranigral transduction promotes functional regeneration in the lesioned nigrostriatal system. J Neurosci 2000;20:4686–4700.
101. Wang L, Muramatsu S, Lu Y et al. Delayed delivery of AAV-GDNF prevents nigral neurodegeneration and promotes functional recovery in a rat model of Parkinson's disease. Gene Ther 2002; 9:381–389.
102. Gash DM, Zhang Z, Ovadia A et al. Functional recovery in parkinsonian monkeys treated with GDNF. Nature 1996;380:252–255.

103. Kordower JH, Emborg ME, Bloch J et al. Neurodegeneration prevented by lentiviral vector delivery of GDNF in primate models of Parkinson's disease. Science 2000;290:767–773.
104. Kordower JH, Palfi S, Chen EY et al. Clinicopathological findings following intraventricular glial-derived neurotrophic factor treatment in a patient with Parkinson's disease. Ann Neurol 1999;46:419–424.
105. Hyman C, Hofer M, Barde YA et al. BDNF is a neurotrophic factor for dopaminergic neurons of the substantia nigra. Nature 1991;350:230–232.
106. Beck KD, Knusel B, Winslow JW et al. Pretreatment of dopaminergic neurons in culture with brain-derived neurotrophic factor attenuates toxicity of 1-methyl-4-phenylpyridinium. Neurodegeneration 1992;1:27–36.
107. Spina MB, Squinto SP, Miller J, Lindsay RM, Hyman C. Brain-derived neurotrophic factor protects dopamine neurons against 6-hydroxydopamine and N-methyl-4-phenylpyridinium ion toxicity: involvement of the glutathione system. J Neurochem 1992;59:99–106.
108. Frim DM, Uhler TA, Galpern WR et al. Implanted fibroblasts genetically engineered to produce brain-derived neurotrophic factor prevent 1-methyl-4-phenylpyridinium toxicity to dopaminergic neurons in the rat. Proc Natl Acad Sci USA 1994;91:5104–5108.
109. Tsukahara T, Takeda M, Shimohama S, Ohara O, Hashimoto N. Effects of brain-derived neurotrophic factor on 1-methyl-4-phenyl-1,2,3,6-tetrahydropyridine-induced parkinsonism in monkeys. Neurosurgery 1995;37:733–739.
110. Levivier M, Przedborski S, Bencsics C, Kang UJ. Intrastriatal implantation of fibroblasts genetically engineered to produce brain-derived neurotrophic factor prevents degeneration of dopaminergic neurons in a rat model of Parkinson's disease. J Neurosci 1995;15:7810–7820.
111. Vucic D, Kaiser WJ, Harvey AJ, Miller LK. Inhibition of reaper-induced apoptosis by interaction with inhibitor of apoptosis proteins (IAPs). Proc Natl Acad Sci USA 1997;16:10183–10188.
112. Simon PD, Vorwerk CK, Mansukani SS et al. Bcl-2 gene therapy exacerbates excitotoxicity. Hum Gene Ther 1999;10:1715–1720.
113. Eberhardt O, Coelln RV, Kugler S et al. Protection by synergistic effects of adenovirus-mediated X-chromosome-linked inhibitor of apoptosis and glial cell line-derived neurotrophic factor gene transfer in the 1-methyl-4-phenyl-1,2,3,6-tetrahydropyridine model of Parkinson's disease. J Neurosci 2000;20:9126–9134.
114. McKinnon SJ, Lehman DM, Tahzib NG et al. Baculoviral IAP repeat-containing-4 protects optic nerve axons in a rat glaucoma model. Mol Ther 2002;5:780–787.
115. Garcia I, Martinou I, Tsujimoto Y, Martinou JC. Prevention of programmed cell death of sympathetic neurons by the bcl-2 proto-oncogene. Science 1992;258:302–304.
116. Allsopp TE, Wyatt S, Paterson HF, Davies AM. The proto-oncogene bcl-2 can selectively rescue neurotrophic factor-dependent neurons from apoptosis. Cell 1993;73:295–307.
117. Offen D, Ziv I, Panet H et al. Dopamine-induced apoptosis is inhibited in PC12 cells expressing bcl-2. Cell Mol Neurobiol 1997;17:289–304.
118. Azzouz M, Hottinger A, Paterna JC et al. Increased motoneuron survival and improved neuromuscular function in transgenic ALS mice after intraspinal injection of an adeno-associated virus encoding bcl-2. Hum Mol Genet 2000;9:803–811.
119. Yamada M, Natsume A, Mata M et al. Herpes simplex virus vector-mediated expression of bcl-2 protects spinal motor neurons from degeneration following root avulsion. Exp Neurol 2001;168:225–230.
120. Blömer U, Kafri T, Randolph-Moore L et al. Bcl-xL protects adult septal cholinergic neurons from axotomized cell death. Proc Natl Acad Sci USA 1998;95:2603–2608.
121. Qin H, Srinivasula SM, Wu G et al. Structural basis of procaspase-9 recruitment by the apoptotic protease-activating factor 1. Nature 1999;399:549–557.
122. Mochizuki H, Hayakawa H, Migita M et al. An AAV-derived Apaf-1 dominant negative inhibitor prevents MPTP toxicity as antiapoptotic gene therapy for Parkinson's disease. Proc Natl Acad Sci USA 2001;98:10918–10923.
123. Sawada H, Ibi M, Kihara T et al. Estradiol protects mesencephalic dopaminergic neurons from oxidative stress-induced neuronal death. J Neurosci Res 1998;54:707–719.
124. Singer CA, Figueroa-Masot XA, Batchelor RH et al. The mitogen-activated protein kinase pathway mediates estrogen neuroprotection after glutamate toxicity in primary cortical neurons. J Neurosci 1999;19:2455–2463.
125. Sawada H, Ibi M, Kihara T et al. Estradiol protects dopaminergic neurons in a MPP(+) Parkinson's disease model. Neuropharmacology 2002;42:1056–1064.

126. Callier S, Morissette M, Grandbois M, Pelaprat D, Di Paolo T. Neuroprotective properties of 17beta-estradiol, progesterone, and raloxifene in MPTP C57Bl/6 mice. Synapse 2001;41:131–138.
127. Dubal DB, Shughrue PJ, Wilson ME et al. Estradiol modulates bcl-2 in cerebral ischemia: a potential role for estrogen receptors. J Neurosci 1999;19:6385–6393.
128. Levites Y, Amit T, Youdim MB, Mandel S. Involvement of protein kinase C activation and cell survival/cell cycle genes in green tea polyphenol, (–)-epigallocatechin-3-gallate neuroprotective action. J Biol Chem 2002;277:30574–30580.
129. Levites Y, Weinreb O, Maor G, Youdim MB, Mandel S. Green tea polyphenol (-)-epigallocatechin-3-gallate prevents N-methyl-4-phenyl-1,2,3,6-tetrahydropyridine-induced dopaminergic neurodegeneration. J Neurochem 2001;78:1073–1082.
130. Ferger B, Spratt C, Earl CD et al. Effects of nicotine on hydroxyl free radical formation *in vitro* and on MPTP-induced neurotoxicity *in vivo*. Naunyn Schmiedebergs Arch Pharmacol 1998;358:351–359.
131. Maggio R, Riva M, Vaglini F et al. Striatal increase of neurotrophic factors as a mechanism of nicotine protection in experimental parkinsonism. J Neural Transm 1997;104:1113–1123.
132. Costa G, Abin-Carriquiry JA, Dajas F. Nicotine prevents striatal dopamine loss produced by 6-hydroxydopamine lesion in the substantia nigra. Brain Res 2001;888:336–342.
133. Gorell JM, Rybicki BA, Johnson CC, Peterson EL. Smoking and Parkinson's disease: a dose–response relationship. Neurology 1999;52:115–119.
134. Fowler JS, Volkow ND, Wang GJ et al. Inhibition of monoamine oxidase B in the brains of smokers. Nature 1996;379:733–736.
135. Haack DG, Baumann RJ, McKean HE, Jameson HD, Turbek JA. Nicotine exposure and Parkinson's disease. Am J Epidemiol 1981;114:191–200.
136. Behmand RA, Harik SI. Nicotine enhances 1-methyl-4-phenyl-1,2,3,6-tetrahydropyridine neurotoxicity. J Neurochem 1992;58:776–779.

SECTION 7

PHYSICAL THERAPIES IN PARKINSON'S DISEASE

14
Physical Therapy in Parkinson's Disease

Mara Lugassy and Jean-Michel Gracies

INTRODUCTION

The movement disturbances characteristic of Parkinson's disease (PD), such as hypometria, bradykinesia, rigidity, and disturbed postural control, can have a significant impact on functioning and quality of life. Typical functional difficulties resulting from these motor impairments range from dressing or rising from a chair to maintaining balance and initiating gait.[1,2] Since the emergence of levodopa in the late 1960s, pharmacological therapy has been the primary management strategy of these symptoms. However, medication regimens are unable to completely control the disease in the long term, because dyskinesias, fluctuations of the medication's efficacy, and cognitive difficulties invariably occur after a number of years.[3] Over the past decades, there has been increasing awareness as to the potential role of physical therapy, and investigations have been carried out to evaluate techniques that may alleviate the main functional disabilities of patients with PD. Despite this expanded interest, surveys show that only 3–29% of PD patients regularly consult with a paramedical therapist, such as a physical, occupational, or speech therapist.[4]

A large variety of physical therapy methods have been evaluated in PD. The approach to therapy in an individual patient may be governed at the most basic level by the stage of the disease. In individuals with mild to moderate disease, who are ambulatory and have retained a certain degree of physical independence, therapy may focus on the *teaching of exercises* directly designed to delay or prevent the aggravation of the motor impairment in PD, with the goal of maintaining or even increasing functional capacities. At the other end of the spectrum, in an individual with compromised ambulation and significant disability due to advanced PD, the therapeutic focus may shift from the teaching of exercises to the *teaching of compensation strategies* allowing preservation of as much functional independence as possible. These strategies include adaptation of the home environment, both to lessen the effects of impairment and to optimize safety.

Most studies investigating physical exercises have been carried out in subjects with mild to moderate PD – that is, up to Hoehn and Yahr stage 3.[5–10] This chapter first covers mild to moderate PD, before considering procedures for advanced stages of PD.

SHORT-TERM EFFECTS OF PHYSICAL EXERCISES ON DOPAMINE METABOLISM

Exercise intensity may affect dopaminergic metabolism in PD. In unmedicated PD patients, one hour of strenuous walking reduces the dopamine transporter availability in the medial striatum (caudate) and in the mesocortical dopaminergic system – as measured using positron emission tomography (PET) scans – which has been considered highly suggestive of increased endogenous dopamine release.[11] In addition, exogenous levodopa seems to be better absorbed during moderate-intensity endurance exercise, as measured using maximal levodopa concentrations in plasma.[12]

The beneficial effect of exercise on the dopamine metabolism in PD patients has been recently supported by two compelling studies in animal models. Rodents with unilateral depletion of striatal dopamine display a marked preferential use of the ipsilateral forelimb. After casting of the unaffected forelimb in unilaterally 6-hydroxy dopamine (6-OHDA)-lesioned rats, the enforced use of the affected forelimb spares its function as well as the dopamine remaining in the lesioned striatum.[13] There was a negative correlation in this study between the time from lesion to immobilization (i.e. to enforced use), and the degree of behavioral and neurochemical sparing. This may suggest the importance of initiating an exercise regimen early in the course of PD. In another recent study in which rats were exposed to either MPTP or 6-OHDA to induce behavioral and neurochemical loss analogous to the situation in PD, the animals that were exercised on a treadmill for 10 days post-lesion demonstrated no behavioral deficits, and showed significant sparing of striatal dopamine, its metabolites, and dopamine transporter levels, compared to lesioned animals that had remained sedentary.[14]

TRAINING TECHNIQUES

Several types of exercise techniques have been evaluated with regard to their impact on motor deficits in mild to moderate PD. Few studies have been controlled, and much of the evidence is anecdotal or relies on open trials. The strongest line of evidence to date supports the benefit of lower-limb resistance training in PD patients, particularly for balance and gait.

Resistance Training

The majority of PD patients experience balance disturbances and increased risk of falls in the course of their illness,[15] and a major goal of physical therapy should be the improvement of postural control and the prevention of falls.[16] In a recent open-label study, 40 PD patients at Hoehn and Yahr stage 3 and 20 healthy age-matched controls underwent a 30-day program comprising a variety of physical therapies including regular physical activity, aerobic strengthening, muscle positioning and lengthening exercises.[17] Physical therapy resulted in significant improvement in tandem stance, one-leg stance, and step test – all tests of balance – in the PD group.

Important risk factors for falls in PD are the muscle atrophy and the decrease in physical conditioning that may result from activity reduction.[18] There is a proven relationship between decreased lower-limb muscle strength and impaired balance in PD, as muscle weakness in the lower extremities may limit the ability to mount appropriate postural adjustments when balance is challenged.[19] A controlled study addressed the effects of lower-limb resistance training in PD, in which patients were randomized to two groups. The first group underwent 30-minute sessions, three times a week for 10 weeks, of standard balance rehabilitation exercises including practicing standing on foam and weight-shifting exercises. The second group underwent the same balance training, and in addition received tri-weekly high intensity resistance training sessions focusing on plantar flexion, as well as knee extension and flexion. Subjects who received balance training increased their lower-extremity strength (composite score from knee extensor, flexor and plantar flexor strength) by only 9%, while subjects who underwent additional resistance training increased their strength by 52%. Balance training merely increased the subjects' ability to maintain balance. This effect was significantly greater and lasted longer in the group undergoing additional lower-limb resistance training.[10]

Improvement in lower-limb muscle strength in PD may also improve gait. In an open protocol, 14 PD patients and 6 normal controls underwent an 8-week course of resistance training, twice a week, with exercises including leg press, calf raise, leg curl, leg extension, and abdominal crunches. Lower-limb strength and gait were assessed in the practically defined levodopa "off" state (i.e. off medication for at least 12 hours) before and after the training period, showing gains in strength in the PD patients that were similar to those of the control subjects, and improvement on quantitative measures of gait such as stride length, gait velocity, and postural angles.[18]

Attentional Strategies and Sensory Cueing

It is a common clinical observation that increased attention or effort may allow improvements of remarkable magnitude in motor tasks performed by PD patients.[20] This observation has contributed to the development of cueing, an increasingly prevalent concept in the field of physical therapy in PD, in which external visual or auditory cues are used to enhance performance. It has been hypothesized that the basal ganglia, which normally discharge in bursts during the preparation of well-learned motor sequences, provide phasic cues to the supplementary motor area, activating and deactivating the cortical subunits corresponding to a given motor sequence.[2] In PD, the internal cues provided by the basal ganglia are no longer appropriately supplied. Thus, restoration of phasic activation of the premotor cortex might be facilitated by external means.

Auditory Cueing

Use of auditory cueing has gained popularity over the past decade.[21] Experimental conditions involving the use of auditory cues for button-pressing tasks have shown that added external auditory information dramatically reduces initiation and execution time and improves motor sequencing.[22,23] In the clinical setting, auditory cueing is most often used in the form of rhythmic auditory stimulation (RAS) during gait, in which patients pace their walking to either a metronome beat or a rhythmic beat embedded in music. PD patients using such rhythmic cues set at rates of 107.5% and 115% of their baseline walking cadence are able to correspondingly increase the cadence and mean velocity of their gait.[24]

A study of a 3-week home-based gait-training program revealed that PD patients trained with RAS in the form of metronome pulsed patterns embedded into the beat structure of music improved gait velocity, stride length, and step cadence compared to subjects receiving gait training without RAS or no gait training at all.[25] Additional research indicated that these gait improvements occur regardless of whether the patient is on or off medication at the time of training.[26]

Combination of Auditory Cueing with Attentional Strategies

Auditory cueing may also be involved in attentional strategies such as the use of verbal instruction sets. In one controlled study in PD, gait was analyzed during trials of natural walking interspersed with randomized conditions in which subjects were verbally instructed to increase either arm swing, or step size, or walking speed. In addition to being able to improve any of these variables in response to specific instructions, hearing only one of these instructions was associated with an improvement in the other gait variables as well.[27]

Visual Cueing

Since the classic experiments by Martin,[28] a number of studies have shown that stride length can be improved by visual cueing, in the form of horizontal lines marked on the floor, which the patient is encouraged to step over. In a series of experiments, Morris et al.[29] demonstrated that PD patients using such horizontal floor markers as visual cues were able to normalize their stride length, velocity and cadence, an effect that persisted for two hours after the intervention. It was noted that while transverse lines of a color contrasting to the floor and separated by an appropriate width are effective for this purpose, zig-zag lines or lines parallel to the walking direction are not. These visual cues might function by supplying a now deficient well-learned motor program in providing external visual information on the appropriate stride length.[21] Similar improvement in stride length and gait velocity are possible using sensory mounted light devices attached to the chest to provide a visual stimulus on the floor over which the patient must step.[30] However, such sensory mounted light devices increase attentional demand and perceived effort of walking, which suggest that static cues are more effective in improving gait while minimizing effort. Finally, there are suggestions that benefit from cueing techniques might be optimal in earlier stages of the disease.[30]

Combination of Visual Cueing with Attentional Strategies

Gait improvement also occurs when, instead of using horizontal markers on the floor, an attentional strategy is used with instructions to simply visualize the length of stride that subjects should take while walking.[29] Whether gait is assisted by direct visual cueing or by such attentional visualization strategy, the benefit is reversed when patients are given additional tasks to do while walking, distracting attention from the gait.[29] Thus, direct visual cues and visualization exercises may both function by focusing *attention* on the gait, such that walking ceases to be a primarily automatic task delegated to the deficient basal ganglia.[29]

Active Mobilization and Stretch

In an open study, 20 PD patients underwent hour-long bi-weekly rehabilitation sessions over the course of 5 weeks, including active mobilization exercises of the trunk, lower limbs, and spinal segments, with the goal of improving movement coordination and avoiding postural disturbances.[31] At the end of the training period, subjects showed improvement in transfers from supine to sitting, sitting to supine, supine rolling, and rising from a chair. Axial mobility may also affect function in PD. There is a significant association between reduced axial rotation and functional reach (maximal reach without taking a step forward) independent of disease state.[32] A controlled study confirmed that physical intervention targeted on improving spinal flexibility improves functional reach in PD.[33]

It has been hypothesized that muscle stiffness alone may be a factor of functional impairment in PD, particularly in the lower limb with respect to shortened stride length and altered gait pattern.[30] Aggressive stretch programs might have the propensity to decrease muscle stiffness. However, stretch alone as a therapy technique has not been systematically evaluated as a method to improve motor function in PD. In one controlled study in which passive stretch was a component of a standard therapy including other motor tasks and balance training, an improvement in rigidity was observed as compared to baseline. This effect had disappeared 2 months after study completion, which suggests that standard therapy programs should probably be continued in the long term, or at least repeated frequently.[34]

Treadmill Training

Treadmill training has been increasingly used in the rehabilitation of patients with spinal cord injury, hemiparesis, and other gait disorders.[35] However, the literature on treadmill training in PD must be analyzed with caution. Some studies have recently suggested that treadmill training might increase walking speed and stride length in PD.[36–38] However, while these studies compared treadmill with non-treadmill training, they were not controlled for the walking speed used in the training. In particular, the non-treadmill training did not involve specific requirements of gait velocity, step cadence, or stride length. Under these circumstances, the positive effects seen after treadmill use may have been the effects of a higher energy, or a higher walking speed used on the treadmill training.

Further, it was demonstrated earlier that, in healthy subjects, walking on a treadmill results in smaller steps than when walking on the ground at the same speed.[39] This finding is particularly relevant to the PD patient population, in which decreased stride length is a fundamental characteristic. In a study which did control for walking speed by having subjects walk first on the ground and then on a treadmill set at the same speed, both PD patients and age-matched controls showed higher stride frequency and shorter stride lengths in the treadmill condition.[40] These effects were more pronounced in the PD patients. Thus, the typical pathological gait characteristics of PD may be accentuated when walking on a treadmill.[40]

Long-term Effects of Physical Therapy

The exact duration of the effects of programs of physical exercise in PD remains unknown. Open studies have reported motor improvements lasting 6 weeks to 6 months after physical therapy was discontinued.[7,41,42] This might underscore the importance of physical therapy not as one event limited in time, but as a continuous or repetitive effort, so that its benefits might be maintained and perhaps accumulated and strengthened over time.

Other benefits from exercise in PD have been suggested, involving in particular an increased sense of wellbeing and an improved quality of life.[41] An observational study reported that mortality was higher by a hazard ratio of 1.8 amongst PD patients who did not exercise regularly compared with patients who did.[6] However, the odds ratios were not adjusted for major health factors, such as cardiovascular disease, lung disease, smoking, or obesity.

Long-term Effects of Cueing

In addition to having greater effects on motor function than physical therapy without cueing,[25,26] the use of cueing may extend the duration of the effects of therapy. In a single-blind prospective study, 20 PD patients were randomized to two physical therapy groups.[9] The first group underwent a 6-week program of posture control exercises, passive and active stretching, and walking exercises, while the second group combined the same regimen with a variety of visual, auditory, and proprioceptive cueing techniques. Although both groups showed improvement on activities of daily living and motor ability (UPDRS) at the end of the program, the group without sensory cue training had returned to baseline at a 6-week follow-up, while the group trained with cueing techniques was still improved at that visit. While it remains uncertain whether all the involved types of sensory cueing or only specific types were associated with this benefit, the learning of new motor strategies associated with cueing may have caused the lasting improvement.[9]

Emotional Arousal, Group Therapy, and Use of Motivational Processes

Attempts at increasing cortical excitability in PD have involved, in addition to external sensory inputs, the use of emotional arousal. Pacchetti and colleagues compared standard physical therapy (passive stretching exercises, motor tasks, gait and balance training) with music therapy, involving choral singing, voice exercises, and rhythmic and free body expression, both administered in weekly group sessions in a randomized, prospective controlled study.[34] The improvement of bradykinesia, emotional wellbeing, activities of daily living, and quality-of-life scores was greater in the music therapy group, while rigidity was the only measure that was more improved in the standard physical therapy group. These effects dissipated at a 2-month follow-up. The improvement in bradykinesia associated with music therapy may have resulted from external rhythmic cues or from the affective arousal induced by the music, influencing motivational processes.[34]

In that study, training, both in the physical therapy and music therapy arms, occurred in a group setting. It has been theorized that physical therapy in group sessions might enhance socialization and motivation, but group therapy has not been systematically compared with individual therapy, and group therapy studies have not been controlled. In their study, Pachetti and colleagues did not observe any increase in emotional function or quality of life in the standard physical therapy group.[34] In open studies of group physical therapy in PD, subjects have reported subjective impressions of benefit in motor symptoms and quality of life, but there was no improvement in quantitative measures of motor function.[43,44]

RECOMMENDATIONS FOR PHYSICAL EXERCISE IN MILD TO MODERATE PD

Schedule

While most protocols of the literature have involved supervised exercise sessions one to three times per week,[4] we recommend that exercise schedule be intensified and expanded from organized physical therapy sessions into a daily event, with a time window (1–1.5 hours) consistently devoted to this activity every day. Controlled studies have indeed demonstrated that PD patients can improve performance on complex motor tasks with intense repeated practice – an effect that persists days after the practice trials have ended.[45,46] Similar principles of repetition can be applied to daily physical exercise.

It has been suggested that such exercises should be performed during the levodopa "on" state, in order to optimize their execution.[15] However, this is not supported by evidence, and the opposite strategy may also be suggested; i.e. the performance of physical exercises during the early-morning "off" phase for example, which might improve dopamine availability and possibly delay the need for the first daily pill.[11,12] Finally, for exercises to be effectively replicated at home, it is probably optimal to teach them as early as possible in the course of the disease.

Types of Exercises

We recommend alternating between two types of exercises in a practice session of a patient with mild to moderate PD: *active* exercises, consisting of series of light-resistance rapid alternating movements, and *passive* exercises, consisting of periods of limb and trunk posturing, achieving passive stretch as well as cardiorespiratory rest.

Upper Body

In the upper body, the phasic light-resistance exercises may involve lightweight lifting, particularly focusing on strengthening shoulder abductors and shoulder flexors, as these exercises also involve the spinal extensors, which are typically hypoactive in PD (Figure 14.1). These active exercises should enhance activity of the spinal extensors and thus improve the stooped posture typical of PD. In contrast, stretching postures should focus on stretching the muscle groups that tend to "close" the body: horizontal and vertical adductors at the shoulder, flexors and pronators at the elbow, flexors at the wrist and fingers.

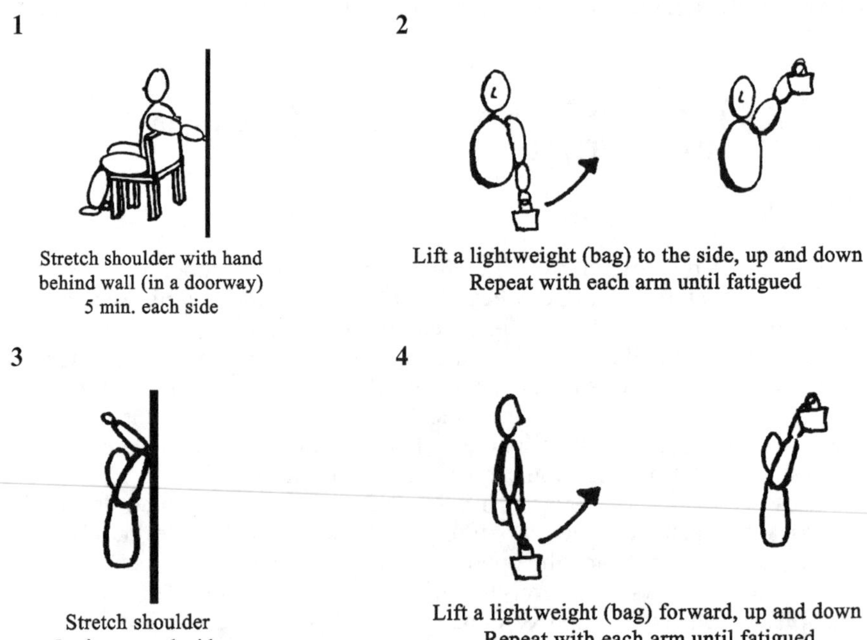

FIGURE 14.1 Stretches and exercises for the upper body.

Each series of lightweight lifting should be pursued for about a minute, whereas each stretching posture should be maintained for about 5–10 minutes (3–5 minutes on each side).

Lower Body

In the lower body, passive exercises should again focus on the muscles that tend to adopt a shortened position in PD, particularly the hamstrings and the hip adductors. The active exercises should primarily focus on sit-to-stand and walking practice (Figure 14.2).

- *Sit-to-stand*: Patients should repeat a series of sit-to-stand exercises every day, ideally as many as possible in a continuous series. This should lead to hip and knee extensor strengthening, which may improve sit-to-stand ability and walking balance.
- *Walking*: Patients should not focus on the speed achieved while walking but on their stride length. Ideally the patient selects a specific distance that should be covered every day, and counts the steps taken to walk that distance. Each day, the patient should try to walk the same distance with as few steps as possible. When stride length improvement over that distance is maximized (i.e. the number of steps taken cannot be further improved), the same process should be restarted on a new, longer distance.

In terms of walking in conditions other than a flat ground, treadmill walking versus walking in swimming pool have not been compared in controlled studies,

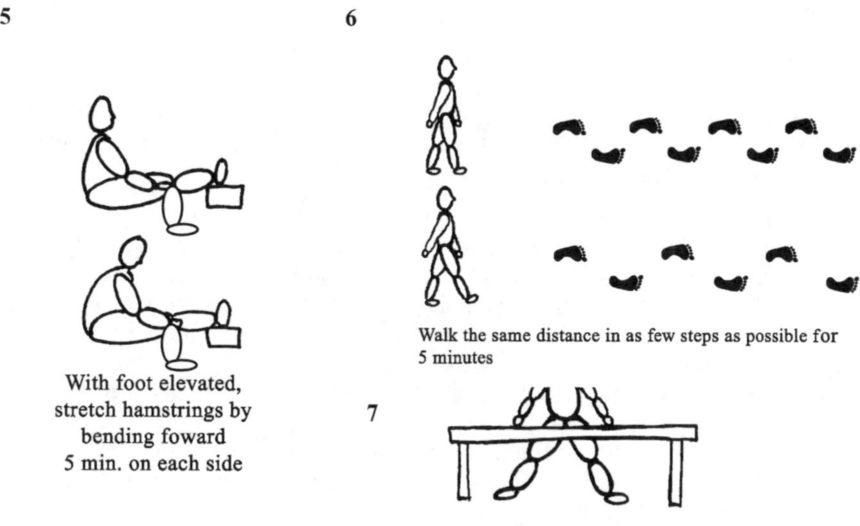

FIGURE 14.2 Stretches and exercises for the lower body.

but we would hypothesize that walking against the viscous resistance of water should maximize work on hip flexion and ankle push-off, and thus better improve stride length than work on a treadmill, which might lead to opposite results.

COMPENSATION STRATEGIES IN ADVANCED STAGES OF PD

The Role of Discipline

As PD progresses and motor function deteriorates, patients become significantly less mobile, and therefore less able to perform daily self-initiated exercises such as active movements against resistance and walking. While the goal of physical therapy remains to optimize functional independence, the method gradually shifts towards teaching strategies to patients and caregivers to compensate for worsening motor impairments. Omitting some of these strategies may jeopardize activities such as walking or swallowing, with potentially serious consequences. The emphasis on a strict patient *discipline* thus becomes even more important than in the early stages, as the patient must now consistently apply the compensation strategies learned in therapy.

One fundamental compensatory strategy in advanced PD involves increasing the amount of attention and effort the patient directs toward any given activity. Motor activities such as walking, talking, writing, and standing up are no longer automatic, and should no longer be taken for granted. The individual with advanced PD must learn to *want* to do each of these activities and actively concentrate on them, possibly even to mentally rehearse them as a new task each time, as opposed to just *doing them*. This corresponds to a major change in daily functioning. Such change can be achieved only with a clear understanding by the therapist and/or the caregiver of:

- the fundamental difference between automatic and consciously controlled movements
- the need to succeed in having patients switch to conscious movement control for virtually all daily motor activities, particularly those that healthy subjects view as the most natural.

We develop examples of these changes in daily strategies below.

However, teaching and maintaining such discipline can become a highly challenging proposition in advanced PD, depending on the presence of depression, on mental deterioration (impairment in memory and in executive functions), and on the motivation of the patient to improve his or her own quality of life.[47] Depression is a common feature of PD particularly in advanced stages[47,48] and is characterized by hopelessness, pessimism, as well as decreased motivation and drive.[49] This may undermine the motivation to practice or to change daily living strategies. Apathy and abulia (lack of drive and initiative) can also be prominent symptoms in PD, independent of depression, and occur with greater frequency than in patients of similar disability level from other causes.[50] In these cases, the caregiver should become the primary object of the teaching and the person responsible for applying the discipline of the various compensation strategies.

Strategies for Freezing Episodes

In advanced PD, episodes of freezing, characterized by a blockade of motor activity especially when encountering obstacles or constricted spaces, can constitute a significant problem, occurring in up to one-third of patients.[51] Management may consist primarily of behavioral strategies. As mentioned in the previous section, one can teach the patient how to substitute external auditory, visual, or proprioceptive cues to replace the deficient internal motor cues normally provided by the basal ganglia.[1] Specific attentional strategies might also be useful (see below).

Sensory Cues

Several techniques have been used to alleviate freezing episodes through external visual input. Visual markers can be placed in the home in areas where freezing episodes are common, such as doorways and narrow hallways. These may include horizontal markers on the floor over which the individual is instructed to step, or a dot on the wall on which the patient is instructed to focus in the event of freezing. If the patient is accompanied, the other person may place a foot in front of the patient, which the patient then steps over.[1] Inverted walking sticks, with the handle used as a horizontal visual cue at the level of the foot, have also been investigated as a potential means to improve freezing.[52] Results have been inconsistent, with some subjects showing worsening of freezing while using such walking stick, and others showing improvement.[5,52] Additionally, caution must be used with inverted sticks in PD patients, as these sticks may cause tripping and increase the risk of falls.[52]

Acoustic cues can be used to decrease freezing. PD patients may carry a metronome, which can be switched on during a freezing episode to emit an auditory beat. Such external cues may be sufficient to initiate movement.

Attentional Strategies

A number of changes in motor behavior have been suggested to potentially alleviate freezing episodes when they occur. These include:

- focusing on swaying from side to side, transferring the bodyweight from one leg to the other[1]
- singing, whistling, loudly saying "go" or "left, right, left right," clapping, or saying a rhyme and stepping off at the last word (behavioral strategies that have the additional advantage of generating auditory cues)[1]
- cue cards posted on the walls of freezing-prone areas, with instructions such as "go" or "large step"[1]
- the one-step-only technique (distraction from the functional or social goal).

Success with a method using a deep-breathing relaxation technique has been noted in a patient who had failed several other techniques to reduce freezing episodes.[53]

It is often noted that, during an episode of freezing, the more the patient worries about the functional end-goal of walking (freeing the elevator entry for other people to come out, moving out of a crowded store through a narrow exit, entering the doctor's office, etc.), the more difficult it may become to do so, particularly as others may look on. The emotional stress associated with the social function of walking in these situations makes the freezing episode worse. At the Mount Sinai Movement Disorders Clinic we attempt to have the patient disconnect for a short while from the social and functional goal of walking forward again, to instead focus analytically on the walking technique. Walking is normally a smooth succession of steps. The patient is asked to focus only on achieving one elementary unit of walking – one step only. One single step should not have any significant social role, as it is usually not sufficient to enter or exit a crowded place.

In practice, the first stage is to *stop trying to walk*. The patient may then *take a deep breath* to mark a pause in the effort and achieve better relaxation. Finally the patient should concentrate on taking *one big step only* – as opposed to walking – and specifically on the hip, knee, and foot movements required to achieve this one step. Clinical experience shows that when the first step is achieved the second and third steps naturally follow.

Movement Planning and Attention

Switching from Automatic Movements to Consciously Controlled Movements

To enhance movement in advanced PD, patients can be taught – or repeatedly reminded – to mentally rehearse each movement before it is executed, and to pay close attention to the movement while it is being performed. For example, in crowded environments where the risk for freezing episodes or tripping increases, the patient should think ahead and plan the most direct route through the obstacles.

Turning around while walking is another difficult task in advanced PD, which may lead to falls. Before turning, the patient should focus on the individual leg movements that are required to effectively turn the body around. Also, it is recommended to accomplish the turn over a wide arc instead of swiveling.[1]

More generally, PD patients often have difficulty maintaining balance secondary to slow righting reactions (recruitment of the appropriate axial muscles) in response to a challenge to equilibrium. Therefore, it is possible to apply to standing balance the above principle of conscious control of tasks that used to be performed well automatically. Patients may be taught to focus their attention on balance whenever they perform an activity involving standing. The purpose is to be in a state of alertness, and readiness to respond to threats of balance, and thus promptly implement the necessary actions to restore equilibrium.[2]

Motor Subunits

It is beneficial for the PD patient to treat long movement sequences not as a whole, but to break them down as a series of component parts or subunits. With this strategy, each subunit is considered and performed as if it were itself a whole movement. This strategy is partly used in the one-step-only technique to alleviate freezing.

Focusing on each subunit of a motor sequence may be particularly effective for multijoint actions such as reaching and grasping, thus facilitating activities such as feeding and dressing, or whole-body activities such as standing up from a bed or a chair.[2] For example, to stand up from a bed, the patient should first mentally rehearse the entire movement, and then break the motor sequence down into a series of subunits, including bending the knees, turning the head, reaching both arms in the desired direction, turning the body, swinging the legs over the bed, and then finally sitting up.[1] A similar strategy can be used for rising from a chair. The patient is encouraged to mentally rehearse the sequence, then to wriggle forward to the front of the seat, make sure the feet are placed back underneath the chair, lean forward, push on the legs and straighten up the back to actually stand up. In a recent open study, PD patients trained with these techniques as part of a 6-week physical therapy home regimen showed significant improvement in their ability to transfer in and out of chairs and beds.[54]

Avoidance of Dual-task Performance

The set-shifting difficulties that are common in advanced PD prevent efficient and rapid switches in concentration between two motor tasks attempted simultaneously.[47] It is thus beneficial in PD to avoid as much as possible having to perform two tasks at the same time.

In a study comparing 12 PD patients with 12 age-matched healthy controls, subjects performed two 10-m walking trials, one freely and one while carrying a tray with four glasses on it. While the gait performance changed only minimally across conditions in controls, the PD patients showed decreased walking speed and stride length while carrying the tray.[8] In another study, single-set instructions to increase either walking speed, arm swing, or stride length (all contributors to efficient walking) resulted in improvement not only of the specific variable upon which the patient had focused, but in the other gait variables as well. However, when subjects were instructed to count aloud while walking (an activity that is not a direct component of the walking movement), these gait improvements did not occur.[27] In this particular paradigm, the acoustic cue provided by the loud counting – that could have been expected to help walking – may have been counteracted by the distraction from the walking movements caused by the additional cognitive task. A more recent study confirms that dual-task performance worsens gait in PD with an equal impairment whether the secondary task is motor or cognitive in nature.[55]

Dual-task performance appears to effect standing balance as well, particularly in PD patients with a prior history of falls.[56,57] In a study comparing 24 PD patients and 20 age-matched controls, there were no differences in postural stability between groups when subjects simply stood on a platform, but PD patients showed significantly greater postural instability compared to controls when given additional tasks, either cognitive or motor.[57]

It has been hypothesized that PD patients may compensate for their deficits in walking or balance by using cortically mediated conscious cognitive processes to overcome the defective basal ganglia activation. When attention is diverted from maintaining equilibrium, the balancing deficits are accentuated.[56] Therefore, PD patients should be instructed to avoid carrying out dual tasks and to instead focus on one task at a time. For example, while walking, patients should be encouraged to avoid carrying objects, talking or thinking about other matters, and instead focus attention towards each individual step and on increasing the stride length.[1] To prevent loss of balance and falls, PD patients should avoid standing while performing complex motor or cognitive tasks such as showering, dressing, or conversing.[58]

MODIFICATION OF THE HOME ENVIRONMENT

In advanced PD, attention should be paid to the home environment, with the goal of maintaining independence and ensuring safety from falls. Because narrow constricted spaces and obstacles can induce freezing episodes and place individuals at risk for tripping and falling, care should be taken to create clear, wide spaces with a minimum of low-lying obstacles in the home setting. In addition, to assist with difficulties in transferring from a lying or sitting to a standing position, higher chairs, toilet seats, and beds can be beneficial as they reduce the energy requirements to raise the center of gravity. Finally, to assist with difficulties with turning in bed, sheets made of satin in the upper part (to allow the body to slide) and of cotton in the lower part (to allow the heels to grip on it and initiate the turning movement) may be used.

AMBULATION ASSISTIVE DEVICES

While walkers are meant to improve walking stability and prevent falls in general and particularly in orthopedic conditions, their impact in a neurological disease such as PD is questionable. The arguments for or against a walker should be weighed on a case-by-case basis, as the use of walkers may worsen gait and increase the risk of tripping or falling.[1,52]

A recent study evaluated the acute effects of standard walkers and wheeled walkers as compared to unassisted walking in PD.[59] Both wheeled and standard walkers significantly slowed gait compared to unassisted walking, while the standard walker also increased freezing. In addition to potentially exacerbating posture and balance difficulties, walkers may also become deleterious in individuals whose steps have become faster and shorter: when the frame advances too far in front of the feet, the person may bend over too far and possibly fall.[1]

However, the main issue with walkers may not be their acute effects on freezing, gait slowing, or the possibility of forward falls, but the possibility of posture and balance impairment caused by chronic use of these devices. By chronically providing passive forward support, walkers may decondition the forward righting reactions required during inadvertent backward sways, and aggravate or even induce a clinical syndrome of retropulsion. This risk has not been established in a prospective study, but anecdotal evidence has been sufficiently prevalent in our center and others[1] that leads us to limit the chronic use of walkers in PD to a minimum in our clinics.

The use of a cane without objectively verifying a positive effect on gait parameters and without providing specific training to the patient is also questionable. Patients with PD often handle canes improperly, carrying them around instead of using them as a support. This is particularly problematic in this condition, as the use of a cane becomes a form of dual-task performance, involving the simultaneous activities of walking and carrying an object. As described above, performing additional tasks while walking can result in gait deterioration. However, it should be recognized that patients may sometimes feel more comfortable using a cane for walking outdoors or in public places, not for the supposed increase in stability that the cane may provide, but as a social signal helping to be recognized by others as someone walking slowly or with a handicap.

Whether a cane or a walker is considered, the indication should be determined objectively and accurately: psychological reassurance, social signal, objective improvement in stability, reduction in energy consumption during gait, etc. Whichever indication(s) are assumed, patients should be tested with and without the assistive device at the clinic to obtain a rigorous assessment of the acute impact of the device on freezing episodes, walking speed, and stride length. Finally, regardless of the acute effects observed at the clinic, the potential effects of a chronic use of these devices should also be considered, particularly with the use of walkers. An assistive device is not necessarily meant to be used indefinitely. One may consider the temporary use of an assistive device in acute periods, such as after deep brain stimulation, or during a period of intensive medication adjustments with risks of walking instability due to excess levodopa and dyskinesias, or after an orthopedic injury such as a hip fracture.

CONCLUSIONS

Interest in physical therapy for patients with Parkinson's disease has grown over recent years. Questions remain as to the most effective regimens. While a number of studies have explored specific treatment options, they are complicated by heterogeneous treatment methods, different outcome measures, and varying time frames of analysis.[4] Many studies have also been limited by inadequate randomization methods, and lack of convincing sham treatments. The latter two are a particular problem in physical therapy research, as unlike in pharmacological studies, neither the therapist nor the patient can be blinded to the arm of the trial.[4] In the future, larger, randomized, sham-controlled studies with staged follow-up will be necessary to determine for each program the benefits, the duration, and the appropriate frequency of training.

To optimize motor function, we provide personal recommendations consisting of strict programs of daily home exercises in the mild to moderate stages of the disease, and the teaching – to the patient and then to the caregiver – of compensation strategies in the late stages.

Acknowledgments

We are grateful to Jerri Chen for her excellent work in illustrating some of the exercises recommended in this chapter.

REFERENCES

1. Morris ME, Iansek R, Kirkwood BR. Moving Ahead With Parkinson's: a Guide to Improving Mobility in People With Parkinson's. Australia: Kingston Centre, 1995.
2. Morris ME, Iansek R. Characteristics of motor disturbance in Parkinson's disease and strategies for movement rehabilitation. Hum Mov Sci 1996;15:649–669.
3. Olanow CW. The scientific basis for the current treatment of Parkinson's disease. Annu Rev Med 2004;55:41–60.
4. Deane K, Ellis-Hill C, Jones D et al. Systematic review of paramedical therapies for Parkinson's disease. Mov Disord 2002;17:984–991.
5. Dietz MA, Goetz CG, Stebbins GT. Evaluation of a modified inverted walking stick as a treatment for parkinsonian freezing episodes. Mov Disord 1990;5:243–247.
6. Kuroda K, Tatara K, Takatorige T, Shinsho F. Effects of physical exercise on mortality in patients with Parkinson's disease. Acta Neurol Scand 1992;86(1):55–59.
7. Comella CL, Stebbins GT, Brown-Toms N, Goetz CG. Physical therapy and Parkinson's disease: a controlled clinical trial. Neurology 1994;44(3 pt 1):376–378.
8. Bond JM, Morris M. Goal-directed secondary motor tasks: their effects on gait in subjects with Parkinson disease. Arch Phys Med Rehabil 2000;81:110–116.
9. Marchese R, Diverio M, Zucci F, Lentino C, Abbruzzese G. The role of sensory cues in the rehabilitation of parkinsonian patients: a comparison of two physical therapy protocols. Mov Disord 2000;15:879–883.
10. Hirsch MA, Toole T, Maitland CG, Rider RA. The effects of balance training and high-intensity resistance training on persons with idiopathic Parkinson's disease. Arch Phys Med Rehabil 2003;84:1109–1117.
11. Ouchi Y, Kanno T, Okada H et al. Changes in dopamine availability in the nigrostriatal and mesocortical dopaminergic systems by gait in Parkinson's disease. Brain 2001;124:784–792.
12. Reuter I, Harder S, Engelhardt M, Baas H. The effects of exercise on pharmacokinetics and pharmacodynamics of levodopa. Mov Disord 2000;15:862–868.
13. Tillerson JL, Cohen AD, Philhower J et al. Forced limb-use effects on the behavioral and neurochemical effects of 6-hydroxydopamine. J Neurosci 2001;21:4427–4435.
14. Tillerson JL, Caudle WM, Reveron ME, Miller GW. Exercise induces behavioral recovery and attenuates neurochemical deficits in rodent models of Parkinson's disease. Neuroscience 2003;119:899–911.
15. Koller WC, Glatt S, Vetere-Overfield B, Hassanein R. Falls and Parkinson's disease. Clin Neuropharmacol 1989;12:98–105
16. Pélissier J, Pérennou D. Exercises program and rehabilitation of motor disorders in Parkinson's disease. Rev Neurol (Paris) 2000;156(suppl. 2 pt 2):190–200.
17. Stankovic I. The effect of physical therapy on balance of patients with Parkinson's disease. Int J Rehabil Res 2004;27(1):53–57.
18. Scandalis TA, Bosak A, Berliner JC, Helman LL, Wells MR. Resistance training and gait function in patients with Parkinson's disease. Am J Phys Med Rehabil 2001;80:38–43.
19. Toole T, Park S, Hirsch MA, Lehman DA, Maitland CG. The multicomponent nature of equilibrium in persons with parkinsonism: a regression approach. J Neural Transm Gen Sect 1996;103:561–580.
20. Muller V, Mohr B, Rosin R et al. Short term effects of behavioral treatment on movement initiation and postural control in Parkinson's disease: a controlled clinical study. Mov Disord 1997;12:306–314.
21. Rubinstein TC, Giladi N, Hausdorff JM. The power of cueing to circumvent dopamine deficits: a review of physical treatment of gait disturbances in Parkinson's disease. Mov Disord 2002;17:1148–1160.
22. Georgiou N, Iansek R, Bradshaw JL et al. An evolution of the role of internal cues in the pathogenesis of parkinsonian hypokinesia. Brain 1993;116:1575–1587.
23. Kritikos A, Leahy C, Bradshaw JL et al. Contingent and non-contingent auditory cueing in Parkinson's disease. Neuropsychologia 1995;33:1193–1203.
24. Howe TE, Lovegreen B, Cody FW, Ashton VJ, Oldham JA. Auditory cues can modify the gait of persons with early-stage Parkinson's disease: a method for enhancing parkinsonian walking performance? Clin Rehabil 2003;17:363–367.
25. Thaut MH, McIntosh GC, Rice RR et al. Rhythmic auditory stimulation in gait training for Parkinson's disease patients. Mov Disord 1996;11:193–200.

26. McIntosh GC, Brown SH, Rice RR, Thaut MH. Rhythmic auditory-motor facilitation of gait patterns in patients with Parkinson's disease. J Neurol Neurosurg Psychiatry 1997;62:22–26.
27. Behrman AL, Teitelbaum P, Cauraugh JH. Verbal instructional sets to normalize the temporal and spatial gait variables in Parkinson's disease. J Neurol Neurosurg Psychiatry 1998;65:580–582.
28. Martin JP. Locomotion and the basal ganglia. In: Martin JP, The Basal Ganglia and Posture. London: Pitman Medical, 1967.
29. Morris ME, Iansek R, Matyas TA, Summers JJ. Stride length regulation in Parkinson's disease normalization strategies and underlying mechanisms. Brain 1996;119:551–568.
30. Lewis GN, Byblow WD, Walt SE. Stride length regulation in Parkinson's disease: the use of extrinsic, visual cues. Brain 2000;123:2077–2090.
31. Viliani T, Pasquetti P, Magnolfi S et al. Effects of physical training on straightening-up processes in patients with Parkinson's disease. Disabil Rehabil 1999;21(2):68–73.
32. Schenkman M, Morey M, Kuchibhatla M. Spinal flexibility and balance control among community-dwelling adults with and without Parkinson's disease. J Gerontol A: Biol Sci Med Sci 2000;55:M441–445.
33. Schenkman M, Cutson TM, Kuchibhatla M et al. Exercise to improve spinal flexibility and function for people with Parkinson's disease: a randomized, controlled trial. J Am Geriatr Soc 1998;46:1207–1216.
34. Pacchetti C, Mancini F, Aglieri R et al. Active music therapy in Parkinson's disease: an integrative method for motor and emotional rehabilitation. Psychosom Med 2000;62:386–393.
35. Hesse S, Werner C, von Frankenberg S, Bardeleben A. Treadmill training with partial body weight support after stroke. Phys Med Rehabil Clin N Am 2003;14(1 suppl.):s111–123.
36. Miyai I, Fujimoto Y, Ueda Y et al. Treadmill training with body weight support: its effects on Parkinson's disease. Arch Phys Med Rehabil 2000;81:849–852.
37. Miyai I, Fujimoto Y, Yamamoto H et al. Long-term effect of body weight-supported treadmill training in Parkinson's disease: a randomized controlled trial. Arch Phys Med Rehabil 2002;83:1370–1373.
38. Pohl M, Rockstroh G, Ruckriem S, Mrass G, Mehrholz J. Immediate effects of speed-dependent treadmill training on gait parameters in early Parkinson's disease. Arch Phys Med Rehabil 2003;84:1760–1766.
39. Murray MP, Spurr GB, Sepic SB, Gardner GM, Mollinger LA. Treadmill vs. floor walking: kinematics, electromyogram, and heart rate. Eur J Appl Physiol 1995;59:87–91.
40. Zijlstra W, Rutgers AWF, Van Weerden TW. Voluntary and involuntary adaptation of gait in Parkinson's disease. Gait Posture 1998;7(1):53–63.
41. Reuter I, Engelhardt M, Stecker K, Baas H. Therapeutic value of exercise training in Parkinson's disease. Med Sci Sports Exerc 1999;31:1544–1549.
42. Pellecchia MT, Grasso A, Biancardi LG et al. Physical therapy in Parkinson's disease: an open long-term rehabilitation trial. J Neurol 2004;251:595–598.
43. Pedersen SW, Oberg B, Insulander A, Vretman M. Group training in parkinsonism: quantitative measurements of treatment. Scand J Rehabil Med 1990;22:207–211.
44. Lokk J. The effects of mountain exercise in Parkinson's persons: a preliminary study. Arch Gerontol Geriatr 2000;31(1):19–25.
45. Behrman AL, Cauraugh JH, Light KE. Practice as an intervention to improve speeded motor performance and motor learning in Parkinson's disease. J Neurol Sci 2000;174:127–136.
46. Soliveri P, Brown RG, Jahanshahi M, Marsden CD. Effect of practice on performance of a skilled motor task in patients with Parkinson's disease. J Neurol Neurosurg Psychiatry 1992;55:454–460.
47. Gracies JM, Olanow CW. Dementia in Parkinson's disease. In: Charney DS, Nestler EJ (eds), The Neurobiology of Mental Illness, 2nd edn. Oxford: Oxford University Press, 2003, pp. 896–916.
48. McDonald WM, Richard IH, DeLong MR. Prevalence, etiology and treatment of depression in Parkinson's disease. Biol Psychiatry 2003;54:363–375.
49. Brown RG, MacCarthy B, Gotham AM, Der GJ, Marsden CD. Depression and disability in Parkinson's disease: a follow-up of 132 cases. Psychol Med 1988;18(1):49–55.
50. Pluck GC, Brown RG. Apathy in Parkinson's disease. J Neurol Neurosurg Psychiatry 2002;73:636–642.
51. Giladi N, McMahon D, Przedborski S et al. Motor blocks in Parkinson's disease. Neurology 1992;42:333–339.
52. Kompoliti K, Goetz CG, Leurgans S, Morrissey M, Siegel IM. "On" freezing in Parkinson's disease: resistance to visual cue walking devices. Mov Disord 2000;15:309–312.

53. Macht M, Ellgring H. Behavioral analysis of the freezing phenomenon in Parkinson's disease: a case study. J Behav Ther Exper Psychiatry 1999;30:241–247.
54. Nieuwboer A, De Weerdt W, Dom R et al. The effect of a home physiotherapy program for persons with Parkinson's disease. J Rehabil Med 2001;33:266–272.
55. O'Shea S, Morris ME, Iansek R. Dual task interference during gait in people with Parkinson's disease: effects of motor versus cognitive secondary tasks. Phys Ther 2002;82:888–897.
56. Morris M, Iansek R, Smithson F, Huxham F. Postural instability in Parkinson's disease: a comparison with and without a concurrent task. Gait Posture 2000;12(3):205–216.
57. Marchese R, Bove M, Abbruzzese G. Effect of cognitive and motor tasks on postural stability in Parkinson's disease: a posturographic study. Mov Disord 2003;18:652–658.
58. Morris ME. Movement disorders in people with Parkinson's disease: a model for physical therapy. Phys Ther 2000;80:578–597.
59. Cubo E, Moore C, Leurgans S, Goetz CG. Wheeled and standard walkers in Parkinson's disease patients with gait freezing. Parkinsonism Rel Disord 2003;10:9–14.

SECTION 8

FUTURE THERAPIES FOR PARKINSON'S DISEASE

15

Novel Therapeutic Approaches to the Treatment of Parkinson's Disease

Peter Jenner

INTRODUCTION

The major pathology of Parkinson's disease (PD) responsible for the onset of the motor deficits centers on cell loss in the zona compacta of substantia nigra (SNc) and subsequent striatal dopamine depletion.[1] Dopaminergic cell loss also occurs in the ventral tegmental area and other nuclei causing dopamine depletion in limbic and cortical regions and elsewhere.[2] However, pathological change in PD occurs on a more widespread basis throughout the hind-, mid- and forebrain. Although pathology may not be as extensive as in the SNc, significant cell loss occurs in the dorsal motor nucleus of the vagus, raphé nuclei, locus coeruleus, pedunculopontine nucleus, and ventral forebrain. Involvement of such diverse cell groups leads not only to disruption of dopaminergic transmission, but also to alterations in 5-HT, norepinephrine (noradrenaline), acetylcholine, GABA, glutamate, and a range of neuropeptides.[3] The widespread biochemical changes occurring in the brain in PD may explain the complex symptomatology of the disorder, although it is not known how most of the degenerative changes in non-dopaminergic cells contribute to either motor or non-motor symptoms. PD is normally considered as a primary degeneration of SNc and as a motor disorder with other components of the illness being secondary to these deficits. However, pathological change may originate in the brainstem, explaining the early loss of olfactory function, and then spread forward to affect nuclei in the mid- and forebrain.[4,5] This may also explain why many patients with PD have a history of anxiety and depression prior to the onset of motor symptoms.[6] All of these findings lead to the concept that PD may require treatment through a range of different pharmacological entities affecting many different neurotransmitter systems in a variety of brain areas to achieve control of all components of the disorder.

Current treatment of PD is based largely on dopamine replacement therapy in the form of levodopa or dopamine agonist drugs.[7] At this time only anticholinergics and glutamate antagonists, such as amantadine, are employed as non-dopaminergic treatments for motor symptoms. The success of dopamine replacement therapy on the motor deficits of PD has led to dopamine systems becoming the focus of the search for novel treatments. Dopaminergic drugs can control the motor symptoms of PD in the early stages of the illness with an improvement in activities of daily living and increase in life expectancy. However, they invariably induce acute side-effects such as nausea, vomiting, and hypotension, and long-term motor complications, including a loss of drug efficacy (wearing off), and unpredictable motor responses ("on"/"off," freezing) and the onset of involuntary movements (dyskinesia).[8] In older patients with PD, drug-related psychosis may also develop. However, there are both motor and non-motor symptoms of PD that do not respond to current dopaminergic treatment. PD is also characterized by bladder dysfunction, constipation, sweating, drooling, speech and swallowing difficulties, and postural instability, as well as sleep disturbance and excessive daytime somnolence. Neuropsychiatric disorders such as anxiety, depression, panic attacks, and cognitive decline are common. Pathological changes in non-dopaminergic systems probably must make a significant contribution to these components of the illness.

Hence, novel therapeutic approaches are required to overcome the problems associated with treating these components of PD and to avoid common complications of drug treatment. These need to be effective throughout the course of the illness without loss of effect, fail to prime basal ganglia for the appearance of dyskinesia, or to provoke established involuntary movements and without provoking psychosis. In addition, they should not exhibit the acute peripheral side-effects caused by current dopaminergic drugs, and they should be effective on the motor and non-motor symptoms of PD that currently do not respond to medication. In this regard, it is likely that new approaches to treatment will have to alter transmission in non-dopaminergic systems and to be effective in areas of the brain other than the striatum. Combining multiple pharmacological actions into a single molecule also would be advantageous, allowing simultaneous treatment of different components of the illness.

This chapter reviews some of the novel approaches to the treatment of PD that are currently under development. However, having an effective experimental model of PD is key to the assessment of potential drug candidates prior to their clinical evaluation. Probably the most effective model of PD to date has been the MPTP-treated primate, so initially its role in the development of novel therapeutic strategies is discussed.

THE MPTP-TREATED PRIMATE MODEL OF PARKINSON'S DISEASE

The selective nigral toxicity of MPTP (1-methyl-4-phenyl-1,2,3,6-tetrahydropyridine) has allowed the creation of a highly effective model of PD in primates.[9–11] Administration of MPTP to a variety of primate species causes SNc degeneration accompanied by depletion of caudate–putamen dopamine content and the onset of motor symptoms, including akinesia, bradykinesia, rigidity, and postural abnormalities – although rest tremor is rarely observed. MPTP treatment does not, however, induce a syndrome that is identical to PD in man since pathology is restricted to SNc and does not extend into other brain nuclei, it is not progressive, and it is not accompanied by Lewy body formation.[12] Nevertheless, it is the predictive nature of the response of MPTP-treated primates to drug treatment that makes the model so useful.[13] All drugs currently used to treat PD are able to reverse motor deficits in MPTP-treated primates, and this has led to its use in the assessment of novel therapeutic strategies and non-dopaminergic approaches for potential clinical use. Importantly, repeated administration of levodopa to MPTP-treated animals rapidly induces dyskinesia that closely resembles that occurring in PD.[14–18] The rapid appearance of involuntary movements relates to extensive nigral cell degeneration induced by MPTP treatment which lowers the threshold of levodopa exposure needed for dyskinesia induction.[17,19] Repeated levodopa administration also induces a shortening of drug effect that resembles "wearing-off," and other treatment-related complications such as "on"/"off" and "freezing" episodes can occur.[20,21] Following acute levodopa challenge, animals also exhibit "beginning-of-dose worsening" and "end-of-dose deterioration." So, the MPTP model not only allows for the assessment of the therapeutic effects of novel treatments for PD, but can also be used to assess a range of motor complications. In addition, MPTP-treated primates exhibit bladder hyperreflexia and constipation, but to date the model has not been extensively used to investigate non-motor components of MPTP's actions.[22,23] However, it appears that there may be more than a passing resemblance to the non-motor, non-dopaminergic aspects of PD in the symptoms exhibited by MPTP-treated primates.

NEW WAYS OF MANIPULATING THE DOPAMINERGIC SYSTEM IN PD

The success of dopaminergic therapies in the treatment of Parkinson's disease has focused drug development on devising novel approaches through this mechanism. Since the introduction of levodopa, a variety of dopamine agonist drugs such as bromocriptine and pergolide were brought into treatment, followed more recently by the use of pramipexole, ropinirole, and cabergoline.[24–27] Although these compounds selectively act on dopamine receptors, they are not specific in their actions and most interact with other neurotransmitter receptors, in particular norepinephrine (noradrenaline) and serotonin receptors.[28–30] Despite the extensive exploitation of dopaminergic approaches to treatment, there has surprisingly been recent activity to refine the range of therapeutic agents acting through this mechanism. As will become apparent, the dopaminergic system still has much to offer to the treatment of PD.

Dopamine Agonists

Dopamine agonist drugs are commonly used as early monotherapy for the treatment of PD as well as in their more traditional role as adjunctive therapy to levodopa in the later stages of the illness when motor complications have appeared. However, all currently used compounds produce a range of dopaminergic side-effects, so there is a need to refine their actions to focus on pharmacological events related to therapeutic efficacy. The discovery of multiple dopamine receptor subtypes in brain was heralded as a means of achieving this end. Two major dopamine receptor families exist, namely the D1-like and D2-like receptors, and these occur in a range of subtypes (D1, D2, D3, D4, D5). D1- and D2-like receptors have differential localizations and distributions within the brain, suggesting that different pharmacological effects should result from the actions of agonist drugs acting at these sites.[31,32] However, the roles of the different receptor families – and in particular the subtypes of dopamine receptors – in the treatment of PD remains poorly understood (see later).

The result of D2 receptor stimulation is the most clear. This is because all currently used dopamine agonist drugs have a common action on D2-like receptors. Stimulation of D2-like receptors produces antiparkinsonian activity and a low level of dyskinesia induction, but it provokes the expression of established involuntary movements.[33–37] D2 receptor stimulation also induces psychosis and is responsible for acute episodes of nausea, vomiting, hypotension, and endocrine changes. Although the effects of dopamine agonists acting through D2-like receptors is predictable, novel compounds such as sumanirole are currently under development for PD.

Interest in D2-like receptors is now focused on compounds that have low intrinsic activity at these sites and function as partial agonists. A partial agonist will act as a full agonist at D2 receptors in the denervated striatum in PD but will compete with dopamine within the relatively intact mesolimbic and mesocortical regions, so acting as an antagonist. Such molecules will be antiparkinsonian but may also prevent or inhibit psychosis. Partial D2 agonists, such as SLV318 and DAB452, increase locomotor activity and reverse motor disability in MPTP-treated primates, so confirming their potential to be effective in the treatment of PD.[38] Importantly, SLV318 co-administered with levodopa did not potentiate dyskinesia induced by levodopa in previously primed MPTP-treated animals, in contrast to the effect of full D2 agonists. DAB452 and SLV318 also possess 5-HT_{1A} agonist activity that could be useful in treating anxiety and depression occurring in PD. The multiple activities of these drugs would therefore be a major advantage over current approaches to dopaminergic therapy.

In contrast, the role of D1-like receptors in PD is less well understood as there are no selective D1 agonists currently available for clinical use. None of the currently employed dopamine agonists has activity at D1 receptors equivalent to its D2 agonist activity, although both pergolide and apomorphine have some effect on D1 sites.[31] However, D1 agonists, such as JKF83959, ABT431, and A777636, are highly effective in reversing motor dysfunction in MPTP-treated primates.[39–41] Limited clinical trials in PD were undertaken with three D1 selective drugs, namely CY208243, dihydrexidine, and ABT431, and all improved motor symptoms.[42,43] However, these compounds were never fully evaluated owing to either toxicological or bio-availability problems. Surprisingly, there is little current activity on the development of D1-like agonists for PD despite the D1 receptor being a clear target for treatment. Indeed, D1 agonists would be antiparkinsonian with a low propensity to prime for dyskinesia but with the ability to provoke established involuntary movements. D1 agonists also may not induce psychosis since there is not a proven association between this receptor system and schizophrenia. They should not induce nausea, vomiting, hypotension, or endocrine changes as these are all

D2 mediated. In addition, D1-like agonists may improve cognitive function[44] and are known to control hyperreflexia of the bladder at least in MPTP-treated primates.[23] One difficulty is that some D1 agonists have induced seizures in experimental animals; although, through structural change, molecular differentiation can be achieved between those D1 receptors involved in the control of motor dysfunction and those inducing seizures. Indeed, a range of evidence suggests that multiple types of D1 receptors exist within brain that have yet to be differentiated.[45–47] There may also be rapid desensitization of D1 receptors in response to prolonged stimulation as a result of receptor internalization,[48–50] but this may also occur with D2 receptors.[51]

However, these difficulties are not insurmountable and the D1 receptor remains an unexploited target for the treatment of PD which may also be effective in preventing common side-effects and in treating components of the illness that are not presently controlled.

Even less is known about the subtypes of the D1- and D2-like receptor families. D1, D2, D3, D4, and D5 dopamine receptors are found both within the striatum and in other areas of basal ganglia, such as the globus pallidus and subthalamic nucleus.[52,53] Dopamine receptors in these areas of basal ganglia are innervated by fibers arising from the nigrostriatal tract, and this innervation is lost following nigral degeneration.[54,55] How these receptor sites in areas such as the globus pallidus contribute to motor activity is not entirely clear, although their manipulation can alter firing rates.[55–60] There are some data to suggest that D3 and D4 receptors play a role in the control of motor behaviors. For example, selective D3 and D4 agonists directly or indirectly modulate exploratory behavior and locomotor hyperactivity.[61,62] The selective D3 agonist S32504 reverses motor deficits in MPTP-treated primates,[63] and D3 receptors may play a role in the motor complications caused by chronic levodopa treatment. For example, repeated levodopa treatment of rats lesioned with 6-hydroxydopamine (6-OHDA) and MPTP-treated primates causes a proliferation of D3 receptors in striatal areas.[64–66] In MPTP-treated primates, this D3 receptor proliferation is associated with the onset of dyskinesia that can be attenuated by drugs normalizing D3 receptor function.[64] It is not known how D3 receptor activation contributes to the antiparkinsonian activity of currently used agents such as pramipexole and ropinirole, which show some selectivity for this subtype.[29,30]

Drug discovery has focused on producing selective D2 agonists for PD. While this is a predictable means of producing drugs that are clinically effective in PD, it may also explain why dopamine agonists are not as effective as levodopa. Dopamine produced from levodopa presumably acts on all dopamine receptor subtypes, so restricting selectivity to one receptor family may limit therapeutic benefit. For example, there is synergy between D1- and D2-like receptors in the control of motor function, so future approaches based on stimulation of both major receptor families may produce agents of great clinical efficacy, and more closely mimicking the effectiveness of levodopa.[67,68]

Dopamine Reuptake Blockers

Regulating the activity of levodopa or dopamine through the use of decarboxylase inhibitors, monoamine oxidase B inhibitors, and catechol-O-methyl transferase (COMT) inhibitors has been highly successful in treating PD. Perhaps surprisingly, inhibition of dopamine reuptake has not been extensively investigated as a means of maximizing the effects of endogenous and exogenous dopamine release from remaining terminals. Some older clinical literature suggests that dopamine reuptake blockers alone or in conjunction with levodopa can produce some symptomatic improvement in PD.[69–72] However, many drugs employed, such as mazindol or nomifensine, were not particularly potent in blocking the dopamine transporter or were more effective on other monoamine transporters. For example, mazindol is more effective at blocking norepinephrine (noradrenaline) reuptake than it is in inhibiting dopamine reuptake.

More recently, highly potent dopamine reuptake blocking drugs, such as brasofensine and BTS74398, have been described although these also are equipotent on the norepinephrine and serotonin transporters.[73] In MPTP-treated primates these drugs increase locomotor activity and reverse motor disability.[74,75] Importantly, when given alone, they do not provoke established dyskinesia. Similarly, on repeated administration to 6-OHDA lesioned rats, BTS74398 does not sensitize motor behaviors or induce abnormal behaviors, suggesting a lower propensity to prime for dyskinesia compared to levodopa.[76] The effects of BTS74398 are dependent on its dopamine reuptake blocking properties rather than its effect on other monoamine transporters. This is also demonstrated by the ability of the selective dopamine reuptake blocker GBR12539 to reverse motor deficits in the MPTP-treated primate model.[77] Perhaps surprisingly, brasofensine and BTS74398 are more effective in animals with extensive nigral degeneration compared to partially lesioned animals with a significant population of dopaminergic terminals remaining in the striatum. The reasons for this are not clear but it may suggest an extrastriatal site of action, and in line with this hypothesis markers of alterations in striatal output are not affected by repeated BTS74398 administration in 6-OHDA lesioned rats.[78]

There has been little clinical evaluation of the new generation of monoamine uptake inhibitors and so it is not possible to correlate the findings in 6-OHDA lesioned rats and MPTP-treated primates with therapeutic efficacy. However, the data available suggest that they should have an antiparkinsonian effect coupled to a lower ability to induce involuntary movements.[79]

Continuous Dopaminergic Stimulation

The current concept of dyskinesia induction in PD implicates a loss of the tonic stimulation of dopamine receptors that occurs under normal physiological conditions and its replacement by supra-physiological pulsatile stimulation that causes alterations in striatal output leading to overactivity of the subthalamic nucleus.[80] This hypothesis has led to the development of the concept of continuous dopaminergic stimulation (CDS) as a means of providing a more physiological replacement of dopaminergic neurotransmission in PD through the use of long-acting dopamine agonists.[81]

Discontinuous or pulsatile stimulation of dopamine receptors by short-acting drugs is proposed as being more likely to pertubate striatal output in a manner leading to dyskinesia induction than the use of continuous dopamine receptor stimulation using long-acting dopaminergic agents. In support of CDS, clinical investigations of dopamine agonist drugs such as ropinirole, pramipexole, pergolide, and cabergoline, lasting for up to five years, showed monotherapy treatment of early PD to result in a lower incidence of involuntary movements compared to levodopa.[24–27] Even when levodopa rescue was required, the prevalence of dyskinesia was reduced compared to that produced by levodopa treatment.

A major component of the concept of CDS originated from studies of levodopa and dopamine agonists in MPTP-treated primates. In animals with marked nigral denervation, repeated treatment with dopamine agonists, including bromocriptine, pergolide, cabergoline, and ropinirole, induced less dyskinesia than occurs with levodopa.[15,19,35–37,82] Similarly, when ropinirole was administered in combination with levodopa in an agonist dominant combination, less intense dyskinesia was observed compared to the effect of an equally effective antiparkinsonian dose of levodopa alone.[35] So, the ability to induce dyskinesia appears to be dependent on the nature of dopamine receptor stimulation, and in MPTP-treated primates there is some correlation between the duration of antiparkinsonian effect and dyskinesia induction. As a specific example, the repeated administration of a short-acting D2 agonist by subcutaneous injection to MPTP-treated monkeys induced a marked incidence of dyskinesia, whereas the same drug administered by continuous subcutaneous infusion caused a much lower intensity of involuntary movements.[83,84]

However, the correlation between the duration of effect of dopamine agonist drugs and the occurrence of dyskinesia is not perfect. For example, repeated administration of equivalent antiparkinsonian doses of levodopa, pergolide, and apomorphine to MPTP-treated primates showed that both pergolide and apomorphine caused less intense dyskinesia than levodopa.[36] However, in this model pergolide has an antiparkinsonian effect which lasts for some 8–9 hours while apomorphine has a duration of only 1–2 hours. So while CDS may be a key component of the induction of dyskinesia, it is not the only factor responsible for the induction of involuntary movements. Indeed, dopamine agonists may inherently differ from levodopa in the way in which dopaminergic stimulation is achieved and in the mechanism of action underlying their clinical response.

Once priming for dyskinesia has occurred following levodopa administration to MPTP-treated primates or patients with PD, the process appears to be at best persistent if not irreversible.[85,86] In primed MPTP-treated monkeys, or in patients with PD, the acute administration of either levodopa or a dopamine agonist both result in the expression of dyskinesia. In levodopa primed MPTP-treated primates, D2 agonist drugs, and levodopa induce dyskinesia to a similar intensity, while D1 agonists produce less marked involuntary movements.[33,34] However, in clinical evaluation, the D1 agonist ABT431 induced dyskinesia equivalent to that seen with levodopa.[43] Importantly, most of the studies undertaken in MPTP-treated primates have compared dyskinesia induction using dopamine agonists selective for either D-1 or D-2 receptors but this might not be comparable with levodopa's actions. The synergy between the antiparkinsonian effects of selective D1 and D2 agonists may also extend to dyskinesia induction. Indeed, equi-effective antiparkinsonian doses of selective D2 agonists such as bromocriptine and ropinirole produce less intense dyskinesia in MPTP-treated monkeys than do mixed D1/D2 agonists, such as pergolide and apomorphine. This, again, emphasizes the inherent difference between levodopa and dopamine agonist drugs. It also suggests that differences in clinical benefit and side-effect profile may be in part due to receptor selectivity.

CDS suggests that there may be therapeutic strategies that can employ levodopa and avoid dyskinesia induction. In PD, the onset of dyskinesia is related to the total exposure to levodopa and the use of higher doses leads to a greater prevalence and intensity of dyskinesia. So, if levodopa is delivered in a manner avoiding pulsatile stimulation, then the incidence and intensity of dyskinesia should match that produced by early monotherapy with a dopamine agonist. Examination of levodopa dose frequency and brain exposure to pulsatile levodopa treatment in MPTP-treated primates showed a relationship between the amount of levodopa administered and the improvement in motor performance.[87] However, the higher the dose of levodopa used, the more severe was the intensity of dyskinesia induction. Increasing brain exposure to levodopa by combining pulsatile treatment with the COMT inhibitor entacapone increased the reversal of motor disability but potentiated levodopa's induction of dyskinesia.[87]

In contrast, however, the administration of levodopa using a more continuous treatment regimen led to a reduction in dyskinesia intensity.[88] Administration of small divided doses of levodopa in conjunction with entacapone produced less dyskinesia than administration of levodopa given alone or levodopa given in a pulsatile manner as two daily doses to the same total dosage. Surprisingly, the more continuous administration of levodopa resulted in a greater reversal of motor deficits than that produced by other treatments while the dyskinesia observed was of shorter duration. This suggests that the manner in which levodopa is administered and the degree of pulsatility does have a significant effect on therapeutic effect and on motor complications.

Dyskinesia is normally associated with an imbalance between the direct and indirect striatal output pathways, but the duration of the biochemical changes produced is too short to explain the prolonged persistence of priming.[89,90] Rather, priming appears to be due to altered glutamatergic transmission involving improper storage of information in the corticostriatal pathway.[91] Consequently, there are few therapeutic options for treating severe involuntary movements in PD (but see later). However, the intensity of dyskinesia can be reduced using continuous intravenous or intraduodenal or intrajejunal infusions of levodopa or the continuous subcutaneous or intravenous administration of apomorphine.[92–94] Switching from optimal doses of levodopa to high-dose dopamine agonist treatment can also reduce the severity of involuntary movements.[95] In MPTP-treated levodopa primed monkeys, replacement of levodopa treatment with the long-acting dopamine agonist cabergoline decreases dyskinesia intensity with only a minor reduction in antiparkinsonian effect.[96] Chronic treatment with small doses of cabergoline may also prevent the onset of dyskinesia in MPTP-treated monkeys.[97] Similarly, switching levodopa to a dopamine agonist, such as ropinirole or piribedil, causes rapid decline in the intensity of dyskinesia, although this is not linked to a reversal of the priming process.[98,99]

All these data suggest that moving from pulsatile to continuous dopaminergic stimulation may be a means of controlling or reversing dyskinesia in the later stages of PD. This means that dopamine agonists may be useful as early monotherapy for PD, as adjunctive therapy to levodopa in patients exhibiting motor complications and also for prevention of dyskinesia expression in late-stage PD while maintaining clinical efficacy.

Novel Mechanisms for Dopamine Replacement Therapy

The manner in which dopaminergic drugs are delivered affects their therapeutic efficacy and the occurrence of motor complications. As a consequence, there has been assessment of alternative routes of delivery of existing and novel dopaminergic agents. In particular, transdermal administration of dopamine agonists provides a means of producing more continuous dopaminergic stimulation resulting in longer periods of mobility. In MPTP-treated primates, dopamine agonists such as (+)-PHNO and N-0437 are highly effective by application to the skin and by delivery from transdermal patches.[98,99] These drugs are short-acting on oral or systemic administration and are transformed on transdermal delivery into agents that act for 24 hours or longer without evidence of the development of tolerance. However, translating transdermal administration in MPTP-treated primates to patch technology in PD is not without difficulty. For example, (+)-PHNO patches did not produce the expected antiparkinsonian effect because drug flux across the skin was insufficient, although they did allow a reduction in levodopa dosage.[100] More recently, the highly potent but short-acting dopamine agonist rotigotine was shown to produce a prolonged antiparkinsonian effect on transdermal administration in MPTP-treated primates. This translates into a clinically effective monotherapy employing rotigotine patches producing an antiparkinsonian activity that when combined with levodopa allows dose lowering.[101–103]

Other routes of drug delivery in PD may also be of use. Rectal administration can avoid first-past metabolism and provide a means of treating PD following-surgery or in intensive care. Similarly, buccal or sublingual formulations or nasal or buccal sprays or inhalation can deliver drugs in a manner that avoids first past-metabolism, so overcoming bioavailability problems as well as solving swallowing difficulties that occur in some patients with PD. For example, water-soluble pro-drugs of levodopa, such as levodopa methylester and levodopa ethylester, that are rapidly hydrolysed to the parent compound *in vivo* have been utilized in PD.[104–106] The ability of alternative routes of administration to overcome pharmacokinetic problems has been emphasized by the effectiveness of subcutaneous and intravenous infusions of apomorphine.[92,93] Apomorphine has a short duration of effect and poor oral bioavailability, but infusions of apomorphine produce a rapid and robust antiparkinsonian effect and a reduction in motor complications.

NON-DOPAMINERGIC APPROACHES TO THE TREATMENT OF PD

The widespread pathology occurring in PD causes disruption of many transmitter systems other than dopamine (see earlier). How this contributes to the symptomatology of the illness remains unclear, but their manipulation may potentially be important in controlling both motor and non-motor components of PD.[107] The loss of the nigrostriatal pathway and the ensuing depletion of caudate–putamen dopamine content also leads to changes in a range of neurotransmitter systems located in output pathways from basal ganglia. The removal of striatal dopaminergic tone leads to changes in the activity of cholinergic interneurones and the direct and indirect GABAergic output pathways.[108,109] The latter leads to alterations in peptide mediated transmission involving enkephalin, substance P and dynorphin that are co-localized in these efferent neurons and to alterations in opioid receptor density in output targets. As a consequence of alterations in striatal output, overactivity of glutamatergic neurones from the subthalamic nucleus to SNr and to GPi occurs.[110] Glutamatergic transmission is also altered in the corticostriatal pathway and in the input to basal ganglia from the pedunculopontine nucleus.

All of these changes illustrate that a range of neurotransmitters and cell surface receptors can potentially be modulated to control motor function beyond the damaged nigrostriatal pathway and that these systems are potential targets for drug development. This has become a new focus for discovery in PD and in the following sections some of the non-dopaminergic pharmacological approaches to the treatment of the illness are described.[111,112]

Other Monoamine Transmitters

There is considerable evidence of a functional interaction between dopaminergic and noradrenergic systems in the control of motor behavior. Alpha-2 adrenergic (α_2) receptors are present in a number of structures within the basal ganglia. Alpha-2c receptors are found on the cell bodies of medium spiny output neurones from the striatum and in GPe, GPi, and SNr, and may be involved in the control of motor function.[113–117] Alpha-2a receptors are also present in the substantia nigra where they act as autoreceptors on the terminals of efferent fibers.[118] In the striatum, α_{2c} receptors may be the target site of projections from the locus coeruleus, although there is little evidence of their innervation. Alternatively, they may respond to norepinephrine (noradrenaline) formed from levodopa/dopamine, and α_2 adrenergic receptors inhibit the firing of dopaminergic neurones and striatal dopamine release.[119] Importantly, while the α_2 adrenergic antagonist atipamezole had no effect alone, it enhances the effect of levodopa on evoked dopamine release in the rat striatum.[120]

Functional interactions between drugs altering α_2 receptor activity and the dopaminergic system that are related to PD are also evident.[121] The α_2 antagonist idazoxan reduces levodopa-induced dyskinesia in MPTP-treated primates.[122–124] Interestingly, in the same model, idazoxan did not inhibit apomorphine-induced dyskinesia, suggesting mechanistic differences between the ways in which these drugs induce involuntary movements.[125] Recently another α_2 antagonist, fipamezole, was also shown to reduce levodopa-induced dyskinesia while extending its duration of action in MPTP-treated primates.[126]

The clinical benefit to be derived from this approach is currently unclear. Idazoxan reduced levodopa-induced dyskinesia in a phase II clinical study in PD but no effect was found in a phase III investigation.[127,128] This may have resulted from variability in dyskinesia rating between centers involved in the trial rather than from drug failure. In support of an effect on involuntary movements, the antidepressant mirtazapine whose principal action is α_2 receptor antagonism decreases levodopa-induced dyskinesia in PD[129] and currently the results of proof of principle studies with fipamezole are awaited.[130]

The basal ganglia receives a significant serotonergic input from the raphe nuclei and there are many types of 5-HT receptors present in the striatum and other areas of basal ganglia. Serotonergic modulation of dopamine-mediated motor function is well documented, but this has yet to be fully exploited in the treatment of PD. A potential difficulty is that the relationship between the two neurotransmitter systems is complex and the outcome dependent on the extent to which each is activated or inhibited.[131] This implies that it may be difficult to establish the dosing levels of drugs used to manipulate serotonergic activity relative to those of dopaminergic agents used to treat PD. For example, increasing 5-HT transmission by blocking serotonin reuptake with fluoxetine can suppress levodopa-induced dyskinesia in both MPTP-treated primates and in PD.[132,133] However, overall clinical studies suggest that serotonin reuptake inhibitors can decrease, increase, or have no effect on the intensity of involuntary movement and that there may be no difference in the occurrence of dyskinesia in those patients with PD who do and do not receive SSRI treatment.[134]

A major problem is determining which of the multiple serotonin receptors (5-HT_1 to 5-HT_7) is an appropriate target for treating PD. 5-HT_{1A} receptors act as autoreceptors that control the release of serotonin from 5-HT neurones.[135] However, they can also increase the release of dopamine derived from levodopa by decarboxylation in 5-HT neurones.[136] In 6-OHDA lesioned rats, the 5-HT_{1A} agonist sarizotan did not produce rotational behavior but it prevented the shortening of response to levodopa that occurs on chronic treatment, suggesting a potential effect on "wearing-off."[137] In MPTP-treated monkeys, sarizotan had no antiparkinsonian effect when given alone or in combination with levodopa but blocked dyskinesias provoked by levodopa treatment.[137] An effect on dyskinesia is also suggested by the ability of the 5-HT_{1A} agonist tandospirone to suppress dyskinesia in a proportion of patients with PD although it caused a worsening of motor symptoms in the remainder.[138] The 5-HT receptor subtype affected seems to be critical. In a series of experiments in MPTP-treated monkeys there was no effect of 5-$HT_{1B/D}$ receptor agonists and antagonists when administered alone or in combination with levodopa or when given to animals exhibiting levodopa-induced dyskinesia.[139] Focal administration of 5-HT_{2C} agonist and antagonist drugs into rat brain also can manipulate motor function but so far this has not been achieved using peripheral drug administration.[140]

Modulation of Cholinergic and GABAergic Function

Inhibition of cholinergic function in basal ganglia using anticholinergic drugs is an established approach to treating PD that has largely been overlooked in recent times. Interneurones are present in striatum and there is cholinergic input to most regions of the basal ganglia from the pedunculopontine nucleus.[141] Anticholinergic drugs acting on muscarinic receptors are used to treat mild symptoms of PD, particularly tremor, but there has been no recent assessment of their therapeutic potential.[142] They are viewed as old-fashioned drugs of low efficacy and with well-documented side-effects.

However, acute dystonic reactions induced by neuroleptic drugs can be reversed using anticholinergic agents; and in idiopathic torsion dystonia, high-dose anticholinergic therapy can reduce involuntary movements.[143,144] In addition, there are also nicotinic receptors present within the striatum, most notably on the terminals of the dopaminergic neurones, and these serve to modulate dopamine release.[145] Perhaps surprisingly, anticholinergics are highly effective in reversing motor deficits in MPTP-treated common marmosets, contrary to the expectations based on their clinical reputation.[146] Anticholinergics such as trihexyphenidyl may also potentiate the antiparkinsonian effects of levodopa.[147,148] Administration of muscarinic antagonists to MPTP-treated levodopa primed animals induced some chorea but no dystonia, whereas the administration of muscarinic agonists produced some dystonia but no chorea.[146] In animals challenged with levodopa to induce dyskinesia, the co-administration of anticholinergics reduced the dystonic component at the expense of remaining chorea, whereas cholinergic agonists decreased chorea leaving the dystonic elements.[146] All of these data suggest that alteration of cholinergic function through muscarinic receptors in PD can be beneficial in improving motor symptoms and in manipulating involuntary movements.

It would seem reasonable to look at the effects of novel anticholinergics targeting those muscarinic receptor subtypes present in basal ganglia and so avoiding alteration in cortical cholinergic activity that may induce cognitive change. However, there has been little or no recent interest in this approach to PD and it remains to be exploited.[149]

In contrast, the administration of nicotine to MPTP-treated primates had little or no effect on basal motor disability, did not induce dyskinetic symptoms in levodopa-primed animals, and did not alter the ability of levodopa to induce dyskinesia.[146,150] However, specific nicotinic receptor subtypes located in basal ganglia may require stimulation for motor effects to be observed. For example, the selective nicotinic agonist SIB1508Y induces rotational behavior in 6-OHDA lesioned rats.[151] It is also reported to potentiate the effects of levodopa in MPTP-treated primates and to exert a mild antiparkinsonian effect when given alone, although we were unable to replicate these effects in our laboratories.[152] Nicotinic agonists may also prevent priming for dyskinesia since nicotine partially inhibits the sensitization of 6-OHDA lesioned rats to the circling response produced by repeated apomorphine administration.[153] The mechanism of this effect is not clear but it may be due to the ability of nicotine to alter striatal glutamatergic function. Cognitive deficits in PD could also be a target for nicotinic drugs. For example, SIB1508Y appears to improve cognitive function in MPTP-treated primates and to improve object retrieval performance.[154,155] Some care may be necessary using cholinergic approaches to cognitive deficits since the acetylcholine esterase inhibitor rivastigmine can worsen motor performance in PD.[156]

One of the most surprising aspects of the treatment of basal ganglia disease is the lack of agents acting through manipulation of GABAergic mechanisms. GABA-containing neurones make up the major component of the outflow pathways of the striatum and of basal ganglia. Alterations in GABAergic activity are widely accepted as being responsible for the onset of motor symptoms in PD and are also associated with the occurrence of dyskinesia. Dopamine release can be modulated by GABAergic agents, and the focal manipulation of GABA pathways in the striatum, substantia nigra, and output nuclei alters motor behaviors in rodents.[157] This suggests that GABAergic pathways are an obvious target for the treatment of PD, but there seems to have been no serious attempts at utilizing GABA receptors or altering GABAergic transmission for producing novel therapies. Recently, flumazenil, a GABA antagonist, was shown to produce a modest improvement in motor function in an open study of PD without the appearance of any adverse events.[158] There may be a need to target those GABA receptors present in basal ganglia without affecting GABAergic systems elsewhere in the brain, and progress may be dependent on improvements in the identification of subtype selective agents.

Manipulation of Glutamatergic Systems

The overactivity of glutamatergic pathways leading to motor symptoms of PD and the onset of dyskinesia has led to exploration of antagonists of ionotropic and metabotropic receptors as potential therapies.[159] Currently, amantadine is the only glutamate antagonist available for treatment and it has long been used for its mild symptomatic effects in PD. This may relate to amantadine's ability to increase dopamine levels in the striatum and to increase the amount of dopamine derived from levodopa in the striatum of 6-OHDA lesioned rats.[160]

Both NMDA and AMPA receptor antagonists can show antiparkinsonian activity in 6-OHDA lesioned rats and in MPTP-treated primates and synergize with levodopa and dopamine agonist drugs.[161,162] The actions reported have been equivocal, although a recent study in reserpine-treated rats suggests that NMDA antagonists selective for the NR2B receptor are antiparkinsonian.[163] NMDA and AMPA antagonists may also improve response fluctuations in PD based on their ability to prevent a decrease in the duration of response to levodopa occurring on repeated administration to 6-OHDA lesioned rats.[164,165] The clinical utility of this approach is shown by the improvement in motor scores and reduction in "off" time produced by the NMDA antagonist remacemide in PD patients with fluctuations receiving dopaminergic medication.[166] Not only ionotopic receptors may be involved in PD since all striatal neurones also possess group 1 metabotropic receptors and their focal manipulation reverses akinesia in rats.[167] Interestingly, metabotropic receptor antagonists seem to produce their motor effects by altering activity in the striopallidal pathway.[168]

The glutamate antagonist riluzole which acts through blockade of sodium channels appears effective in experimental models of PD, but surprisingly in clinical evaluation its effects have been limited.[169,170] This suggests some disparity in the predictive nature of the preclinical evaluation of glutamate antagonists and their effects in humans which needs to be addressed in future studies.

NMDA antagonists can also suppress dyskinesia in PD. Both amantadine and LY235959 inhibit dyskinesia produced by levodopa administration in MPTP-treated primates without adversely affecting the motor response to levodopa.[171–174] NR2B subunit selective glutamate antagonists may be useful in suppressing dyskinesia and potentiating the therapeutic response to levodopa.[175,176] Amantadine is currently used to suppress involuntary movements in PD patients, although only half of patients respond at doses that do not induce significant side-effects.[177] If more selective glutamate antagonists can be produced that are receptor subtype selective and that do not adversely affect glutamatergic function elsewhere in the brain, then these may be useful as clinical tools for the treatment of PD.

Manipulation of Opiate Receptor Function

Mu, delta, and kappa opioid receptor subtypes are present within the output pathways of basal ganglia and can be utilized to alter motor activity. Alterations in enkephalin, dynorphin, and substance P expression in the direct and indirect output pathways occur in PD and in dyskinesia, and in dyskinetic levodopa-treated patients an increased opioid receptor density is present in globus pallidus.[178–180] In MPTP-treated primates, opioid receptor antagonists reduced levodopa-induced dyskinesia in the order $\mu = \delta > \sigma > \kappa$,[181] but in other studies a potentiation was observed.[182] However, in unilateral MPTP-lesioned common marmosets naloxone also decreased the intensity of dyskinesia produced by levodopa by normalizing the motor response without decreasing antiparkinsonian activity.[183] Similarly, in unilateral 6-OHDA lesioned marmosets, apomorphine-induced circling was reduced by the administration of naloxone resulting in a normalization of motor symmetry.[183] However, clinical efficacy of the approach is unclear with reports of naloxone both inhibiting and having no effect on levodopa-induced dyskinesia in PD.[184,185] The complexity of the situation is further emphasized by clinical and laboratory data showing that opioid agonists can also reduce the intensity of levodopa-induced dyskinesia.[186–188]

Manipulation of Cannabinoid Receptors

Cannabinoid CB-1 receptors are widely localized within the striatum and their stimulation enhances GABAergic transmission.[189,190] CB-1 receptors appear involved in the control of motor function since the cannabinoid receptor agonist nabilone suppresses levodopa-induced dyskinesia in PD.[191] However, the role of cannabinoid drugs is confused since both cannabinoid agonists and antagonists can inhibit dyskinesia in MPTP-treated monkeys[192,193] and modulate the behavioral effects of levodopa in reserpine-treated rats.[194] Significantly, 6-OHDA lesions of the nigrostriatal pathway increase striatal levels of the endocannabinoid anandamide while decreasing the activity of its membrane transporter and hydrolase (FAAH).[195] These alterations in the endocannabinoid system are completely reversed by chronic treatment with levodopa. However, an almost entirely opposite set of findings in 6-OHDA lesioned rats was reported.[196] The data suggest that abnormalities in cannabinoid systems and their modulation would potentially form a new and effective means of controlling the motor symptoms of PD. However, it remains to be determined why both agonists and antagonists seem to be effective and to determine which of these approaches may be therapeutically successful.

Adenosine Receptor Antagonists

There is one area of non-dopaminergic treatments for PD that has received considerable attention in recent years, namely the ability of adenosine A_{2a} receptor antagonists to provide symptomatic benefit.[197,198] Interest in the A_{2a} receptor stems from its selective localization to basal ganglia and specifically to the indirect output pathway.[199] Adenosine-2A receptors are localized on the medium spiny neurones projecting from the striatum to GPe and modulate the activity of these neurones so as to alter the release of GABA.[200–202] This occurs at the striatal level and also through the modulation of presynaptic GABA release in GPe. However, A_{2a} antagonists also affect the release of acetylcholine from striatal cholinergic interneurones and release dopamine from the nigrostriatal tract.[202] There is a close interaction between A_{2a} receptors and D2 dopamine receptors such that these may form tetramers, and there is also a close association between A_{2a} receptors and glutamate receptors forming a complex functional interaction that controls the release of glutamate from the corticostriatal pathway.[205,206] The control of glutamatergic activity appears complex as the A_{2a} antagonist SCH58261 increases glutamate release in the 6-OHDA lesioned striatum but decreases glutamate release in the intact striatum.[205] The ability of adenosine antagonists to alter the activity of indirect output pathway is shown by their ability to alter preproenkephalin (PPE) mRNA expression in both 6-OHDA lesioned rodents and in animals treated with haloperidol.[206,207] The increases in PPE mRNA produced by these treatments are reversed by the administration of the selective antagonists KW6002 or SCH58261. In contrast, neither of these drugs has any effect on the expression of preprotachygkinin (PPT) mRNA which is an index of activity of the direct output pathway.

There is also clear evidence of the functional activity of adenosine antagonists in experimental models associated with PD. For example, A_{2a} antagonists, including KW6002 and KF17837, increase locomotor activity in MPTP-treated or reserpinized mice and reverse haloperidol-induced catalepsy.[208–210] Importantly, KW6002 and SCH58261 potentiate rotational behavior produced by levodopa or dopamine agonist drugs in the unilateral 6-OHDA lesioned rat.[211–213] Another A_{2a} antagonist GSC was shown to reverse, but not prevent, the decrease in the duration of rotational behavior observed on long-term administration of levodopa to 6-OHDA lesioned rats. This suggests that such compounds might be important, not only in controlling the symptoms of PD, but in preventing "wearing-off" seen on chronic treatment. In addition, there may be synergism between A_{2a} antagonists and levodopa since SCH58261 in combination with levodopa produces a reversal of reserpine-induced rigidity in rats that is greater than that produced by either drug alone.[214] Adenosine-2A antagonists also have effects in rodent models associated with levodopa-induced dyskinesia. In 6-OHDA lesioned rats exposed to repeated levodopa treatments so as to exhibit abnormal movements, KW6002 reversed motor disability without evoking their appearance.[206] Although KW6002 produced an additive reduction in motor disability when administered with levodopa, it did not increase the intensity of the abnormal movements.

Perhaps the best evidence for a potential role of adenosine antagonists in PD is seen in the MPTP-treated primate model. KW6002 produced a dose-related increase in motor activity after oral administration accompanied by a corresponding decrease in motor disability.[215] The effects were of long duration exceeding that produced by levodopa and most dopamine agonist drugs and were not associated with tolerance when KW6002 was administered at a maximally effective dose for 28 days. Importantly, in MPTP-treated primates that have been primed with levodopa to exhibit dyskinesia, KW6002 given at a maximal antiparkinsonian dose did not provoke involuntary movements either on acute administration or on repeated treatment for 28 days.

When the effects of co-administration of KW6002 were examined in conjunction with levodopa, or with a D2 agonist drug, additive antiparkinsonian effects were observed.[216] However, importantly when levodopa or the D2 agonist were re-administered 24 or 48 hours following the initial administration of KW6002, the same additive effects were observed. This suggests that adenosine antagonists can produce alterations in the activity of the indirect output pathway linked to modulation through A_{2a} receptors which are prolonged and that last beyond the time over which the drug will be present in brain. Again, the increase in locomotor activity and reversal of motor disability produced by KW6002 given in conjunction with levodopa was not associated with an increased expression of involuntary movements.[216] If anything there was a lessening of dyskinesia intensity when KW6002 was repeatedly administered with levodopa. These findings suggest that in patients with PD, adenosine antagonists should produce an additive antiparkinsonian response in combination with currently used dopaminergic therapies but without enhancing dyskinesia intensity as currently occurs when a dopamine agonist is added to levodopa treatment. Other findings also suggest that KW6002 may prevent or delay the priming process that leads to the induction of involuntary movements induced by long-term administration in otherwise drug-naive MPTP-treated primates.[215,216] Because KW6002 produces additive effects when administered with levodopa, it should allow a reduction in dosage of levodopa and hence a reduction in dopaminergic side-effects. Importantly, A_{2a} antagonists may also be effective in the management of neuropsychiatric disease, particularly anxiety and depression, because some A_{2a} receptors are localized to limbic areas and to the hippocampus and amigdala. KW6002 would then be effective against the motor symptoms of PD and the high incidence of anxiety and depression associated with this disorder. Finally, A_{2a} antagonists may act as neuroprotective agents because they are able to protect the nigrostriatal pathway against 6-OHDA and MPTP toxicity and so may influence the progression of PD.[217] It may well be worth exploring the neuroprotective potential of adenosine antagonists in PD in view of the apparent relationship between lowered prevalence of PD and caffeine intake.[218,219]

To date the clinical efficacy of A_{2a} antagonists remains to be proven, but early clinical evaluation of KW6002 showed it to be effective in the control of motor symptoms.[220,221] This has been identified as an ability to cause a reduction in "off" time in patients receiving optimal dopaminergic therapy as well as an ability to potentiate the effects of suboptimal infusions of levodopa. Surprisingly, in those patients receiving optimal dopaminergic therapy KW6002 caused an increase in "on" time-related non-troublesome dyskinesia, and this requires some explanation in view of the preclinical evidence of its lack of effect on involuntary movements. In this respect, the recent finding that A_{2a} receptor density is increased in the striopallidal pathway in PD in those patients exhibiting dyskinesia but not in those without involuntary movements is of interest.

CONCLUSIONS

There is a need to improve upon the current pharmacological treatment of PD so as to maintain long-term control of the illness, and also to enable relief of motor and non-motor symptoms that do not respond to current dopaminergic therapies. Despite the extensive investigation of the role of dopaminergic systems in PD, it appears that there may still be novel therapeutic approaches that can be targeted at this neurotransmitter system and which may provide an improvement in symptomatic control coupled to a reduction in the side-effect profile of drug treatment. Indeed, some of these approaches may also have an effect on components of the illness that are not currently controlled by using actions at dopamine receptor subtypes that are not currently a targeted in PD.

However, the future treatment of PD may well lie in the use of non-dopaminergic pharmacological approaches. This area has only recently started to be fully explored but it already seems that there are many different neuronal targets within the basal ganglia that could be effectively used to alter motor output from the basal ganglia. Indeed, more new approaches have been suggested by the recent description of the ability of the anticonvulsant drugs zonizamide and leviteracetam to improve motor symptoms in PD.[222–224] While non-dopaminergic approaches look extremely promising for the future treatment of PD, we will have to await the outcome of extensive clinical investigation of most of the novel pharmacological targets to establish their efficacy in treating the illness and to verify the predictability of the preclinical models. Non-dopaminergic therapies may avoid many of the common side-effects that are associated with the current dopaminergic approaches to PD, but it is certain that by acting through other neuronal systems they will bring their own range of unwanted effects to the treatment of the disease.

Overall, the future for pharmacological approaches to the treatment of PD appears extremely bright and there is much innovation and activity attempting to produce novel therapeutic strategies. This must be to the advantage of both the physician treating patients with PD and to the improvement of the quality of life of those with PD.

REFERENCES

1. Ehringer H, Hornykiewicz O. Distribution of noradrenaline and dopamine (3-hydroxytyramine) in the human brain and their behavior in diseases of the extrapyramidal system. Klin Wochenschr 1960;38:1236–1239.
2. Jellinger K. The pathology of parkinsonism. In: Marsden CD, Fahn S (eds), Movement Disorders, 2nd edn. Sevenoaks: Butterworth, 1987, pp. 124–165.
3. Agid Y, Javoy-Agid F, Ruberg M. Biochemistry of neurotransmitters in Parkinson's disease. In: Marsden CD, Fahn S (eds), Movement Disorders, 2nd edn. Sevenoaks: Butterworth, 1987, pp. 166–230.
4. Braak H, Del Tredici K, Rub U et al. Staging of brain pathology related to sporadic Parkinson's disease. Neurobiol Aging 2003;24:197–211.
5. Doty RL, Golbe LI, McKeown DA et al. Olfactory testing differentiates between progressive supranuclear palsy and idiopathic Parkinson's disease. Neurology 1993;43:962–965.
6. Leentjens AF, Van den AM, Metsemakers JF, Lousberg R, Verhey FR. Higher incidence of depression preceding the onset of Parkinson's disease: a register study. Mov Disord 2003;18:414–418.
7. Olanow CW, Tatton WGJP. Mechanisms of cell death in Parkinson's disease. In: Jankovic J, Tolosa E (eds), Parkinson's Disease and Movement Disorders. Philadelphia: Lippincott Williams & Wilkins, 2002, pp. 39–59.
8. Obeso JA, Linazasoro G, Gorospe A, Rodriguez MC, Lera G. Complications associated with chronic levodopa therapy in Parkinson's disease. In: Olanow CW, Obeso JA (eds), Beyond the Decade of the

Brain: Dopamine Agonists in Early Parkinson's Disease. Tunbridge Wells: Wells Medical, 1997, pp. 11–35.
9. Burns RS, Chiueh CC, Markey SP et al. A primate model of parkinsonism: selective destruction of dopaminergic neurons in the pars compacta of the substantia nigra by N-methyl-4-phenyl-1,2,3,6-tetrahydropyridine. Proc Natl Acad Sci USA 1983;80:4546–4550.
10. Jenner P, Rupniak NM, Rose S et al. 1-Methyl-4-phenyl-1,2,3,6-tetrahydropyridine-induced parkinsonism in the common marmoset. Neurosci Lett 1984;50:85–90.
11. Langston JW, Forno LS, Rebert CS, Irwin I. Selective nigral toxicity after systemic administration of 1-methyl-4-phenyl-1,2,5,6-tetrahydropyrine (MPTP) in the squirrel monkey. Brain Res 1984;292:390–394.
12. Jenner P, Marsden CD. MPTP-induced parkinsonism: a model of Parkinson's disease and its relevance to the disease process. In: Jankovic J, Tolosa E (eds), Parkinson's Disease and Movement Disorders. Baltimore: Williams & Watkins, 1993, pp. 55–75.
13. Jenner P. The contribution of the MPTP-treated primate model to the development of new treatment strategies for Parkinson's disease. Parkinsonism Relat Disord 2003;9:131–137.
14. Arai N, Isaji M, Miyata H et al. Differential effects of three dopamine receptor agonists in MPTP-treated monkeys. J Neural Transm Park Dis Dement Sect 1995;10:55–62.
15. Bedard PJ, Di Paolo T, Falardeau P, Boucher R. Chronic treatment with levodopa, but not bromocriptine, induces dyskinesia in MPTP-parkinsonian monkeys: correlation with [3H]spiperone binding. Brain Res 1986;379:294–299.
16. Boyce S, Clarke CE, Luquin R et al. Induction of chorea and dystonia in parkinsonian primates. Mov Disord 1990;5:3–7.
17. Di Monte DA, McCormack A, Petzinger G et al. Relationship among nigrostriatal denervation, parkinsonism, and dyskinesias in the MPTP primate model. Mov Disord 2000;15:459–466.
18. Pearce RK, Jackson M, Smith L, Jenner P, Marsden CD. Chronic L-dopa administration induces dyskinesias in the 1-methyl-4-phenyl-1,2,3,6-tetrahydropyridine-treated common marmoset (*Callithrix jacchus*). Mov Disord 1995;10:731–740.
19. Jenner P. Factors influencing the onset and persistence of dyskinesia in MPTP-treated primates. Ann Neurol 2000;47:S90–99.
20. Blanchet PJ, Grondin R, Bedard PJ. Dyskinesia and wearing-off following dopamine D1 agonist treatment in drug-naive 1-methyl-4-phenyl-1,2,3,6-tetrahydropyridine-lesioned primates. Mov Disord 1996;11:91–94.
21. Kuoppamaki M, Al Barghouthy G, Jackson M et al. Beginning-of-dose and rebound worsening in MPTP-treated common marmosets treated with levodopa. Mov Disord 2002;17:1312–1317.
22. Albanese A, Jenner P, Marsden CD, Stephenson JD. Bladder hyperreflexia induced in marmosets by 1-methyl-4-phenyl-1,2,3,6-tetrahydropyridine. Neurosci Lett 1988;87:46–50.
23. Yoshimura N, Mizuta E, Kuno S, Sasa M, Yoshida O. The dopamine D1 receptor agonist SKF 38393 suppresses detrusor hyperreflexia in the monkey with parkinsonism induced by 1-methyl-4-phenyl-1,2,3,6-tetrahydropyridine (MPTP). Neuropharmacology 1993;32:315–321.
24. Oertel W. Pergolide vs L-dopa. Mov Disord 2000;15:S4.
25. Parkinson Study Group. Pramipexole vs levodopa as initial treatment for Parkinson's disease. J Am Med Assoc 2000;284:1931–1938.
26. Rascol O, Brooks DJ, Korczyn AD et al. A five-year study of the incidence of dyskinesia in patients with early Parkinson's disease who were treated with ropinirole or levodopa. 056 Study Group. N Engl J Med 2000;342:1484–1491.
27. Rinne UK, Bracco F, Chouza C et al. Early treatment of Parkinson's disease with cabergoline delays the onset of motor complications: results of a double-blind levodopa controlled trial. The PKDS009 Study Group. Drugs 1998;55(Suppl. 1):23–30.
28. Millan MJ, Maiofiss L, Cussac D et al. Differential actions of antiparkinson agents at multiple classes of monoaminergic receptor. I: A multivariate analysis of the binding profiles of 14 drugs at 21 native and cloned human receptor subtypes. J Pharmacol Exp Ther 2002;303:791–804.
29. Newman-Tancredi A, Cussac D, Audinot V et al. Differential actions of antiparkinson agents at multiple classes of monoaminergic receptor. II: Agonist and antagonist properties at subtypes of dopamine D(2)-like receptor and alpha(1)/alpha(2)-adrenoceptor. J Pharmacol Exp Ther 2002;303:805–814.
30. Newman-Tancredi A, Cussac D, Quentric Y et al. Differential actions of antiparkinson agents at multiple classes of monoaminergic receptor. III: Agonist and antagonist properties at serotonin, 5-HT(1) and 5-HT(2), receptor subtypes. J Pharmacol Exp Ther 2002;303:815–822.

31. Perachon S, Schwartz JC, Sokoloff P. Functional potencies of new antiparkinsonian drugs at recombinant human dopamine D1, D2 and D3 receptors. Eur J Pharmacol 1999;366:293–300.
32. Schwartz J-C, Giros B, Martres M-P, Sokoloff P. The dopamine receptor family: molecular biology and pharmacology. Neurosciences 1992;4:99–108.
33. Blanchet P, Bedard PJ, Britton DR, Kebabian JW. Differential effect of selective D-1 and D-2 dopamine receptor agonists on levodopa-induced dyskinesia in 1-methyl-4-phenyl-1,2,3,6-tetrahydropyridine-exposed monkeys. J Pharmacol Exp Ther 1993;267:275–279.
34. Gomez-Mancilla B, Bedard PJ. Effect of D1 and D2 agonists and antagonists on dyskinesia produced by L-dopa in 1-methyl-4-phenyl-1,2,3,6-tetrahydropyridine-treated monkeys. J Pharmacol Exp Ther 1991;259:409–413.
35. Maratos EC, Jackson MJ, Pearce RK, Jenner P. Antiparkinsonian activity and dyskinesia risk of ropinirole and L-dopa combination therapy in drug naive MPTP-lesioned common marmosets (*Callithrix jacchus*). Mov Disord 2001;16:631–641.
36. Maratos EC, Jackson MJ, Pearce RK, Cannizzaro C, Jenner P. Both short- and long-acting D-1/D-2 dopamine agonists induce less dyskinesia than L-dopa in the MPTP-lesioned common marmoset (*Callithrix jacchus*). Exp Neurol 2003;179:90–102.
37. Pearce RK, Banerji T, Jenner P, Marsden CD. De novo administration of ropinirole and bromocriptine induces less dyskinesia than L-dopa in the MPTP-treated marmoset. Mov Disord 1998;13:234–241.
38. Johnston LC, Smith L, Rose S, Jenner P. The novel dopamine D-2 receptor partial agonist, SLV-308, reverses motor disability in MPTP-lesioned common marmosets (*Callithrix jacchus*). Br J Pharmacol 2000;133:134P.
39. Gnanalingham KK, Erol DD, Hunter AJ et al. Differential anti-parkinsonian effects of benzazepine D1 dopamine agonists with varying efficacies in the MPTP-treated common marmoset. Psychopharmacology (Berl) 1995;117:275–286.
40. Shiosaki K, Jenner P, Asin KE et al. ABT-431: the diacetyl prodrug of A-86929, a potent and selective dopamine D1 receptor agonist: in vitro characterization and effects in animal models of Parkinson's disease. J Pharmacol Exp Ther 1996;276:150–160.
41. Taylor JR, Lawrence MS, Redmond DE et al. Dihydrexidine, a full dopamine D-1 agonist, reduces MPTP-induced parkinsonism in monkeys. Eur J Pharmacol 1991;199:380–391.
42. Markstein R, Seilen MP, Vigault JM et al. Pharmacological properties of CY 208-243 a novel D-1 agonist. In: Sandler M, Dahlstrom A, Belkmaker R (eds), Progress in Catecholamine Research. New York: Alan R Liss, 1988, pp. 59–64.
43. Rascol O, Nutt JG, Blin O et al. Induction by dopamine D1 receptor agonist ABT-431 of dyskinesia similar to levodopa in patients with Parkinson disease. Arch Neurol 2001;58:249–254.
44. Abi-Dargham A, Mawlawi O, Lombardo I et al. Prefrontal dopamine D1 receptors and working memory in schizophrenia. J Neurosci 2002;22:3708–3719.
45. O'Sullivan GJ, Roth BL, Kinsella A, Waddington JL. SK&F 83822 distinguishes adenylyl cyclase from phospholipase C-coupled dopamine D1-like receptors: behavioural topography. Eur J Pharmacol 2004;486:273–280.
46. Undie AS, Friedman E. Stimulation of a dopamine D1 receptor enhances inositol phosphates formation in rat brain. J Pharmacol Exp Ther 1990;253:987–992.
47. Waddington JL. Functional interactions between D-1 and D-2 dopamine receptor systems: their role in the regulation of psychomotor behaviour, putative mechanisms, and clinical relevance. J Psychopharmacol 1989;3:54–63.
48. Dumartin B, Caille I, Gonon F, Bloch B. Internalization of D1 dopamine receptor in striatal neurons *in vivo* as evidence of activation by dopamine agonists. J Neurosci 1998;18:1650–1661.
49. Muriel MP, Bernard V, Levey AI et al., Levodopa induces a cytoplasmic localization of D1 dopamine receptors in striatal neurons in Parkinson's disease. Ann Neurol 1999;46:103–111.
50. Muriel MP, Orieux G, Hirsch EC. Levodopa but not ropinirole induces an internalization of D1 dopamine receptors in parkinsonian rats. Mov Disord 2002;17:1174–1179.
51. Ko F, Seeman P, Sun WS, Kapur S. Dopamine D2 receptors internalize in their low-affinity state. Neuroreport 2002;13:1017–1020.
52. Rivera A, Trias S, Penafiel A et al. Expression of D4 dopamine receptors in striatonigral and striatopallidal neurons in the rat striatum. Brain Res 2003;989:35–41.
53. Smith Y, Kieval JZ. Anatomy of the dopamine system in the basal ganglia. Trends Neurosci 2000;23:S28–33.

54. Jan C, Francois C, Tande D et al. Dopaminergic innervation of the pallidum in the normal state, in MPTP-treated monkeys and in parkinsonian patients. Eur J Neurosci 2000;12:4525–4535.
55. Ni Z, Gao D, Bouali-Benazzouz R, Benabid AL, Benazzouz A. Effect of microiontophoretic application of dopamine on subthalamic nucleus neuronal activity in normal rats and in rats with unilateral lesion of the nigrostriatal pathway. Eur J Neurosci 2001;14:373–381.
56. Freeman A, Ciliax B, Bakay R et al. Nigrostriatal collaterals to thalamus degenerate in parkinsonian animal models. Ann Neurol 2001;50:321–329.
57. Galvan A, Floran B, Erlij D, Aceves J. Intrapallidal dopamine restores motor deficits induced by 6-hydroxydopamine in the rat. J Neural Transm 2001;108:153–166.
58. Kreiss DS, Mastropietro CW, Rawji SS, Walters JR. The response of subthalamic nucleus neurons to dopamine receptor stimulation in a rodent model of Parkinson's disease. J Neurosci 1997;17:6807–6819.
59. Ni Z, Bouali-Benazzouz R, Gao D, Benabid AL, Benazzouz A. Intrasubthalamic injection of 6-hydroxydopamine induces changes in the firing rate and pattern of subthalamic nucleus neurons in the rat. Synapse 2001;40:145–153.
60. Ni ZG, Bouali-Benazzouz R, Gao DM, Benabid AL, Benazzouz A. Time-course of changes in firing rates and firing patterns of subthalamic nucleus neuronal activity after 6-OHDA-induced dopamine depletion in rats. Brain Res 2001;899:142–147.
61. Leriche L, Schwartz JC, Sokoloff P. The dopamine D3 receptor mediates locomotor hyperactivity induced by NMDA receptor blockade. Neuropharmacology 2003;45:174–181.
62. Powell SB, Paulus MP, Hartman DS, Godel T, Geyer MA. RO-10-5824 is a selective dopamine D4 receptor agonist that increases novel object exploration in C57 mice. Neuropharmacology 2003;44:473–481.
63. Millan MJ, Di Cara B, Hill M et al. S32504, a novel naphtoxazine agonist at dopamine D3/D2 receptors. II: Actions in rodent, primate, and cellular models of antiparkinsonian activity in comparison to ropinirole. J Pharmacol Exp Ther 2004;309:921–935.
64. Bezard E, Ferry S, Mach U et al. Attenuation of levodopa-induced dyskinesia by normalizing dopamine D3 receptor function. Nat Med 2003;9:762–767.
65. Bordet R, Ridray S, Carboni S et al. Induction of dopamine D3 receptor expression as a mechanism of behavioral sensitization to levodopa. Proc Natl Acad Sci USA 1997;94:3363–3367.
66. Bordet R, Ridray S, Schwartz JC, Sokoloff P. Involvement of the direct striatonigral pathway in levodopa-induced sensitization in 6-hydroxydopamine-lesioned rats. Eur J Neurosci 2000; 12:2117–2123.
67. Carlson JH, Bergstrom DA, Walters JR. Stimulation of both D1 and D2 dopamine receptors appears necessary for full expression of postsynaptic effects of dopamine agonists: a neurophysiological study. Brain Res 1987;400:205–218.
68. Hu XT, White FJ. Loss of D1/D2 dopamine receptor synergisms following repeated administration of D1 or D2 receptor selective antagonists: electrophysiological and behavioral studies. Synapse 1994;17:43–61.
69. Bedard PJ, Parkes JD, Marsden CD. Nomifensine in Parkinson's disease. Br J Clin Pharmacol 1977;4:187–190.
70. Delwaide PJ, Martinelli P, Schoenen J. Mazindol in the treatment of Parkinson's disease. Arch Neurol 1983;40:788–790.
71. Goetz CG, Tanner CM, Klawans HL. Bupropion in Parkinson's disease. Neurology 1984; 34:1092–1094.
72. Park DM, Findley LJ, Hanks G, Sandler M. Nomifensine: effect in Parkinsonian patients not receiving levodopa. J Neurol Neurosurg Psychiat 1981;44:352–354.
73. Cheetham SC, Butler S, Hearson N et al. BTS 74 398: a novel monoamine reuptake inhibitor for the treatment of Parkinson's disease. Br J Pharmacol 1998;123:224.
74. Hansard MJ, Smith LA, Jackson MJ, Cheetham SC, Jenner P. The monoamine reuptake inhibitor BTS 74 398 fails to evoke established dyskinesia but does not synergise with levodopa in MPTP-treated primates. Mov Disord 2004;19:15–21.
75. Pearce RK, Smith LA, Jackson MJ et al. The monoamine reuptake blocker brasofensine reverses akinesia without dyskinesia in MPTP-treated and levodopa-primed common marmosets. Mov Disord 2002;17:877–886.
76. Lane EL, Cheetham SC, Jenner P. Markers of striatal output do not reflect motor behaviour produced by acute and chronic administration of the monoamine uptake inhibitor BTS 74 398. Eur J Neurosci 2005;21:179–186.

77. Hansard MJ, Smith LA, Jackson MJ, Cheetham SC, Jenner P. Dopamine reuptake inhibition and failure to evoke dyskinesia in MPTP-treated primates. Eur J Pharmacol 2002;451:157–160.
78. Lane EL, Cheetham SC, Jenner P. Repeated administration of the monoamine reuptake inhibitor BTS 74 398 induces ipsilateral circling in the 6-hydroxydopamine lesioned rat without sensitising motor behaviours. J Pharmacol Exp Ther 2005;312:1124–1131.
79. Nutt JG, Carter JH, Sexton GJ. The dopamine transporter: importance in Parkinson's disease. Ann Neurol 2004;55:766–773.
80. Olanow W, Schapira AH, Rascol O. Continuous dopamine-receptor stimulation in early Parkinson's disease. Trends Neurosci 2000;23:S117–126.
81. Obeso JA, Olanow CW, Nutt JG. Levodopa motor complications in Parkinson's disease. Trends Neurosci 2000;23:S2–7.
82. Grondin R, Goulet M, Di Paolo T, Bedard PJ. Cabergoline, a long-acting dopamine D2-like receptor agonist, produces a sustained antiparkinsonian effect with transient dyskinesias in parkinsonian drug-naive primates. Brain Res 1996;735:298–306.
83. Bedard PJ, Gomez-Mancilla B, Blanchet P et al. Dopamine agonists as the first line therapy of parkinsonism in MPTP monkeys. In: Olanow CW (ed.), Beyond the Decade of the Brain. Vol. 2: Dopamine Agonists in Early Parkinson's Disease. Tunbridge Wells: Wells Medical, 1997, pp. 101–113.
84. Banchet PJ, Calon F, Martel JC et al. Continuous administration decreases and pulsatile administration increases behavioral sensitivity to a novel dopamine D2 agonist (U-91356A) in MPTP-exposed monkeys. J Pharmacol Exp Ther 1995;272:854–859.
85. Agid Y, Bonnet AM, Ruberg M, Javoy-Agid F. Pathophysiology of L-dopa-induced abnormal involuntary movements. Psychopharmacology Suppl. 1985;2:145–159.
86. Bejjani BP, Arnulf I, Demeret S et al. Levodopa-induced dyskinesias in Parkinson's disease: is sensitization reversible? Ann Neurol 2000;47:655–658.
87. Smith LA, Jackson MJ, Hansard MJ, Maratos E, Jenner P. Effect of pulsatile administration of levodopa on dyskinesia induction in drug-naive MPTP-treated common marmosets: effect of dose, frequency of administration, and brain exposure. Mov Disord 2003;18:487–495.
88. Smith LA, Jackson MJ, Al Barghouthy G et al. Multiple small doses of levodopa plus entacapone produce continuous dopaminergic stimulation and reduce dyskinesia induction in MPTP treated drug-naive primates. Mov Disord 2005; in press.
89. Albin RL, Young AB, Penney JB. The functional anatomy of basal ganglia disorders. Trends Neurosci 1989;12:366–375.
90. DeLong MR. Primate models of movement disorders of basal ganglia origin. Trends Neurosci 1990;13:281–285.
91. Picconi B, Centonze D, Hakansson K et al. Loss of bidirectional striatal synaptic plasticity in L-dopa-induced dyskinesia. Nat Neurosci 2003;6:501–506.
92. Frankel JP, Lees AJ, Kempster PA, Stern GM. Subcutaneous apomorphine in the treatment of Parkinson's disease. J Neurol Neurosurg Psychiat 1990;53:96–101.
93. Manson AJ, Hanagasi H, Turner K et al. Intravenous apomorphine therapy in Parkinson's disease: clinical and pharmacokinetic observations. Brain 2001;124:331–340.
94. Nutt JG, Obeso JA, Stocchi F. Continuous dopamine-receptor stimulation in advanced Parkinson's disease. Trends Neurosci 2000;23:S109–115.
95. Facca A, Sanchez-Ramos J. High-dose pergolide monotherapy in the treatment of severe levodopa-induced dyskinesias. Mov Disord 1996;11:327–329.
96. Hadj TA, Gregoire L, Bangassoro E, Bedard PJ. Sustained cabergoline treatment reverses levodopa-induced dyskinesias in parkinsonian monkeys. Clin Neuropharmacol 2000; 23:195–202.
97. Belanger N, Gregoire L, Tahar AH, Bedard PJ. Chronic treatment with small doses of cabergoline prevents dopa-induced dyskinesias in parkinsonian monkeys. Mov Disord 2003;18:1436–1441.
98. Jackson MJ, Smith LA, Al Barghouthy G, Rose S, Jenner P. Decreased expression of L-dopa induced dyskinesia by switching to ropinirole in MPTP-treated common marmosets. Mov Disord 2005; submitted.
99. Smith L, Jackson MJ, Al Barghouthy G et al. Switching from L-dopa to the long-acting D2/D3 agonist piribedil reduces the expression of dyskinesia in MPTP-treated common marmosets. Mov Disord 2005; submitted.
100. Coleman RJ, Temlett JA, Nomoto N, Quinn NP, Jenner P. The antiparkinsonian effecs of transdermal +PHNO. In: Quinn NP, Jenner P (eds), Disorders of Movement: Clinical, Pharmacological and Physiological Aspects. London: Academic Press, 1989.

101. Fahn S, Parkinson Study Group. Rotigotine transdermal system (SPM-962) is safe and efective as monotherapy in early Parkinson's disease. Parkinsonism Relat Disord 2001;7:S55.
102. Hutton JT, Metman LV, Chase TN et al. Transdermal dopaminergic D(2) receptor agonist therapy in Parkinson's disease with N-0923 TDS: a double-blind, placebo-controlled study. Mov Disord 2001;16:459–463.
103. The Parkinson Study Group. A controlled trial of rotigotine monotherapy in early Parkinson's disease. Arch Neurol 2003;60:1721–1728.
104. Djaldetti R, Inzelberg R, Giladi N et al. Oral solution of levodopa ethylester for treatment of response fluctuations in patients with advanced Parkinson's disease. Mov Disord 2002; 17:297–302.
105. Djaldetti R, Giladi N, Hassin-Baer S, Shabtai H, Melamed E. Pharmacokinetics of etilevodopa compared to levodopa in patients with Parkinson's disease: an open-label, randomized, crossover study. Clin Neuropharmacol 2003;26:322–326.
106. Steiger MJ, Stocchi F, Carta A et al. The clinical efficacy of oral levodopa methyl ester solution in reversing afternoon "off" periods in Parkinson's disease. Clin Neuropharmacol 1991;14:241–244.
107. Bezard E, Brotchie JM, Gross CE. Pathophysiology of levodopa-induced dyskinesia: potential for new therapies. Nat Rev Neurosci 2001;2:577–588.
108. Obeso JA, Rodriguez-Oroz MC, Rodriguez M, DeLong MR, Olanow CW. Pathophysiology of levodopa-induced dyskinesias in Parkinson's disease: problems with the current model. Ann Neurol 2000;47:S22–32.
109. Penney JB, Young AB. Striatal inhomogeneities and basal ganglia function. Mov Disord 1986;1:3–15.
110. Obeso JA, Rodriguez-Oroz MC, Rodriguez M et al. Pathophysiology of the basal ganglia in Parkinson's disease. Trends Neurosci 2000;23:S8–19.
111. Brotchie JM. Adjuncts to dopamine replacement: a pragmatic approach to reducing the problem of dyskinesia in Parkinson's disease. Mov Disord 1998;13:871–876.
112. Jenner P. Pathophysiology and biochemistry of dyskinesia: clues for the development of non-dopaminergic treatments. J Neurol 2000;247(Suppl. 2):II43–50.
113. Holmberg M, Scheinin M, Kurose H, Miettinen R. Adrenergic alpha2C-receptors reside in rat striatal GABAergic projection neurons: comparison of radioligand binding and immunohistochemistry. Neuroscience 1999;93:1323–1333.
114. Kulatunga M, Scheinin M, Kotti T. Coexistence of a2c-adrenoceptor immunoreactivity with GABA, calbindin D28K and parvalbumin immunoreactivity in rat striatal neurons. Soc Neurosci Abstr 1997;23:586.
115. Rosin DL, Talley EM, Lee A et al. Distribution of alpha 2C-adrenergic receptor-like immunoreactivity in the rat central nervous system. J Comp Neurol 1996;372:135–165.
116. Scheinin M, Lomasney JW, Hayden-Hixson DM et al. Distribution of alpha 2-adrenergic receptor subtype gene expression in rat brain. Brain Res Mol Brain Res 1994;21:133–149.
117. Unnerstall JR, Kopajtic TA, Kuhar MJ. Distribution of alpha 2 agonist binding sites in the rat and human central nervous system: analysis of some functional, anatomic correlates of the pharmacologic effects of clonidine and related adrenergic agents. Brain Res 1984;319:69–101.
118. Cathala L, Guyon A, Eugene D, Paupardin-Tritsch D. Alpha2-adrenoceptor activation increases a cationic conductance and spontaneous GABAergic synaptic activity in dopaminergic neurones of the rat substantia nigra. Neuroscience 2002;115:1059–1065.
119. Lahdesmaki J, Sallinen J, MacDonald E, Sirvio J, Scheinin M. Alpha2-adrenergic drug effects on brain monoamines, locomotion, and body temperature are largely abolished in mice lacking the alpha2A-adrenoceptor subtype. Neuropharmacology 2003;44:882–892.
120. Yavich L, Sirvio J, Haapalinna A, Ylinen A, Mannisto PT. Atipamezole, an alpha2-adrenoceptor antagonist, augments the effects of L-dopa on evoked dopamine release in rat striatum. Eur J Pharmacol 2003;462:83–89.
121. Brefel-Courbon C, Thalamas C, Saint Paul HP et al. a2-adrenoceptor antagonists: a new approach to Parkinson's disease? Drug Ther 1998;3:189–207.
122. Colpaert FC, Degryse AD, Van Craenendonck HV. Effects of an alpha 2 antagonist in a 20-year-old Java monkey with MPTP-induced parkinsonian signs. Brain Res Bull 1991;26:627–631.
123. Grondin R, Hadj TA, Doan VD, Ladure P, Bedard PJ. Noradrenoceptor antagonism with idazoxan improves L-dopa-induced dyskinesias in MPTP monkeys. Naunyn Schmiedebergs Arch Pharmacol 2000;361:181–186.

124. Henry B, Fox SH, Peggs D, Crossman AR, Brotchie JM. The alpha2-adrenergic receptor antagonist idazoxan reduces dyskinesia and enhances anti-parkinsonian actions of L-dopa in the MPTP-lesioned primate model of Parkinson's disease. Mov Disord 1999;14:744–753.
125. Fox SH, Henry B, Hill MP et al. Neural mechanisms underlying peak-dose dyskinesia induced by levodopa and apomorphine are distinct: evidence from the effects of the alpha(2) adrenoceptor antagonist idazoxan. Mov Disord 2001;16:642–650.
126. Savola JM, Hill M, Engstrom M et al. Fipamezole (JP-1730) is a potent alpha2 adrenergic receptor antagonist that reduces levodopa-induced dyskinesia in the MPTP-lesioned primate model of Parkinson's disease. Mov Disord 2003;18:872–883.
127. Peyro-Saint-Paul H, Rascol O, Blin O et al. A pilot study of idazoxan, an alpha2 antagonist, in Parkinson's disease. Mov Disord 1996;11:116.
128. Rascol O, Arnulf I, Brefel C et al. L-dopa-induced dyskinesias improvement by an a2 antagonist, idazoxan, in patients with Parkinson's disease. Mov Disord 1991;12:111.
129. Meco G, Fabrizio E, Di Rezze S, Alessandri A, Pratesi L. Mirtazapine in L-dopa-induced dyskinesias. Clin Neuropharmacol 2003;26:179–181.
130. Pact V, Giduz T. Mirtazapine treats resting tremor, essential tremor, and levodopa-induced dyskinesias. Neurology 1999;53:1154.
131. Carter CJ, Pycock CJ. The role of 5-hydroxytryptamine in dopamine-dependent stereotyped behaviour. Neuropharmacology 1981;20:261–265.
132. Durif F, Vidailhet M, Bonnet AM, Blin J, Agid Y. Levodopa-induced dyskinesias are improved by fluoxetine. Neurology 1995;45:1855–1858.
133. Gomez-Mancilla B, Bedard PJ. Effect of nondopaminergic drugs on L-dopa-induced dyskinesias in MPTP-treated monkeys. Clin Neuropharmacol 1993;16:418–427.
134. Gony M, Lapeyre-Mestre M, Montastruc JL. Risk of serious extrapyramidal symptoms in patients with Parkinson's disease receiving antidepressant drugs: a pharmacoepidemiologic study comparing serotonin reuptake inhibitors and other antidepressant drugs. Clin Neuropharmacol 2003;26:142–145.
135. Santiago M, Matarredona ER, Machado A, Cano J. Influence of serotoninergic drugs on in vivo dopamine extracellular output in rat striatum. J Neurosci Res 1998;52:591–598.
136. Yamato H, Kannari K, Shen H, Suda T, Matsunaga M. Fluoxetine reduces L-dopa-derived extracellular DA in the 6-OHDA-lesioned rat striatum. Neuroreport 2001;12:1123–1126.
137. Bibbiani F, Oh JD, Chase TN. Serotonin 5-HT1A agonist improves motor complications in rodent and primate parkinsonian models. Neurology 2001;57:1829–1834.
138. Kannari K, Kurahashi K, Tomiyama M et al. Tandospirone citrate, a selective 5-HT1A agonist, alleviates L-dopa-induced dyskinesia in patients with Parkinson's disease. No To Shinkei 2002; 54:133 –137.
139. Jackson MJ, Al Barghouthy G, Pearce RK et al. Effect of 5-HT1B receptors on motor control in normal and MPTP-treated common marmosets. Pharmacol Biochem Behav 2004;79:391-400.
140. Fox SH, Moser B, Brotchie JM. Behavioral effects of 5-HT2C receptor antagonism in the substantia nigra zona reticulata of the 6-hydroxydopamine-lesioned rat model of Parkinson's disease. Exp Neurol 1998;151:35–49.
141. Woolf NJ, Butcher LL. Cholinergic systems in the rat brain. III: Projections from the pontomesencephalic tegmentum to the thalamus, tectum, basal ganglia, and basal forebrain. Brain Res Bull 1986;16:603–637.
142. Parkes D, Jenner P, Rushton D, Marsden D. Neurological Disorders. London: Springer-Verlag, 1987.
143. Burke RE, Fahn S, Marsden CD. Torsion dystonia: a double-blind, prospective trial of high-dosage trihexyphenidyl. Neurology 1986;36:160–164.
144. Fahn S. High dosage anticholinergic therapy in dystonia. Neurology 1983;33:1255–1261.
145. Rowell PP, Carr LA, Garner AC. Stimulation of [3H]dopamine release by nicotine in rat nucleus accumbens. J Neurochem 1987;49:1449–1454.
146. Banerji T, Pearce RK, Jackson MJ, Jenner P, Marsden CD. Cholinergic manipulation of L-dopa-induced dyskinesias in the MPTP-treated common marmoset (*Callithrix jacchus*). Br J Pharmacol 1996;117:24P.
147. Domino EF, Ni L. Trihexyphenidyl interactions with the dopamine D1-selective receptor agonist SKF-82958 and the D2-selective receptor agonist N-0923 in 1-methyl-4-phenyl-1,2,3,6-tetrahydropyridine-induced hemiparkinsonian monkeys. J Pharmacol Exp Ther 1998;284:307–311.
148. Domino EF, Ni L. Trihexyphenidyl potentiation of L-dopa: reduced effectiveness three years later in MPTP-induced chronic hemiparkinsonian monkeys. Exp Neurol 1998;152:238–242.

149. Brocks DR. Anticholinergic drugs used in Parkinson's disease: an overlooked class of drugs from a pharmacokinetic perspective. J Pharm Pharm Sci 1999;2:39–46.
150. Domino EF, Ni L, Zhang H. Nicotine alone and in combination with L-dopa methyl ester or the D(2) agonist N-0923 in MPTP-induced chronic hemiparkinsonian monkeys. Exp Neurol 1999;158:414–421.
151. Cosford ND, Bleicher L, Herbaut A et al. (S)-(-)-5-ethynyl-3-(1-methyl-2-pyrrolidinyl)pyridine maleate (SIB-1508Y): a novel anti-parkinsonian agent with selectivity for neuronal nicotinic acetylcholine receptors. J Med Chem 1996;39:3235–3237.
152. Pope-Coleman A, Lloyd GK, Schneider JS. The nicotinic receptor agonist SIB-1508Y potentiates L-dopa responses in parkinsonian monkeys. Soc Neurosci Abstr 1996;22:217.
153. Meshul CK, Kamel D, Moore C, Kay TS, Krentz L. Nicotine alters striatal glutamate function and decreases the apomorphine-induced contralateral rotations in 6-OHDA-lesioned rats. Exp Neurol 2002;175:257–274.
154. Schneider JS, Van Velson M, Menzaghi F, Lloyd GK. Effects of the nicotinic acetylcholine receptor agonist SIB-1508Y on object retrieval performance in MPTP-treated monkeys: comparison with levodopa treatment. Ann Neurol 1998;43:311–317.
155. Van-Velson M, Tinker J, Lloyd GK, Menzaghi F, Schneider JS. The nicotinic receptor agonist SIB-1508Y, but not levodopa, improves cognition in chronic MPTP-treated monkeys with and without motor disability. Soc Neurosci Abstr 1997;23:1898.
156. Richard IH, Justus AW, Greig NH, Marshall F, Kurlan R. Worsening of motor function and mood in a patient with Parkinson's disease after pharmacologic challenge with oral rivastigmine. Clin Neuropharmacol 2002;25:296–299.
157. Reavill C, Jenner P, Marsden CD. Gamma-aminobutyric acid and basal ganglia outflow pathways. In: Ciba Foundation Symposium 107: Functions of the Basal Ganglia. London: Pitman, 1984, pp. 164–182.
158. Ondo WG, Hunter C. Flumazenil, a GABA antagonist, may improve features of Parkinson's disease. Mov Disord 2003;18:683–685.
159. Greenmayre JT. Glutamatergic influences on the basal ganglia. Clin Neuropharmacol 2001;24:65–70.
160. Arai A, Kannari K, Shen H et al. Amantadine increases L-dopa-derived extracellular dopamine in the striatum of 6-hydroxydopamine-lesioned rats. Brain Res 2003;972:229–234.
161. Klockgether T, Turski L. NMDA antagonists potentiate antiparkinsonian actions of L-dopa in monoamine-depleted rats. Ann Neurol 1990;28:539–546.
162. Klockgether T, Turski L, Honore T et al. The AMPA receptor antagonist NBQX has antiparkinsonian effects in monoamine-depleted rats and MPTP-treated monkeys. Ann Neurol 1991;30:717–723.
163. Nash JE, Hill MP, Brotchie JM. Antiparkinsonian actions of blockade of NR2B-containing NMDA receptors in the reserpine-treated rat. Exp Neurol 1999;155:42–48.
164. Greenamyre JT, Eller RV, Zhang Z et al. Antiparkinsonian effects of remacemide hydrochloride, a glutamate antagonist, in rodent and primate models of Parkinson's disease. Ann Neurol 1994;35:655–661.
165. Marin C, Jimenez A, Bonastre M, Chase TN, Tolosa E. Non-NMDA receptor-mediated mechanisms are involved in levodopa-induced motor response alterations in Parkinsonian rats. Synapse 2000;36:267–274.
166. Parkinson Study Group. The impact of remacide hydrochloride on levodopa concentrations in Parkinson's disease. Clin Neuropharmacol 1999;22:220–225.
167. Breysse N, Baunez C, Spooren W, Gasparini F, Amalric M. Chronic but not acute treatment with a metabotropic glutamate 5 receptor antagonist reverses the akinetic deficits in a rat model of parkinsonism. J Neurosci 2002;22:5669–5678.
168. Ossowska K, Wardas J, Pietraszek M, Konieczny J, Wolfarth S. The striopallidal pathway is involved in antiparkinsonian-like effects of the blockade of group I metabotropic glutamate receptors in rats. Neurosci Lett 2003;342:21–24.
169. Braz CA, Borges V, Ferraz HB. Effect of riluzole on dyskinesia and duration of the on state in Parkinson disease patients: a double-blind, placebo-controlled pilot study. Clin Neuropharmacol 2004;27:25–29.
170. Jankovic J, Hunter C. A double-blind, placebo-controlled and longitudinal study of riluzole in early Parkinson's disease. Parkinsonism Relat Disord 2002;8:271–276.
171. Blanchet PJ, Konitsiotis S, Chase TN. Amantadine reduces levodopa-induced dyskinesias in parkinsonian monkeys. Mov Disord 1998;13:798–802.

172. Blanchet PJ, Konitsiotis S, Whittemore ER, Zhou ZL, Woodward RM, Chase TN. Differing effects of N-methyl-D-aspartate receptor subtype selective antagonists on dyskinesias in levodopa-treated 1-methyl-4-phenyl-tetrahydropyridine monkeys. J Pharmacol Exp Ther 1999;290:1034–1040.
173. Konitsiotis S, Blanchet PJ, Verhagen L, Lamers E, Chase TN. AMPA receptor blockade improves levodopa-induced dyskinesia in MPTP monkeys. Neurology 2000;54:1589–1595.
174. Papa SM, Chase TN. Levodopa-induced dyskinesias improved by a glutamate antagonist in Parkinsonian monkeys. Ann Neurol 1996;39:574–578.
175. Hadj TA, Gregoire L, Darre A et al. Effect of a selective glutamate antagonist on L-dopa-induced dyskinesias in drug-naive parkinsonian monkeys. Neurobiol Dis 2004;15:171–176.
176. Loschmann PA, De Groote C, Smith L et al. Antiparkinsonian activity of Ro 25-6981, a NR2B subunit specific NMDA receptor antagonist, in animal models of Parkinson's disease. Exp Neurol 2004;187:86–93.
177. Verhagen ML, Del Dotto P et al. Amantadine as treatment for dyskinesias and motor fluctuations in Parkinson's disease. Neurology 1998;50:1323–1326.
178. Morissette M, Grondin R, Goulet M, Bedard PJ, Di Paolo T. Differential regulation of striatal preproenkephalin and preprotachykinin mRNA levels in MPTP-lesioned monkeys chronically treated with dopamine D1 or D2 receptor agonists. J Neurochem 1999;72:682–692.
179. Piccini P, Weeks RA, Brooks DJ. Alterations in opioid receptor binding in Parkinson's disease patients with levodopa-induced dyskinesias. Ann Neurol 1997;42:720–726.
180. Zeng BY, Pearce RK, MacKenzie GM, Jenner P. Alterations in preproenkephalin and adenosine-2a receptor mRNA, but not preprotachykinin mRNA, correlate with occurrence of dyskinesia in normal monkeys chronically treated with L-dopa. Eur J Neurosci 2000;12:1096–1104.
181. Henry B, Fox SH, Crossman AR, Brotchie JM. Mu- and delta-opioid receptor antagonists reduce levodopa-induced dyskinesia in the MPTP-lesioned primate model of Parkinson's disease. Exp Neurol 2001;171:139–146.
182. Samadi P, Gregoire L, Bedard PJ. The opioid agonist morphine decreases the dyskinetic response to dopaminergic agents in parkinsonian monkeys: interaction between dopamine and opioid systems. Neurobiol Disease 2004;16:246-253
183. Klintenberg R, Svenningsson P, Gunne L, Andren PE. Naloxone reduces levodopa-induced dyskinesias and apomorphine-induced rotations in primate models of parkinsonism. J Neural Transm 2002;109:1295–1307.
184. Sandyk R, Snider SR. Naloxone treatment of L-dopa-induced dyskinesias in Parkinson's disease. Am J Psychiat 1986;143:118.
185. Trabucchi M, Bassi S, Frattola L. Effect of naloxone on the "on-off" syndrome in patients receiving long-term levodopa therapy. Arch Neurol 1982;39:120–121.
186. Berg D, Becker G, Reiners K. Reduction of dyskinesia and induction of akinesia induced by morphine in two parkinsonian patients with severe sciatica. J Neural Transm 1999;106:725–728.
187. Samadi P, Gregoire L, Bedard PJ. The opioid agonist morphine decreases the dyskinetic response to dopaminergic agents in parkinsonian monkeys. Neurobiol Dis 2004;16:246–253.
188. Vermeulen RJ, Drukarch B, Sahadat MC et al. Morphine and naltrexone modulate D2 but not D1 receptor induced motor behavior in MPTP-lesioned monkeys. Psychopharmacology (Berl) 1995;118:451–459.
189. Mailleux P, Parmentier M, Vanderhaeghen JJ. Distribution of cannabinoid receptor messenger RNA in the human brain: an in-situ hybridization histochemistry with oligonucleotides. Neurosci Lett 1992;143:200–204.
190. Maneuf YP, Nash JE, Crossman AR, Brotchie JM. Activation of the cannabinoid receptor by delta 9-tetrahydrocannabinol reduces gamma-aminobutyric acid uptake in the globus pallidus. Eur J Pharmacol 1996;308:161–164.
191. Sieradzan KA, Fox SH, Hill M et al. Cannabinoids reduce levodopa-induced dyskinesia in Parkinson's disease: a pilot study. Neurology 2001;57:2108–2111.
192. Brotchie JM. The neural mechanisms underlying levodopa-induced dyskinesia in Parkinson's disease. Ann Neurol 2000;47:S105–112.
193. Fox SH, Henry B, Hill M, Crossman A, Brotchie J. Stimulation of cannabinoid receptors reduces levodopa-induced dyskinesia in the MPTP-lesioned nonhuman primate model of Parkinson's disease. Mov Disord 2002;17:1180–1187.
194. Segovia G, Mora F, Crossman AR, Brotchie JM. Effects of CB1 cannabinoid receptor modulating compounds on the hyperkinesia induced by high-dose levodopa in the reserpine-treated rat model of Parkinson's disease. Mov Disord 2003;18:138–149.

195. Maccarrone M, Gubellini P, Bari M et al. Levodopa treatment reverses endocannabinoid system abnormalities in experimental parkinsonism. J Neurochem 2003;85:1018–1025.
196. Ferrer B, Asbrock N, Kathuria S, Piomelli D, Giuffrida A. Effects of levodopa on endocannabinoid levels in rat basal ganglia: implications for the treatment of levodopa-induced dyskinesias. Eur J Neurosci 2003;18:1607–1614.
197. Kase H, Richardson PJ, Jenner P (eds). Adenosine Receptors and Parkinson's Disease. London: Academic Press, 2000.
198. Kase H. New aspects of physiological and pathophysiological functions of adenosine A2A receptor in basal ganglia. Biosci Biotechnol Biochem 2001;65:1447–1457.
199. Svenningsson P, Hall H, Sedvall G, Fredholm BB. Distribution of adenosine receptors in the postmortem human brain: an extended autoradiographic study. Synapse 1997;27:322–335.
200. Mori A, Shindou T. Physiology of adenosine receptors in the striatum regulation of striatal projection neurons. In: Kase H, Richardson PJ, Jenner P (eds), Adenosine Receptors and Parkinson's Disease. London: Academic Press, 2000.
201. Ochi M, Koga K, Kurokawa M et al. Systemic administration of adenosine A(2A) receptor antagonist reverses increased GABA release in the globus pallidus of unilateral 6-hydroxydopamine-lesioned rats: a microdialysis study. Neuroscience 2000;100:53–62.
202. Richardson PJ, Kurokawa M. Regulation of neurotransmitter release in basal ganglia by adenosine receptor agonists and antagonists *in vitro* and *in vivo*. In: Kase H, Richardson PJ, Jenner P (eds), Adenosine Receptors and Parkinson's Disease. London: Academic Press, 2000.
203. Morelli M, Acquas E, Ongini E. Dopamine–adenosine interactions. In: Di Chiara G (ed.), Handbook of Experimental Pharmacology. Berlin: Springer-Verlag, 2002, pp. 135–150.
204. Nash JE, Brotchie JM. A common signaling pathway for striatal NMDA and adenosine A2a receptors: implications for the treatment of Parkinson's disease. J Neurosci 2000;20:7782–7789.
205. Corsi C, Pinna A, Gianfriddo M et al. Adenosine A2A receptor antagonism increases striatal glutamate outflow in dopamine-denervated rats. Eur J Pharmacol 2003;464:33–38.
206. Lundblad M, Vaudano E, Cenci MA. Cellular and behavioural effects of the adenosine A2a receptor antagonist KW-6002 in a rat model of L-dopa-induced dyskinesia. J Neurochem 2003;84:1398–1410.
207. Wardas J, Pietraszek M, Dziedzicka-Wasylewska M. SCH 58261, a selective adenosine A2A receptor antagonist, decreases the haloperidol-enhanced proenkephalin mRNA expression in the rat striatum. Brain Res 2003;977:270–277.
208. Hauber W, Neuscheler P, Nagel J, Muller CE. Catalepsy induced by a blockade of dopamine D1 or D2 receptors was reversed by a concomitant blockade of adenosine A(2A) receptors in the caudate-putamen of rats. Eur J Neurosci 2001;14:1287–1293.
209. Shiozaki S, Ichikawa S, Nakamura J et al. Actions of adenosine A2A receptor antagonist KW-6002 on drug-induced catalepsy and hypokinesia caused by reserpine or MPTP. Psychopharmacology (Berl) 1999;147:90–95.
210. Wardas J, Konieczny J, Lorenc-Koci E. SCH 58261, an A(2A) adenosine receptor antagonist, counteracts parkinsonian-like muscle rigidity in rats. Synapse 2001;41:160–171.
211. Carta AR, Pinna A, Tronci E, Morelli M. Adenosine A2A and dopamine receptor interactions in basal ganglia of dopamine denervated rats. Neurology 2003;61:S39–43.
212. Koga K, Kurokawa M, Ochi M, Nakamura J, Kuwana Y. Adenosine A(2A) receptor antagonists KF17837 and KW6002 potentiate rotation induced by dopaminergic drugs in hemi-Parkinsonian rats. Eur J Pharmacol 2000;408:249–255.
213. Pinna A, Fenu S, Morelli M. Motor stimulant effects of the adenosine A2A receptor antagonist SCH 58261 do not develop tolerance after repeated treatments in 6-hydroxydopamine-lesioned rats. Synapse 2001;39:233–238.
214. Wardas J. Synergistic effect of SCH 58261, an adenosine A2A receptor antagonist, and L-dopa on the reserpine-induced muscle rigidity in rats. Pol J Pharmacol 2003;55:155–164.
215. Kanda T, Jackson MJ, Smith LA et al. Adenosine A2A antagonist: a novel antiparkinsonian agent that does not provoke dyskinesia in parkinsonian monkeys. Ann Neurol 1998;43:507–513.
216. Kanda T, Jackson MJ, Smith LA et al. Combined use of the adenosine A(2A) antagonist KW-6002 with L-DOPA or with selective D1 or D2 dopamine agonists increases antiparkinsonian activity but not dyskinesia in MPTP-treated monkeys. Exp Neurol 2000;162:321–327.
217. Ikeda K, Kurokawa M, Aoyama S, Kuwana Y. Neuroprotection by adenosine A2A receptor blockade in experimental models of Parkinson's disease. J Neurochem 2002;80:262–270.
218. Checkoway H, Powers K, Smith-Weller T et al. Parkinson's disease risks associated with cigarette smoking, alcohol consumption, and caffeine intake. Am J Epidemiol 2002;155:732–738.

219. Hernan MA, Takkouche B, Caamano-Isorna F, Gestal-Otero JJ. A meta-analysis of coffee drinking, cigarette smoking, and the risk of Parkinson's disease. Ann Neurol 2002;52:276–284.
220. Hauser RA, Hubble JP, Truong DD. Randomized trial of the adenosine A(2A) receptor antagonist istradefylline in advanced PD. Neurology 2003;61:297–303.
221. Sherzai A, Bara-Jimenez W, Gillespie M et al. Adenosine A2a antagonist treatment of Parkinson's disease. Neurology 2002;58:A667.
222. Bezard E, Brotchie J, Crossman A et al. Levetiracetam (Keppra) reduces L-dopa-induced choreic dyskinesia in the MPTP-lesioned macaque. Presented at the 55th Annual Meeting of the American Academy of Neurology, 2003.
223. Brotchie J, Bezard E, Crossman A et al. The antiepileptic levetiracetam (Keppra) modifies the process of priming for L-dopa-induced dyskinesia in the MPTP-lesioned nonhuman primate. Presented at the 55th Annual Meeting of the American Academy of Neurology, 2003.
224. Murata M. Novel therapeutic effects of the anti-convulsant, zonisamide, on Parkinson's disease. Curr Pharm Des 2004;10:687–693.

Index

Page numbers in italic, e.g. *215*, refer to figures. Page numbers in bold, e.g. **191**, denote entries in tables.